Arteriogenesis and
Therapeutic Neovascularization

Arteriogenesis and Therapeutic Neovascularization

Special Issue Editors

Elisabeth Deindl
Paul H. A. Quax
Thomas Schmitz-Rixen

MDPI • Basel • Beijing • Wuhan • Barcelona • Belgrade • Manchester • Tokyo • Cluj • Tianjin

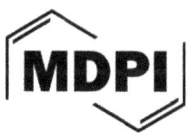

Special Issue Editors

Elisabeth Deindl
Walter-Brendel-Centre of
Experimental Medicine
Germany

Paul H. A. Quax
Leiden University Medical
Center
The Netherlands

Thomas Schmitz-Rixen
Goethe-University Hospital
Frankfurt am Main
Germany

Editorial Office
MDPI
St. Alban-Anlage 66
4052 Basel, Switzerland

This is a reprint of articles from the Special Issue published online in the open access journal *Cells* (ISSN 2073-4409) (available at: https://www.mdpi.com/journal/cells/special_issues/arteriogenesis_neovascularization).

For citation purposes, cite each article independently as indicated on the article page online and as indicated below:

LastName, A.A.; LastName, B.B.; LastName, C.C. Article Title. *Journal Name* **Year**, *Article Number*, Page Range.

ISBN 978-3-03936-593-7 (Hbk)
ISBN 978-3-03936-594-4 (PDF)

Cover image courtesy of Elisabeth Deindl (Artist Xenia Deindl).

© 2020 by the authors. Articles in this book are Open Access and distributed under the Creative Commons Attribution (CC BY) license, which allows users to download, copy and build upon published articles, as long as the author and publisher are properly credited, which ensures maximum dissemination and a wider impact of our publications.

The book as a whole is distributed by MDPI under the terms and conditions of the Creative Commons license CC BY-NC-ND.

Contents

About the Special Issue Editors vii

Elisabeth Deindl and Paul H. A. Quax
Arteriogenesis and Therapeutic Angiogenesis in Its Multiple Aspects
Reprinted from: *Cells* 2020, *9*, 1439, doi:10.3390/cells9061439 1

Kerstin Troidl, Christian Schubert, Ann-Kathrin Vlacil, Ramesh Chennupati, Sören Koch, Jutta Schütt, Raghav Oberoi, Wolfgang Schaper, Thomas Schmitz-Rixen, Bernhard Schieffer and Karsten Grote
The Lipopeptide MALP-2 Promotes Collateral Growth
Reprinted from: *Cells* 2020, *9*, 997, doi:10.3390/cells9040997 5

Ilze Bot, Daniël van der Velden, Merel Bouwman, Mara J. Kröner, Johan Kuiper, Paul H. A. Quax and Margreet R. de Vries
Local Mast Cell Activation Promotes Neovascularization
Reprinted from: *Cells* 2020, *9*, 701, doi:10.3390/cells9030701 19

Nicolas Ricard, Jiasheng Zhang, Zhen W. Zhuang and Michael Simons
Isoform-Specific Roles of ERK1 and ERK2 in Arteriogenesis
Reprinted from: *Cells* 2020, *9*, 38, doi:10.3390/cells9010038 33

Manuel Lasch, Amelia Caballero Martinez, Konda Kumaraswami, Hellen Ishikawa-Ankerhold, Sarah Meister and Elisabeth Deindl
Contribution of the Potassium Channels $K_V1.3$ and $K_{Ca}3.1$ to Smooth Muscle Cell Proliferation in Growing Collateral Arteries
Reprinted from: *Cells* 2020, *9*, 913, doi:10.3390/cells9040913 51

Özgür Uslu, Joerg Herold and Sandip M. Kanse
VEGF-A-Cleavage by FSAP and Inhibition of Neo-Vascularization
Reprinted from: *Cells* 2019, *8*, 1396, doi:10.3390/cells8111396 67

Zhiyong Lei, Timothy D. Klasson, Maarten M. Brandt, Glenn van de Hoek, Ive Logister, Caroline Cheng, Pieter A. Doevendans, Joost P. G. Sluijter and Rachel H. Giles
Control of Angiogenesis via a VHL/miR-212/132 Axis
Reprinted from: *Cells* 2020, *9*, 1017, doi:10.3390/cells9041017 85

Reginald V.C.T. van der Kwast, Paul H.A. Quax and A. Yaël Nossent
An Emerging Role for isomiRs and the microRNA Epitranscriptome in Neovascularization
Reprinted from: *Cells* 2020, *9*, 61, doi:10.3390/cells9010061 97

Laura Parma, Hendrika A. B. Peters, Fabiana Baganha, Judith C. Sluimer, Margreet R. de Vries and Paul H. A. Quax
Prolonged Hyperoxygenation Treatment Improves Vein Graft Patency and Decreases Macrophage Content in Atherosclerotic Lesions in ApoE3*Leiden Mice
Reprinted from: *Cells* 2020, *9*, 336, doi:10.3390/cells9020336 119

Tilman Ziegler, Farah Abdel Rahman, Victoria Jurisch and Christian Kupatt
Atherosclerosis and the Capillary Network; Pathophysiology and Potential Therapeutic Strategies
Reprinted from: *Cells* 2020, *9*, 50, doi:10.3390/cells9010050 137

Diego Caicedo, Pablo Devesa, Clara V. Alvarez and Jesús Devesa
Why Should Growth Hormone (GH) Be Considered a Promising Therapeutic Agent for Arteriogenesis? Insights from the GHAS Trial
Reprinted from: *Cells* **2020**, *9*, 807, doi:10.3390/cells9040807 . . . . **151**

Johanna Vogel, Daniel Niederer, Georg Jung and Kerstin Troidl
Exercise-Induced Vascular Adaptations under Artificially Versus Pathologically Reduced Blood Flow: A Focus Review with Special Emphasis on Arteriogenesis
Reprinted from: *Cells* **2020**, *9*, 333, doi:10.3390/cells9020333 . . . . **183**

Florian Simon, Markus Udo Wagenhäuser, Albert Busch, Hubert Schelzig and Alexander Gombert
Arteriogenesis of the Spinal Cord—The Network Challenge
Reprinted from: *Cells* **2020**, *9*, 501, doi:10.3390/cells9020501 . . . . **195**

About the Special Issue Editors

Elisabeth Deindl (Dr.) graduated at the ZMBH in Heidelberg, Germany, where she worked on hepatitis B viruses. Thereafter, she joined the lab of Wolfgang Schaper at the Max-Planck-Institute in Bad Nauheim, where she started to decipher the molecular mechanisms of arteriogenesis. After a short detour on stem cells, she again focused on arteriogenesis, becoming a leading expert in the field. By using a peripheral model of arteriogenesis, she demonstrated that collateral artery growth is a matter of innate immunity, and presented a blueprint of sterile inflammation, which is locally triggered by extracellular RNA.

Paul H. A. Quax (Ph.D.) completed his Ph.D. at the University of Leiden, the Netherlands, on the role of plasminogen activators in tissue remodeling. He continued working on this topic in relation to vascular remodeling, first at the Gaubius Laboratory TNO, and later at the Leiden University Medical Center, as a professor in experimental vascular medicine. His interest in arteriogenesis was driven by the lack of therapeutic options for patients with peripheral arterial disease. Therapeutic arteriogenesis and angiogenesis induced by gene therapy, growth factors, modulation of inflammatory and immune response, but also by the modulation of microRNAs and other noncoding RNAs in small animal models, are topics of his research.

Thomas Schmitz-Rixen (MD, Ph.D.) completed his Ph.D. at the University of Cologne, Germany, on the role of immunosuppression after vascular allotransplantation. As a professor of vascular surgery in Frankfurt/M, he joined the lab of Wolfgang Schaper at the Max-Planck-Institute in Bad Nauheim, to look into the molecular mechanism of arteriogenesis. He developed an animal model of fast and intense collateralization in the lower extremities and the brain. His recent topics of research in therapeutic arteriogenesis, both in humans and animal models, are related to the role of microRNA.

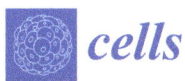

Editorial

Arteriogenesis and Therapeutic Angiogenesis in Its Multiple Aspects

Elisabeth Deindl [1,*] and Paul H. A. Quax [2,*]

1. Walter-Brendel-Centre of Experimental Medicine, University Hospital, Ludwig-Maximilians-University, 81377 Munich, Germany
2. Department of Surgery, Einthoven Laboratory for Experimental Vascular Medicine, Leiden University Medical Center, 2300 RC Leiden, The Netherlands
* Correspondence: elisabeth.deindl@med.uni-muenchen.de (E.D.); p.h.a.quax@lmuc.nl (P.H.A.Q.); Tel.: +49-89-2180-76504 (E.D.); +31-71-526-1584 (P.H.A.Q.)

Received: 5 June 2020; Accepted: 9 June 2020; Published: 10 June 2020

Arteriogenesis, also frequently called collateral formation or even therapeutic angiogenesis, comprises those processes that lead to the formation and growth of collateral blood vessels that can act as natural bypasses to restore blood flow to distal tissues in occluded arteries. Both in coronary occlusive artery diseases as well as in peripheral occlusive arterial disease, arteriogenesis may play an important role in the restoration of blood flow. Despite the big clinical potential and the many promising clinical trials on arteriogenesis and therapeutic angiogenesis, the exact molecular mechanisms involved in the multifactorial processes of arteriogenesis are still not completely understood. In this inflammatory-driven vascular remodeling process, many cell types, both vascular cells and immune cells, many cytokines and growth factors, as well as various noncoding RNAs may be involved. Consequently, many questions regarding the exact molecular mechanisms involved in the regulation of the arteriogenic response still need to be answered, and these answers will contribute to defining new therapeutic options.

This Special Issue of *Cells* is devoted to all aspects of arteriogenesis, collateral formation and therapeutic angiogenesis. It contains articles that collectively provide a balanced, state-of-the-art view on various aspects of arteriogenesis and the underlying regulation of vascular remodeling.

As indicated above, arteriogenesis is an inflammatory-driven vascular remodeling process and Toll-like receptors (TLRs), especially TLR4, are known to be involved in arteriogenesis. Troidl et al., demonstrate that after the induction of hind limb ischemia in mice, the lipopeptide and TLR2/6 ligand macrophage-activating protein of 2-kDA (MALP-2) increased the growth of pre-existing collateral arteries in the upper hind limb, along with intimal endothelial cell proliferation in the collateral wall and pericollateral macrophage accumulation. In addition, MALP-2 increased capillary density in the lower hind limb. These promising results with the TLR2/6 ligand MALP-2 illustrate the potential to promote peripheral blood flow recovery by collateral artery growth by enhancing the inflammatory response [1].

The role of inflammation and immune cells in arteriogenesis is also illustrated by Bot el al., who extended the studies on the role of mast cells in arteriogenesis and collateral formation and demonstrated that local mast cell activation increased blood flow through the hind limb, due an increase in the diameter of the collaterals, as well as in the number of CD31$^+$ capillaries. Together, these data illustrate that locally activated mast cell contribute to arteriogenesis and angiogenesis [2].

The induction of angiogenesis by vascular endothelial growth factor (VEGF) is well established, and the VEGF stimulation of endothelial cells encompasses a complex series of events that include the activation of various intracellular signaling cascades. Of these, the activation of ERK1/2 has been directly linked to the extent of arteriogenesis. Little is known about the individual contribution of ERK isoforms to this process. Ricard et al. focused on the role of ERK1/2 isoforms in adult arteriogenesis. The induction of acute hind limb ischemia resulted in excessive but poorly functional arteriogenesis in mice with a global deletion of Erk1, whereas mice with an endothelial-specific deletion of Erk2 exhibited a decreased arteriogenesis. They generated a floxed ERK1 mouse line and conditionally deleted the gene in macrophages, endothelial, and smooth muscle cells. While the endothelial or macrophage deletions of ERK1 failed to recapitulate the phenotype of the ERK1$^{-/-}$ mice, the combined deletion of Erk1 in endothelial cells and macrophages came close to the phenotype in global Erk1 null mice. This shows that endothelial and macrophage ERK1 is critical to endothelial/macrophage crosstalk and effective adult arteriogenesis [3].

The importance of smooth muscle cell (SMC) proliferation in arteriogenesis is demonstrated by Lasch et al., They investigated the functional relevance of the potassium channels $K_V1.3$ and $K_{Ca}3.1$ for SMC proliferation in arteriogenesis and showed convincingly that the modulation of the potassium channel $K_V1.3$ contributes to SMC proliferation in arteriogenesis, whereas $K_{Ca}3.1$ is more likely to be involved in vasodilation [4].

VEGF is a key factor for endothelial cell proliferation and migration, as well as recruitment of pericytes and vessel assembly. VEGF can be modulated in many ways. In this Special Issue, Uslu et al., study the effects of FSAP (factor-VII-activating protease) on VEGF. The stimulatory effects of $VEGF_{165}$ on endothelial cell proliferation, migration, and signal transduction were not altered by FSAP (factor-VII-activating protease) in vitro. However, FSAP inhibited $VEGF_{165}$-mediated angiogenesis in the matrigel model in vivo, showing the role of the environment of growth-factor-mediated neovascularization [5].

Hypoxia and the (lack of) HIF1α degradation by the von Hippel-Lindau (VHL) protein complex are key determinants for VEGF activity in neovascularization. Lei et al. demonstrate very elegantly how the VHL/miR-212/miR-132 axis can play a crucial role the control of angiogenesis and that a scarcity of functional pVHL induces excessive vascular outgrowth, which is further enhanced by miR-212/132 expression, providing an exciting target for the modulation of angiogenesis [6].

MicroRNAs are small noncoding RNAs that post-transcriptionally regulate the expression of groups of target genes. However, these microRNAs can be modified themselves too, with all related consequences for processes they regulate like arteriogenesis and angiogenesis. Recent studies have revealed that many microRNAs have variants with altered terminal sequences, known as isomiRs. Additionally, endogenous microRNAs have been identified that carry biochemically modified nucleotides, revealing a dynamic microRNA epitranscriptome. Van der Kwast et al., provide in this Special Issue an overview on the mechanisms of how both types of microRNA alterations are dynamically regulated in response to ischemia and are able to influence angiogenesis and arteriogenesis [7].

The impact of hypoxia is studied by Parma et al. in their studies on intraplaque angiogenesis in lesion in murine vein grafts that are hypoxic and show profound angiogenesis in the plaque. Resolving the hypoxia by treatment of the mice with carbogen gas (95% oxygen) only had a short effect on the hypoxia in the tissue. However, this study demonstrates that long-term carbogen treatment did improve vein graft patency and plaque stability and reduced intraplaque macrophage accumulation via ROS-mediated DNA damage and apoptosis, but failed to have long-term effects on hypoxia and intraplaque angiogenesis [8].

The relation of atherosclerosis and the microvasculature is discussed in the review paper by Ziegler et al., in this Special Issue. They describe how atherosclerotic risk factors have their impact on capillary networks and that this is an element that is frequently forgotten in the current therapeutic revascularization strategies. They advocate that the microcirculatory changes during atherosclerosis, such as capillary rarefaction, warrant further investigation [9].

In the review by Caicedo et al., evidence for the involvement of the proangiogenic hormones of the growth hormone (GH)/IGF-I axis in arteriogenesis dealing with the arterial occlusion and making of them a potential therapy is described. All the elements that trigger the local and systemic production of GH/IGF-I, as well as their possible roles both in physiological and pathological conditions, are analyzed. Moreover, they describe the use of GH in the GHAS trial, in which GH or a placebo were administrated to patients suffering from critical limb ischemia with no option for revascularization [10].

Exercise training is the most promising and is the first step in the treatment of patients with peripheral arterial diseases. In their paper, Vogel et al. describe exercise-induced vascular adaptations under pathologically reduced blood flow and compare this to changes after artificially reduced blood flow. Major similarities include the overall ischemic situation, the changes in microRNA (miRNA) expression, and the increased production of nitric oxide synthase (NOS) with their associated arteriogenesis after training with blood flow restriction [11].

Last but not least, we address a specific form of arteriogenesis in this Special Issue. A huge collateral network protects the central nervous system from ischemia. Patients are at risk of spinal cord ischemia during (endovascular) aortic aneurysm repair surgery. However, predicting which patient will develop postoperative problems is difficult. One possible reason for this is the rather unknown arteriogenesis of the spinal cord blood supply. The review of Simon et al. aims to illuminate arteriogenesis in general, with the focus on the special needs of the spinal cord blood supply [12].

We believe that the papers in this Special Issue, each addressing a specific aspect of arteriogenesis and therapeutic angiogenesis, will help us to better understand the underlying mechanisms and will help to promote arteriogenesis and therapeutic angiogenesis effectively in patients with vascular occlusive diseases.

References

1. Troidl, K.; Schubert, C.; Vlacil, A.K.; Chennupati, R.; Koch, S.; Schütt, J.; Oberoi, R.; Schaper, W.; Schmitz-Rixen, T.; Schieffer, B.; et al. The lipopeptide MALP-2 promotes collateral growth. *Cells* **2020**, *9*, 997. [CrossRef] [PubMed]
2. Bot, I.; Velden, D.V.; Bouwman, M.; Kröner, M.J.; Kuiper, J.; Quax, P.H.A.; de Vries, M.R. Local mast cell activation promotes neovascularization. *Cells* **2020**, *9*, 701. [CrossRef] [PubMed]
3. Ricard, N.; Zhang, J.; Zhuang, Z.W.; Simons, M. Isoform-specific roles of ERK1 and ERK2 in arteriogenesis. *Cells* **2020**, *9*, 38. [CrossRef] [PubMed]
4. Lasch, M.; Caballero Martinez, A.; Kumaraswami, K.; Ishikawa-Ankerhold, H.; Meister, S.; Deindl, E. Contribution of the potassium channels $K_V 1.3$ and $K_{Ca} 3.1$ to smooth muscle cell proliferation in growing collateral arteries. *Cells* **2020**, *9*, 913. [CrossRef] [PubMed]
5. Uslu, Ö.; Herold, J.; Kanse, S.M. VEGF-A-cleavage by FSAP and inhibition of neovascularization. *Cells* **2019**, *8*, 1396. [CrossRef] [PubMed]
6. Lei, Z.; Klasson, T.D.; Brandt, M.M.; van de Hoek, G.; Logister, I.; Cheng, C.; Doevendans, P.A.; Sluijter, J.; Giles, R.H. Control of angiogenesis via a VHL/miR-212/132 axis. *Cells* **2020**, *9*, 1017. [CrossRef] [PubMed]
7. van der Kwast, R.V.C.T.; Quax, P.H.A.; Nossent, A.Y. An emerging role for isomiRs and the microRNA epitranscriptome in neovascularization. *Cells* **2020**, *9*, 61. [CrossRef] [PubMed]
8. Parma, L.; Peters, H.A.B.; Baganha, F.; Sluimer, J.C.; de Vries, M.R.; Quax, P.H.A. Prolonged hyperoxygenation treatment improves vein graft patency and decreases macrophage content in atherosclerotic lesions in ApoE3*Leiden mice. *Cells* **2020**, *9*, 336. [CrossRef] [PubMed]
9. Ziegler, T.; Abdel Rahman, F.; Jurisch, V.; Kupatt, C. Atherosclerosis and the capillary network; pathophysiology and potential therapeutic strategies. *Cells* **2020**, *9*, 50. [CrossRef] [PubMed]
10. Caicedo, D.; Devesa, P.; Alvarez, C.V.; Devesa, J. Why should growth hormone (GH) be considered a promising therapeutic agent for arteriogenesis? Insights from the GHAS trial. *Cells* **2020**, *9*, 807. [CrossRef] [PubMed]
11. Vogel, J.; Niederer, D.; Jung, G.; Troidl, K. Exercise-induced vascular adaptations under artificially versus pathologically reduced blood flow: A focus review with special emphasis on arteriogenesis. *Cells* **2020**, *9*, 333. [CrossRef] [PubMed]
12. Simon, F.; Wagenhäuser, M.U.; Busch, A.; Schelzig, H.; Gombert, A. Arteriogenesis of the spinal cord—the network challenge. *Cells* **2020**, *9*, 501. [CrossRef] [PubMed]

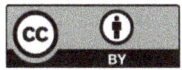

© 2020 by the authors. Licensee MDPI, Basel, Switzerland. This article is an open access article distributed under the terms and conditions of the Creative Commons Attribution (CC BY) license (http://creativecommons.org/licenses/by/4.0/).

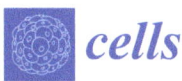

Article

The Lipopeptide MALP-2 Promotes Collateral Growth

Kerstin Troidl [1,2,*], Christian Schubert [2], Ann-Kathrin Vlacil [3], Ramesh Chennupati [1], Sören Koch [3], Jutta Schütt [3], Raghav Oberoi [3], Wolfgang Schaper [1], Thomas Schmitz-Rixen [2], Bernhard Schieffer [3] and Karsten Grote [3]

1. Max-Planck-Institute for Heart and Lung Research, 61231 Bad Nauheim, Germany; ramesh.chennupati@mpi-bn.mpg.de (R.C.); wolfgang.schaper@mpi-bn.mpg.de (W.S.)
2. Department of Vascular and Endovascular Surgery, University Hospital Frankfurt, 60488 Frankfurt, Germany; christian.schubert@mpi-bn.mpg.de (C.S.); schmitz-rixen@em.uni-frankfurt.de (T.S.-R.)
3. Cardiology and Angiology, Philipps-University Marburg, 35043 Marburg, Germany; ann-kathrin.koch@staff.uni-marburg.de (A.-K.V.); Kochsoe@students.uni-marburg.de (S.K.); j.lamle@gmx.de (J.S.); oberoi.raghav@gmail.com (R.O.); bernhard.schieffer@staff.uni-marburg.de (B.S.); grotek@staff.uni-marburg.de (K.G.)
* Correspondence: kerstin.troidl@mpi-bn.mpg.de

Received: 6 April 2020; Accepted: 14 April 2020; Published: 16 April 2020

Abstract: Beyond their role in pathogen recognition and the initiation of immune defense, Toll-like receptors (TLRs) are known to be involved in various vascular processes in health and disease. We investigated the potential of the lipopeptide and TLR2/6 ligand macrophage activating protein of 2-kDA (MALP-2) to promote blood flow recovery in mice. Hypercholesterolemic apolipoprotein E (Apoe)-deficient mice were subjected to microsurgical ligation of the femoral artery. MALP-2 significantly improved blood flow recovery at early time points (three and seven days), as assessed by repeated laser speckle imaging, and increased the growth of pre-existing collateral arteries in the upper hind limb, along with intimal endothelial cell proliferation in the collateral wall and pericollateral macrophage accumulation. In addition, MALP-2 increased capillary density in the lower hind limb. MALP-2 enhanced endothelial nitric oxide synthase (eNOS) phosphorylation and nitric oxide (NO) release from endothelial cells and improved the experimental vasorelaxation of mesenteric arteries ex vivo. In vitro, MALP-2 led to the up-regulated expression of major endothelial adhesion molecules as well as their leukocyte integrin receptors and consequently enhanced the endothelial adhesion of leukocytes. Using the experimental approach of femoral artery ligation (FAL), we achieved promising results with MALP-2 to promote peripheral blood flow recovery by collateral artery growth.

Keywords: TLR2/6; femoral artery ligation; blood flow recovery; collateral growth

1. Introduction

Cardiovascular diseases are still one of the most common causes of morbidity and mortality worldwide. In this regard, atherosclerosis—a chronic inflammatory disease of the arteries—has long been identified as the underlying cause that could ultimately lead to fatal events such as myocardial infarction, strokes [1] and also to peripheral artery disease (PAD) [2]. Atherosclerosis is characterized as a progressing process of plaque growth in the arterial vessel wall that develops in the setting of hyperlipidemia and goes along with vascular lumen stenosis, plaque rupture and erosion [3]. The growth of pre-existing collateral arteries (also termed as arteriogenesis) represents an endogenous mechanism of bypassing occluded vessels and is an important adaptive response to maintain or restore arterial perfusion [4]. Arteriogenesis occurs in tissues near to arterial stenosis whereas down-stream ischemic regions undergo angiogenesis, which is the growth of new capillaries. Collateral growth is driven by hemodynamic forces such as shear stress [5,6] and wall stress and leads to initial vasodilation due to increased levels of nitric oxide [7]. It is the reason why significant stenoses of main arteries may remain asymptomatic in patients for some time. However, in most cases, collateral growth could not ensure sufficient blood supply to the affected region, which becomes ischemic over time. Therefore, developing therapeutic approaches to improve this process is certainly desirable.

Just like atherosclerosis, collateral growth is critically driven by inflammatory processes. Chemokines, such as CC-chemokine ligands (CCL)2, and adhesion molecules, such as intercellular adhesion molecules (ICAM)-1, mediate the recruitment and accumulation of mainly monocytes into the arterial wall at sites of collateral growth. The proliferation of endothelial cells and smooth muscle cells subsequently lead to the lumen size expansion of the affected collateral artery [8]. In recent years, we have successfully used the Toll-like receptor (TLRs) 2/6 agonist macrophage activating protein of 2-kDA (MALP-2) to boost inflammatory processes and promote adaptive and regenerative mechanisms. TLRs belong to the class of pattern recognition receptors which were initially discovered on mammalian immune cells and recognize conserved pathogen-associated molecular patterns in order to initiate the immune response and combat bacterial infections [9]. In addition, an important role of TLRs has emerged later in many physiological as well as pathophysiological processes. For example, during atherogenesis, pattern recognition receptors such as TLRs are involved in the induction of inflammatory processes in response to exogenous and endogenous ligands which arise after necrotic cell death or extracellular matrix degradation [10]. MALP-2 is a common diacylated bacterial lipopeptide which is recognized by a heterodimer of TLR2 and TLR6 and was originally described as a potent activator of macrophages [11–13]. We recently reported that a single application of MALP-2 triggers beneficial vascular effects such as angiogenesis [14], endothelial wound healing and the inhibition of neointima formation following vascular injury [15]. Additionally, we observed the augmented angiogenic potential of mesenchymal stem cells after MALP-2 treatment in a sheep model of tissue engineering [16]. Given the importance of inflammatory processes for collateral growth—and because we had already established vascular cells as suitable target cells for MALP-2—we next investigated the potential of MALP-2 to promote blood flow recovery after the experimental ligation of the femoral artery by collateral growth in mice.

2. Materials and Methods

2.1. Reagents and Antibodies

The macrophage-activating lipopeptide of 2 kDa (MALP-2) was synthesized and purified as described before [11]. Fibronectin was purchased from Promocell (Heidelberg, Germany), calcein-AM from eBioscience (San Diego, CA, USA), 4′,6-diamidino-2-phenylindole (DAPI) from Sigma-Aldrich (Munich, Germany). Phenylephrine (PE), acetylcholine (ACh), noradrenaline and N-Nitroarginine methyl ester (L-NAME) were purchased from Sigma-Aldrich. Indomethacin was obtained from Alfa Aaesar (Thermo Fisher Scientific, Waltham, MA, USA), sodium nitroprusside from Honeywell (Seelze, Germany) and U46619 from Cayman Chemical (Ann Arbor, MI, USA). Antibodies for immunofluorescence against CD68, CD31 and Ki67 were from Abcam (Cambridge, UK) and against α-SMA-Cy3 were from Sigma-Aldrich. Antibodies for Western blot against VCAM-1 and β-Actin were from Santa Cruz (Dallas, TX, USA) and against p-AKT (S473), AKT, p-eNOS (S1177) and eNOS were from Cell Signaling Technology (Danvers, MA, USA). Appropriate secondary antibodies for immunofluorescence and Western blot were purchased from Thermo Fisher Scientific (Waltham, MA, USA).

2.2. Mice and Cells

The animal handling and all experimental procedures were in accordance with the guidelines from Directive 2010/63/EU of the European Parliament on the protection of animals used for scientific purposes and were approved by the Animal Care and Use Committee of the state Hessen (approval reference numbers V54-19c20/15-B2/1152 (23.05.17); B2-1077 (29.07.16)). For femoral artery ligation

(FAL), 8–12-week-old male C57BL/6 and BALB/c mice were purchased from Charles River (Sulzfeld, Germany). Six to ten-week-old male Apoe-deficient mice with a C57BL/6 background from our own breeding were fed a high fat diet (HFD, 21% butterfat, 1.5% cholesterol, Ssniff, Soest, Germany) for 12 weeks and operated on thereafter. Adductor muscles were isolated from the left and right upper hind limbs of 10-week-old male C57BL/6 mice, cut into 1–2 mm pieces with fine scissors and 4 pieces were placed in a well of a 96-well plate for ex vivo stimulation with MALP-2. The endothelial MyEnd cell line was grown in Dulbecco's modified Eagle medium (DMEM, Gibco, Darmstadt, Germany) with 10% fetal calf serum (FCS, PAN-Biotech, Aidenbach, Germany) and 1% penicillin/streptomycin (100 U/mL and 100 mg/mL, Sigma-Aldrich). The MyEnd cells showed typical endothelial properties and, as they grew to complete confluence, were highly positive for the endothelial marker CD31 and expressed the MALP-2 receptors TLR2 and TLR6 (Figure S1). The monocyte/macrophage cell line J774A.1 was grown in DMEM-Glutamax (Gibco) with 10% FCS and 1% penicillin/streptomycin (P/S).

2.3. Experimental Femoral Artery Ligation (FAL)

The mice were subjected to FAL as described elsewhere [17]. During the surgical procedure, the mice were under general anesthesia with isoflurane (2.5% for induction, 1.5–2.0% maintenance). After the FAL, the mice were intravenously injected with MALP-2 (1 µg in 125 µL phosphate-buffered saline (PBS) per mouse) or vehicle control (125 µL PBS). For postoperative analgesia, carprofen (5 mg/kg body weight) was subcutaneously injected once prior to surgery. The contralateral leg served as the control. After the termination of experiments, the mice were euthanized by an anesthetic overdose.

2.4. Laser Speckle Imaging

The perfusion of the hind paws was assessed using a laser speckle imaging device (moorFLPI-2; software for acquisition and MoorFLPI Review V5.0 for evaluation, Moor Instruments, Axminster, UK) on a heating plate (37 °C) before the FAL (d0 pre), immediately after (d0 post), and d3, d7 and d10 after the FAL.

2.5. Histology and Immunohistochemistry

The mice were perfused with 10 mL of a vasodilation buffer (100 µg adenosine, 1 µg sodium nitroprusside, 0.05% bovine serum albumin in PBS, pH 7.4), followed by 10 mL of 3% paraformaldehyde post mortem. Tissue from the ligated left and the not ligated right adductor muscles was harvested and placed in 15% sucrose in PBS for 4 h and overnight at 4 °C in 30% sucrose in PBS. The tissue was cryopreserved in Tissuetek (Sakura Finetek, Staufen, Germany) and cut into 8 µm cryosections. A morphometric analysis was performed using haematoxilin-eosin staining to evaluate the dimensions of the collateral arteries with the help of ImageJ software (National Institutes of Health, Bethesda, MD, USA). The cryosections were fixed with 5% paraformaldehyde and stained with antibodies against Ki-67, CD31, α-SMA or CD68. The slides were covered with Mowiol (Sigma-Aldrich) and analyzed with a confocal microscope (Leica SP5, Leica, Wetzlar, Germany).

2.6. Organ Chamber Experiments (Wire Myography)

The male C57BL/6 mice of 10–12 weeks were killed by CO_2/O_2 inhalation. The mesenteric artery was dissected free from surrounding fat and connective tissue and directly mounted in a wire myograph (Danish Myo Technology, Aarhus, Denmark) containing Krebs solution (119 mM NaCl, 4.7 mM KCl, 2.5 mM $CaCl_2 \cdot 2H_2O$, 1.17 mM $MgSO_4 \cdot 7H_2O$, 20 mM $NaHCO_3$, 1.18 mM KH_2PO_4, 0.027 mM EDTA, 11 mM glucose). Mesenteric arterial segments (2 mm) were distended to the diameter at which maximal contractile responses to 10 µM noradrenaline could be obtained. The maximal relaxing response to acetylcholine (ACh, 10 µM) was recorded during a contraction induced by 10 µM noradrenaline; arterial segments which showed less than 85% relaxation were discarded from the experiments.

2.7. Real-Time PCR

For the analysis of the mRNA expression, the total RNA was isolated using RNA-Solv®Reagent (Omega Bio-tek, Norcross, GA, USA) following the manufacturer's instructions and reverse-transcribed with SuperScript reverse transcriptase, oligo(dT) primers (Thermo Fisher Scientific), and deoxynucleoside triphosphates (Promega, Mannheim, Germany). Real-time PCR was performed in duplicates in a total volume of 20 µL using Power SYBR green PCR Master Mix (Thermo Fisher Scientific) on a Step One Plus Real-Time PCR System (Applied Biosystems, Foster City, CA, USA) in 96-well PCR plates (Applied Biosystems). The SYBR Green fluorescence emissions were monitored after each cycle. For normalization, the expression of glyceraldehyde 3-phosphate dehydrogenase as housekeeper was determined in duplicates. The gene expression was calculated using the $2^{-\Delta\Delta Ct}$ method. The PCR primers were obtained from Microsynth AG (Balgach, Switzerland) and are available upon request.

2.8. Enzyme-Linked Immunosorbent Assay (ELISA)

The supernatant from cultured tissue pieces of the adductor muscles of C57BL/6 mice was analyzed for CCL2, GM-CSF, IL-1α and TNF-α using a mouse-specific ELISA from R&D Systems (Minneapolis, MN, USA) according to the manufacturer's protocol with the help of an Infinite M200 PRO plate reader (TECAN Instruments, Maennedorf, Switzerland).

2.9. Western Blot

The total protein was extracted with a buffer that contained 150 mM NaCl, 1% Triton X-100, 0.5% sodium deoxycholate, 0.1% SDS and 50 mM Tris that was supplemented with a protease inhibitor cocktail (Roche, Penzberg, Germany). The total protein content was measured using a protein quantitation assay (Thermo Fisher Scientific) according to the manufacturer's protocol. The total protein (20 µg) was loaded onto 10% denaturing SDS gel and transferred to 0.45 mm polyvinylidene fluoride membranes (GE Healthcare, Little Chalfont, UK) for immunoblotting. The membranes were blocked with 5% nonfat dry milk (Sigma-Aldrich) and probed with primary antibodies against VCAM-1, β-Actin, p-AKT, AKT, p-eNOS and eNOS, followed by horseradish peroxidase–labeled secondary antibodies. Proteins were detected using a chemiluminescence substrate (Bio-Rad Laboratories, Hercules, USA). The results were documented on a Chemo-star imaging system (INTAS, Göttingen, Germany). The signal intensity of the chemiluminescence was quantified using Quantity One software (Bio-Rad).

2.10. Griess Assay

The MyEnd cells were plated in fibronectin-coated wells of a 96-well plate (TPP, Trasadingen, Switzerland) in DMEM with 10% FCS and 1% P/S and grown to complete confluence. The cells were starved in DMEM with 1% FCS and 1% P/S for 16 h and stimulated with MALP-2 (1 µg/mL) for 2 h. The NO levels in each well were measured using a Griess reagent (Sigma-Aldrich) according to the manufacturer's instructions.

2.11. Adhesion Assay

The MyEnd cells were plated in fibronectin-coated wells of a 48-well plate (TPP) in DMEM with 10% FCS and 1% P/S and grown to complete confluence. The cells were starved in DMEM with 1% FCS and 1% P/S for 16 h and stimulated with MALP-2 (1 µg/mL) for 6 h. In parallel, J774A.1 cells were labeled with 5 µM of calcein-AM (Invitrogen, Carlsbad, CA, USA). according to the manufacturer's instructions. After stimulation, the MyEnd cells were washed twice with 500 µL of PBS per well; 0.5×10^6 labeled J774A.1 cells in 500 µL of DMEM with 1% FCS were added per well and co-cultured for 1 h in 5% CO_2 at 37 °C. After co-incubation, each well was washed three times with 500 µL of PBS and 10 high powerfield (HPF) digital images were taken using an Axio Vert.A1 microscope equipped with an AxioCam MRm camera (Carl Zeiss, Microimaging, Jena, Germany). The adhered calcein-AM-labeled J774A.1 cells per HPF image were counted using ImageJ software.

2.12. Statistical Analysis

All the data are represented as means ± SEM. The data were compared using the 2-tailed Student t-test for independent samples or by a 1-way ANOVA followed by the Tukey multiple comparison test (GraphPad Prism, version 6.05; GraphPad Software, La Jolla, CA, USA). A value of $P < 0.05$ was considered statistically significant. The numbers of independent experiments are indicated in each figure legend. The real-time PCR was performed in technical duplicates.

3. Results

3.1. MALP-2 Improved Perfusion Recovery and Collateral Growth in the Hind Limb Following FAL in Hypercholesterolemic Apoe-Deficient Mice

Based on our previous findings [14–16], we hypothesized that MALP-2 is capable of promoting collateral growth. To analyze the functional effects of systemic MALP-2 application in this regard, the mouse FAL model was applied sequentially to two different wild-type mice strains (C57BL/6 and BALB/c) and additionally to Apoe-deficient mice (Apoe-KO) on a high fat diet (HFD) for 12 weeks. Laser Speckle perfusion measurements were performed prior to and after surgery as well as on days 3 and 7 and, for Apoe-KO mice, on day 10. Following the left FAL, the ratio of left hind limb perfusion compared to that of the hind paw of the non-ligated right site dropped to less than 25% in all groups (Figure 1a). The perfusion recoveries of C57BL/6 and BALB/c wild-type mice which received MALP-2 or PBS (control) were found to be similar on day three and day seven post FAL (Figure 1a). However, MALP-2 significantly improved the perfusion recovery of hypercholesterolemic Apoe-KO mice on day three post FAL. The beneficial effect of MALP-2 on perfusion recovery was limited to early time points and returned to control conditions on day 10 post FAL (Figure 1a,b). Since the functional improvement of MALP-2 in the FAL model was limited to Apoe-KO mice on a HFD, we concluded that hypercholesterolemic conditions with compromised vascular functions are required for the observed beneficial effects of MALP-2; we therefore focused on this model in the following analysis.

The remodeling of the collateral arteries was verified by morphometry in cross sections of the left adductors 10 days after the FAL. The MALP-2 application significantly increased the collateral inner diameter as well as the collateral wall area, thus documenting enhanced collateral growth with MALP-2 (Figure 1c). Since collateral growth is critically influenced by hemodynamic forces, we analyzed the atherosclerotic arterial plaque load in the experimental Apoe-KO mice after 12 weeks of the HFD diet. As expected, we detected plaques in the aortic root and in the thoracoabdominal aorta However, the atherosclerotic plaque load was not different between the control and the MALP-2-treated group (Figure S2a,b). Plaques in the femoral artery were only detected in rare cases. In addition, we investigated the collateral arteries, which were found to be highly positive for Oil Red O, indicating lipid deposition in the collateral vascular wall in hypercholesterolemic Apoe-deficient mice (Figure S2c). As expected, this was not the case in parallel-performed control Oil Red O staining in collaterals from C57BL/6 mice (Figure S2c). However, atherosclerotic plaques were not detected, excluding the possibility that plaque morphology itself might influence the hemodynamics and thereby collateral remodeling and growth.

3.2. MALP-2 Increased Pericollateral Macrophage Accumulation, Endothelial Cell Proliferation and Downstream Angiogenesis Following FAL

In order to investigate the influence of MALP-2 on the vascular remodeling process, tissue from the adductor muscles was harvested from hypercholesterolemic Apoe-deficient mice 3, 7 and 10 days following the FAL. In the initial phase, the collateral growth is critically driven by pericollateral macrophage assembly and endothelial proliferation [4,6,18]. MALP-2 significantly increased the macrophage accumulation around the collateral artery on day three after the FAL compared to the control. There was no effect of MALP-2 at later time points (Figure 2a). Likewise, we detected significantly more proliferating endothelial cells in MALP-2-treated mice on days three and seven after the FAL. In general, no proliferating endothelial cells were detected on day 10 (Figure 2b). The stenosis or occlusion of a major arterial conductance vessel entails a reduced blood supply and subsequent ischemia in the downstream supply area. Angiogenesis with an increased capillary density is usually the counteracting adaptive process in tissue ischemia. Therefore, we investigated angiogenesis in the gastrocnemius muscle and found that MALP-2 increased the capillary density on day three and day seven. This was not different anymore on day 10 post FAL (Figure 2c). Our results indicated that the effects of MALP-2 on collateral growth occurred within the first seven days after FAL.

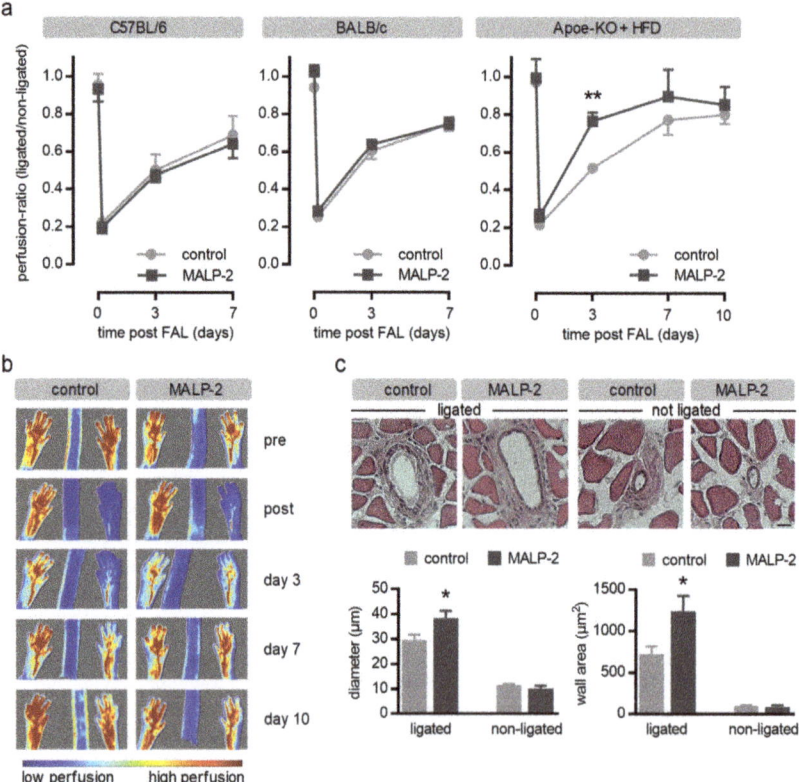

Figure 1. MALP-2 improved the perfusion recovery and collateral growth in the hind limb following femoral artery ligation (FAL) in hypercholesterolemic Apoe-deficient mice. (a) Following the FAL, the perfusion recovery was determined by laser Speckle perfusion imaging for C57BL/6, BALB/c and hypercholesterolemic Apoe-KO mice (12 weeks on a high fat diet (HFD)) treated with MALP-2 or PBS (control) pre/post the FAL, after three and seven days and, in Apoe-KO mice, after 10 days. Data are expressed as the ratio of the ligated and the non-ligated hind limb. ** $P < 0.01$, $N = 4$–7. (b) Representative laser speckle perfusion images indicate the effect of MALP-2 compared to the control (PBS) on perfusion recovery in the ligated hind limbs of Apoe-KO mice pre/post the FAL and after 3, 7 and 10 days. (c) Representative haematoxilin-eosin staining of cross sections of collateral arteries in the adductor muscle of the ligated and the non-ligated hind limbs of hypercholesterolemic Apoe-KO mice treated with MALP-2 or PBS (control) 10 days after the FAL and the corresponding morphometric analysis of the collateral diameter and wall area. Scale bar = 10 µm. * $P < 0.05$ vs. control, $N = 6$–14 collaterals.

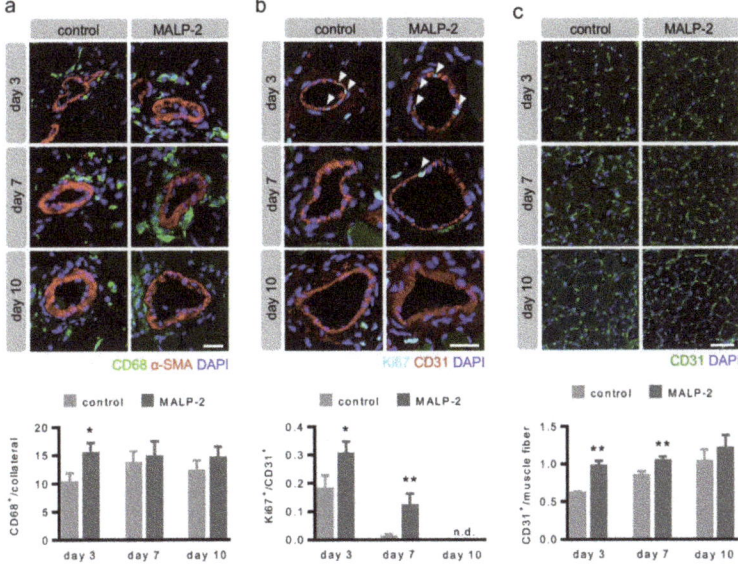

Figure 2. MALP-2 increased pericollateral macrophage accumulation, endothelial cell proliferation and downstream angiogenesis following FAL. This shows the representative immunostaining of cross sections of collateral arteries in the adductor muscle and the calf muscle of the ligated hind limb in hypercholesterolemic Apoe-KO mice treated with MALP-2 and PBS (control) 3, 7 and 10 days after the FAL and the corresponding quantitative analysis. (**a**) CD68 staining to assess the accumulation of macrophages around the collateral (α-SMA indicates the media of the collateral wall). Scale bar = 25 µm. (**b**) Ki67 staining to determine the portion of proliferating CD31-positive collateral endothelial cells (white arrow heads). Scale bar = 25 µm. (**c**) CD31 indicates capillary density in the calf muscle. Scale bar = 50 µm. * $P < 0.05$, ** $P < 0.01$ vs. control, N = up to 20 collaterals, n.d. = not detected.

To explore which factors were potentially involved in the process of MALP-2-induced collateral growth, we stimulated tissue pieces of the adductor muscles from C57BL/6 mice ex vivo with MALP-2. A real-time PCR analysis revealed increased expression levels for the established mediators of collateral growth such as CC-chemokine ligand 2 (*Ccl2*) [19] and granulocyte macrophage colony-stimulating factor (*Gm-csf*) [20] as well as, for the general inflammatory markers, interleukin 1β (*Il-1β*) and tumor necrosis factor-α (*Tnf-α*, Figure 3a). Likewise, the corresponding protein in the supernatant was found to be enhanced (Figure 3b). Das et al. recently reported that the axis of C-X-C motif chemokine ligand 2 (CXCL12, also known as stromal cell-derived factor 1) and its receptor C-X-C motif receptor 4 (CXCR4) is relevant for the injury-induced cardiac collateral growth in neonatal mice and could also be induced by exogenous CXCL12 in adult mice [21]. However, MALP-2 did not induce *Cxcl12* expression ex vivo in the adductor muscle tissue (Figure 3c) or in the cultured MyEnd endothelial cells (Figure 3d), suggesting that this process did not play a role in MALP-2-dependent collateral growth.

3.3. MALP-2 Improved NO-Dependent Vascular Relaxation and Enhanced Endothelial Cell-Derived NO Release

Since endothelial dysfunction may limit collateral growth itself or the beneficial effects of collateral vessels on tissue perfusion, we assessed the effect of MALP-2 on vascular relaxation. To this end, we isolated mesenteric arteries from C57BL/6 mice to perform wire myography. MALP-2 significantly improved acetylcholine (ACh)-induced relaxation of phenylephrine (PE)-preconstricted (10 µM) mesenteric arteries (Figure 4a). To test for differences in endothelium-derived NO release, we inhibited endothelium-dependent hyperpolarization by depolarizing the vessels with high potassium buffers (60 mM K⁺) and by inhibiting cyclooxygenases using indomethacin. Under these conditions, the relaxing responses to ACh could be entirely attributed to NO [22]. The MALP-2 treatment resulted in significantly increased endothelium-derived NO responses (Figure 4b). This effect completely disappeared when the endothelial nitric oxide synthase (eNOS) was additionally blocked with L-NAME (Figure 4c). Furthermore, MALP-2 also significantly improved the relaxation response in thoracic aorta (data not shown). These results demonstrated a crucial role for endothelium-derived NO in MALP-2-dependent vascular relaxation. Moreover, in MyEnd cells, MALP-2 led to a fast and transient increase in the protein kinase B (also known as AKT) phosphorylation (Figure 5a) and eNOS phosphorylation (Figure 5b) and consequently to an increased NO release (Figure 5c).

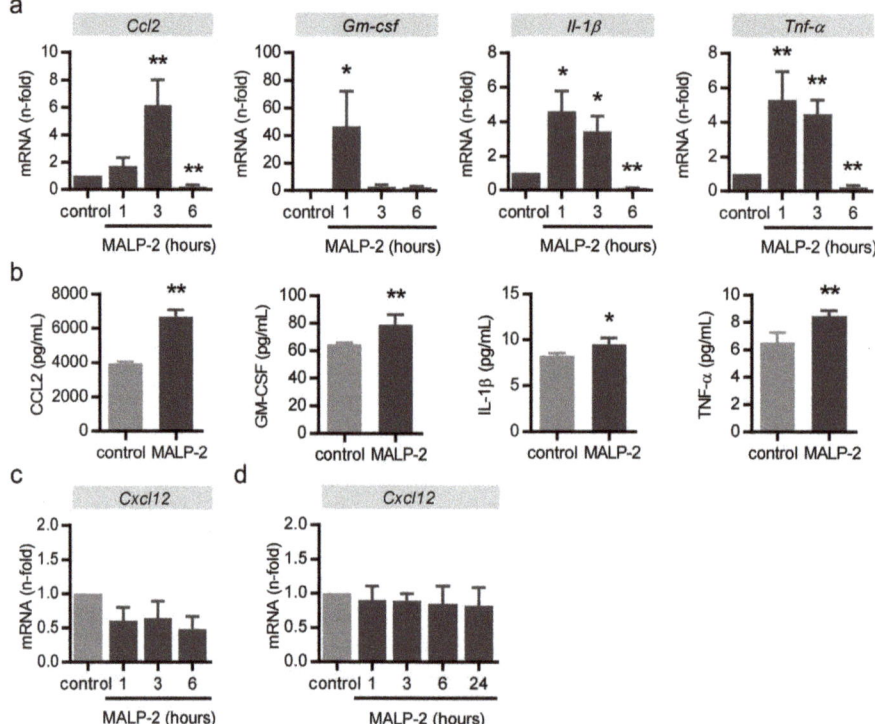

Figure 3. MALP-2 up-regulated inflammatory genes in the upper hind limb muscle. Tissue pieces of the adductor muscles of C57BL/6 mice were isolated and stimulated ex vivo with MALP-2 (1 µg/mL); *Ccl2*, *Gm-csf*, *Il-1β* and *Tnf-α* mRNA levels were analyzed after the indicated times by (**a**) real-time PCR and (**b**) the corresponding protein in the supernatant after 6 h by ELISA. *CXCL12* mRNA levels were analyzed (**c**) in tissue pieces of the adductor muscle of C57BL/6 mice ex vivo and in (**d**) MyEND cells following MALP-2 stimulation (1 µg/mL) after the indicated times by real-time PCR. * $P < 0.05$, ** $P < 0.01$ vs. control, $N = 4$–6.

3.4. MALP-2 Up-Regulated Endothelial Adhesion Molecules and Enhanced the Endothelial Adhesion of Monocytic Cells

Arteriogenesis is a multi-faceted, highly coordinated process involving the endothelial adhesion of monocytes onto endothelial cells [4,6]. To explore the potential underlying mechanism responsible for the positive effects of MALP-2 on collateral growth after FAL, we conducted a series of in vitro experiments. In endothelial MyEnd cells, MALP-2 led to a strong transient increase in the mRNA levels of vascular cell adhesion molecule-1 (*Vcam-1*) after only 1 h (Figure 6a) and slightly delayed to an increase in VCAM-1 protein levels (Figure 6b). The mRNA levels of the other major endothelial adhesion molecules, i.e., intercellular adhesion molecule-1 (*Icam-1*), *E-selectin* and *P-selectin*, were also increased between 1 and 3 h following the MALP-2 stimulation (Figure 6a). In addition, we investigated the mRNA expression of integrin receptors on monocytes/macrophages as counterparts to the endothelial adhesion molecules. Likewise, the mRNA levels of integrin α4β1 (very late antigen-4, *Vla4*), integrin αM (*Itgam*) and E-selectin ligand-1 (*Esl-1*) were slightly and transiently increased in the monocyte/macrophage cell line J774A.1 by MALP-2 (Figure S3). Consequently, the pretreatment of a monolayer of MyEnd cells with MALP-2 almost doubled the number of adherent J774A.1 cells (Figure 6c).

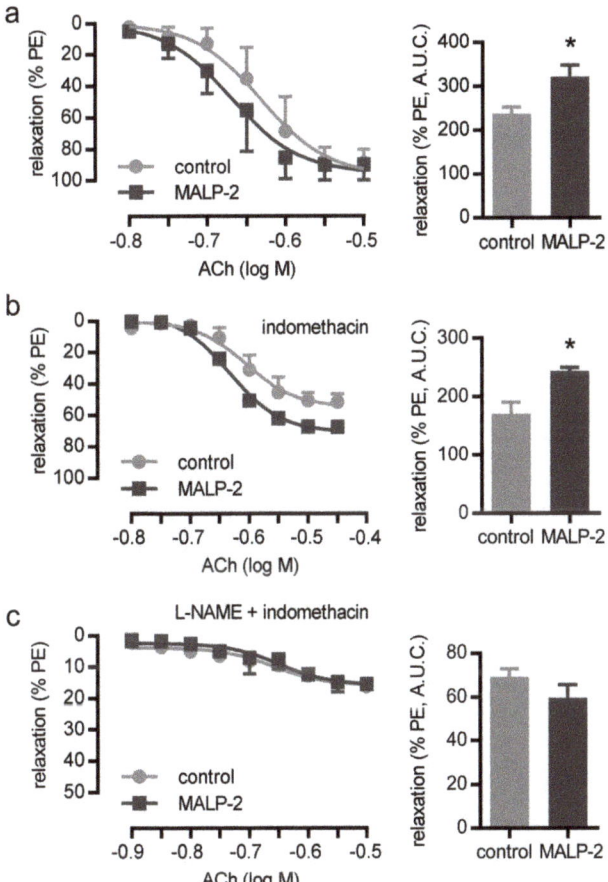

Figure 4. MALP-2 improved NO-dependent vascular relaxation in the mesenteric arteries of C57BL/6 mice. (**a**) The relaxation response to acetylcholine (ACh 0.001–10 µM) during phenylephrine-induced (PE, 10 µM) contraction in mesenteric arteries incubated with MALP-2 or PBS (control), $N = 6$. (**b**) The relaxation response to ACh (0.01–10 µM) during K$^+$-induced (60 mM) contraction in mesenteric arteries incubated with indomethacin (10 µM, COX-inhibitor) and MALP-2 or PBS, $N = 3$. (**c**) The relaxation response to ACh (0.001–10 µM) in the presence of L-NAME (100 µM, NOS inhibitor) and indomethacin (10 µM). A.U.C. = area under the curve, * $P < 0.05$ vs. control, $N = 3$.

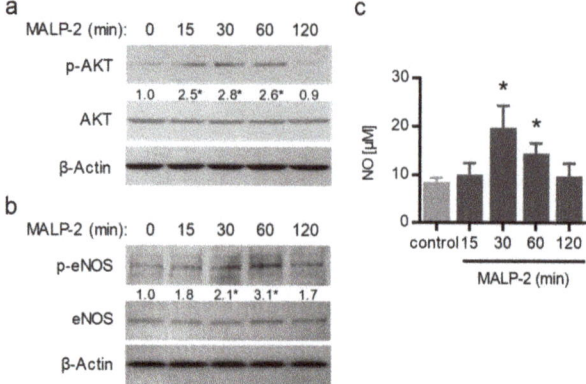

Figure 5. MALP-2 enhanced the endothelial cell-derived NO release. MyEnd cells were stimulated with MALP-2 (1 µg/mL); (**a**) the AKT phosphorylation (p-AKT) as well as (**b**) the eNOS phosphorylation (p-eNOS) were analyzed after the indicated times by Western blot and (**c**) the NO release was analyzed with the Griess reagent. The numbers between panels indicate fold-change vs. unstimulated after normalization to total AKT or eNOS, respectively. β-Actin was used as the loading control. * $P < 0.05$ vs. control, $N = 4$–5.

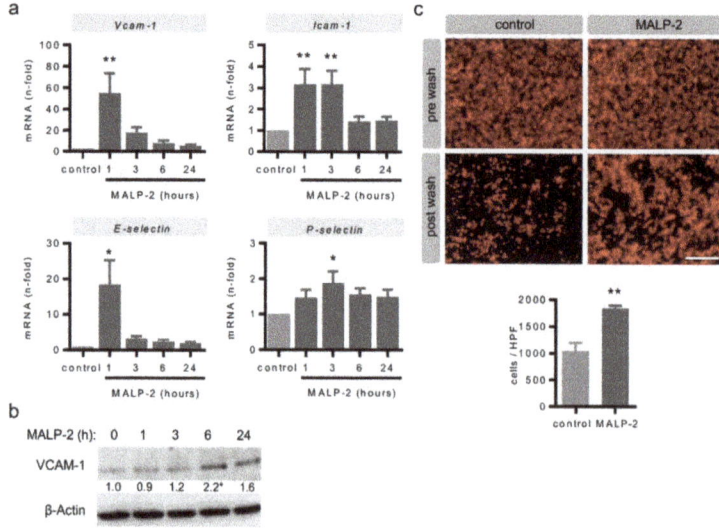

Figure 6. MALP-2 up-regulated endothelial adhesion molecules and enhanced the endothelial adhesion of monocytic cells. (**a**) The MyEnd cells were stimulated with MALP-2 (1 µg/mL) and the VCAM-1, ICAM-1, E-selectin and P-selectin mRNA levels were analyzed after the indicated times by real-time PCR. * $P < 0.05$, ** $P < 0.01$ vs. control, $N = 6$–8. (**b**) The MyEnd cells were stimulated with MALP-2 (1 µg/mL) and the VCAM-1 protein expression was analyzed after the indicated times by Western blot. β-Actin was used as the loading control. The numbers between panels indicate fold-change vs. unstimulated after normalization to β-Actin. * $P < 0.05$ vs. control, $N = 4$–5. (**c**) Fluorescence images depicting calcein-AM-labeled J774A.1 cells on a MyEnd monolayer with or without pretreatment with MALP-2 (1 µg/mL) for 6 h with an additional adhesion time of 1 h and the corresponding quantitative analysis. Pictures before and after washing are shown. Scale bar = 100 µm, ** $P < 0.01$ vs. control, $N = 3$.

4. Discussion

Atherosclerosis, as a chronic inflammatory arterial disease, contributes to the major mortality of cardiovascular diseases worldwide. On the one hand, this is due to acute events such as myocardial infarction and strokes [23], but on the other, this is due to progressive lumen stenosis, which is the main trigger for adaptive arteriogenesis [4–6,18].

In this regard, growing collaterals represent a naturally occurring adaptive bypass system to avoid tissue ischemia. Well-developed collaterals, despite significant stenosis or even the occlusion of major coronary or peripheral arteries, could be the reason why some patients stay asymptomatic over a long period of time [4]. However, collateral growth is usually not sufficient to protect patients against ischemia for all their lives and thus therapies supporting this process are desirable. The model used in this study was a model of hind limb ischemia in mice. Critical limb ischemia represents the most severe form of PAD in patients [24,25]. The highly deadly disease is characterized by pain during walking and even at rest, as well as non-healing ulcers in the lower extremities. If the extent of the femoral artery occlusion due to advanced atherosclerosis becomes too large for percutaneous or surgical interventions, limb amputation remains the only treatment option. Catheter-based angiographic interventions or surgical bypasses are basically emergency procedures for the revascularization of the main artery in order to restore limb perfusion. Similar to these interventions, novel therapies such as cell-based or molecular therapies normally do not promote collateral growth [24,25]. Studies addressing therapeutic arteriogenesis are rare. Some of those investigated the potential of GM-CSF, identified in a rabbit model [20], with different outcomes in patients with coronary artery disease [26] or PAD [27]. Finally, the therapeutic improvement of collateral growth in cardiovascular patients hardly plays a role in clinical practice at present. In the current study, we used the lipopeptide and TLR2/6 ligand MALP-2 to investigate therapeutic arteriogenesis. Over the past few years, we had already demonstrated the high potential of MALP-2 to promote vascular regeneration, such as angiogenesis [14] and endothelial regeneration after vascular wounding [15]. We now identified the possible application of MALP-2 to promote arteriogenesis and uncovered the potential underlying mechanisms. We found that MALP-2 functionally improved perfusion recovery in the hind limb by enhanced collateral growth. The increase in the collateral lumen diameter was driven by augmented pericollateral macrophage accumulation and enhanced endothelial cell proliferation. MALP-2-enhanced the NO release of endothelial cells and improved NO-dependent vasorelaxation as well as endothelial adhesion molecule expression and subsequent monocytic cell adhesion. We had already reported enhanced secretion of GM-CSF from endothelial cells of various origin following MALP-2 stimulation [14,15]. Since the beneficial effect of GM-CSF on collateral growth has already been proven in animal experiments [20] and clinical studies [27], it is conceivable that the observed beneficial effect of MALP-2 on collateral growth is dependent on growth factors such as GM-CSF as well. Of note, we did not see any beneficial effects of MALP-2 application in two commonly used wild-type mouse strains—neither in C57BL/6 mice nor in BALB/c mice, which have known differences in cardiovascular regeneration [28]. As we saw the functional and morphological changes upon MALP-2 treatment that were summarized above exclusively in Apoe-deficient mice on a HFD and not in wild-type mice, we concluded that hypercholesteremic conditions are required for the beneficial MALP-2 effects on arteriogenesis. This conclusion was supported by the observation—to our knowledge, for the first time—that the collaterals were already positive for Oil Red O in this model. The staining demonstrated lipid deposition in the vascular wall of the collaterals, indicating vascular dysfunction. Ultimately, the mouse model used—with compromised vascular function and advanced atherosclerotic plaque load in larger arteries— approximately reflects the situation of cardiovascular patients.

In order to optimize the application route of MALP-2, we tested different variants. Initially, our intention was to choose an application route to bring MALP-2 as close as possible to the pre-existing collaterals after ligation. Therefore, we injected MALP-2 divided into small quantities into the Musculus adductor near to the collaterals. However, at the sites of injection, the tissue was affected in such a manner that subsequent histological analyses were not possible anymore. In addition, we tried to inject directly into the femoral artery proximal to the ligation. This application route proved difficult due to the small dimensions of the vessel. Since we observed increased mortality after the operation, we refrained from using this method. In the end, we chose the widely used intravenous application route (tail vein) for the MALP-2 injection, knowing that the lipophilic substance would be partially absorbed by the endothelium and that only small amounts would enter the target area of the collaterals. Although our approach was successful, there is still room to improve application strategies to bring MALP-2 into close proximity to the collaterals, e.g., in a biodegradable intra-arterial matrigel deposit or similar.

The potential limitations of our study are the same as those that generally apply for experimental studies in mice. The ligation of the femoral artery induces the growth of pre-existing collateral arteries and is therefore widely accepted as a reliable model for arteriogenesis. However, the vascular dimensions and related hemodynamic forces are different to the situation of cardiovascular patients. To substantiate our findings for a potential therapeutic use in promoting collateral growth, experiments in higher animals are needed. In regard to therapeutic angiogenesis, this has been already done in a sheep model of tissue engineering [16]. Moreover, we used just one single dose of MALP-2 (1 µg/mouse) as this was proved to be effective in a previous in vivo study by our group [15]. Dose-response experiments would maybe reveal an even more effective dose. However, based on the data already published, our local animal authorities did not approve dose-finding experiments in this study.

Seemingly, TLR2/6 signaling is particularly suitable in promoting vascular regeneration and adaptation. This is not only documented by our studies [14–16]. Indeed, other TLR2 ligands, such as bacterial peptidoglycan [29] or the proteoglycan versican as an endogenous ligand [30], have been shown to induce angiogenic factors. Likewise, endogenous lipid oxidation productions are capable of promoting angiogenesis [31]. The common principle of our studies is a single bolus injection of MALP-2 to transiently increase inflammation, which could be considered an immunological mechanism to promote regeneration and adaptation. In contrast, long-term application of MALP-2 led to increased circulating inflammatory markers and increased atherosclerosis [32].

In summary, we identified a novel property of the lipopeptide and TLR2/6 ligand MALP-2 to restore blood flow recovery by enhanced collateral growth with possible implications for therapeutic arteriogenesis (Figure S4).

Supplementary Materials: The following are available online at http://www.mdpi.com/2073-4409/9/4/997/s1, Figure S1: Characterization of MyEnd cells, Figure S2: Vascular lipid deposition in hypercholesterolemic Apoe-KO 7 days after FAL and MALP-2 or PBS (control) injection, Figure S3: MALP-2 up-regulates mRNA expression for integrin receptors in J774A.1 cells, Figure S4: Mode of action of MALP-2 in arteriogenesis.

Author Contributions: Conceptualization, K.T. and K.G.; methodology and validation, K.T., C.S., A.-K.V., R.C., S.K., J.S., R.O., K.G.; formal analysis and investigation, K.T and K.G; writing—original draft preparation, K.G.; writing—review and editing, K.T., W.S., T.S.-R., B.S.; supervision, project administration and funding acquisition, K.T. and K.G. All authors have read and agreed to the published version of the manuscript.

Funding: This research was funded by the Anna-Maria and Uwe Karsten Kühl foundation (T188/30462/2017), the B. Braun foundation (BBST-D-18-00021) and the von Behring-Röntgen foundation (62-0002).

Acknowledgments: We thank Daniela Beppler, Silke Brauschke, Brigitte Matzke and Christina Reschke for excellent technical assistance.

Conflicts of Interest: The authors declare no conflict of interest.

References

1. Sanchis-Gomar, F.; Perez-Quilis, C.; Leischik, R.; Lucia, A. Epidemiology of coronary heart disease and acute coronary syndrome. *Ann. Transl. Med.* **2016**, *4*, 256. [CrossRef] [PubMed]
2. Fowkes, F.G.; Aboyans, V.; Fowkes, F.J.; McDermott, M.M.; Sampson, U.K.; Criqui, M.H. Peripheral artery disease: Epidemiology and global perspectives. *Nat. Rev. Cardiol.* **2017**, *14*, 156–170. [CrossRef] [PubMed]
3. Hansson, G.K.; Libby, P.; Tabas, I. Inflammation and plaque vulnerability. *J. Intern. Med.* **2015**, *278*, 483–493. [CrossRef] [PubMed]

4. Seiler, C.; Stoller, M.; Pitt, B.; Meier, P. The human coronary collateral circulation: Development and clinical importance. *Eur. Heart J.* **2013**, *34*, 2674–2682. [CrossRef]
5. Pipp, F.; Boehm, S.; Cai, W.J.; Adili, F.; Ziegler, B.; Karanovic, G.; Ritter, R.; Balzer, J.; Scheler, C.; Schaper, W.; et al. Elevated fluid shear stress enhances postocclusive collateral artery growth and gene expression in the pig hind limb. *Arterioscler. Thromb. Vasc. Biol.* **2004**, *24*, 1664–1668. [CrossRef]
6. Eitenmuller, I.; Volger, O.; Kluge, A.; Troidl, K.; Barancik, M.; Cai, W.J.; Heil, M.; Pipp, F.; Fischer, S.; Horrevoets, A.J.; et al. The range of adaptation by collateral vessels after femoral artery occlusion. *Circ. Res.* **2006**, *99*, 656–662. [CrossRef]
7. Troidl, K.; Tribulova, S.; Cai, W.-J.; Rüding, I.; Apfelbeck, H.; Schierling, W.; Troidl, C.; Schmitz-Rixen, T.; Schaper, W. Effects of endogenous nitric oxide and of DETA NONOate in arteriogenesis. *J. Cardiovasc. Pharmacol.* **2010**, *55*, 153–160. [CrossRef]
8. Shireman, P. The chemokine system in arteriogenesis and hind limb ischemia. *J. Vasc. Surg.* **2007**, *45*, A48–A56. [CrossRef]
9. O'Neill, L.A.; Golenbock, D.; Bowie, A.G. The history of Toll-like receptors—redefining innate immunity. *Nat. Rev. Immunol.* **2013**, *13*, 453–460. [CrossRef]
10. Lundberg, A.M.; Hansson, G.K. Innate immune signals in atherosclerosis. *Clin. Immunol.* **2010**, *134*, 5–24. [CrossRef]
11. Mühlradt, P.F.; Kiess, M.; Meyer, H.; Sussmuth, R.; Jung, G. Isolation, structure elucidation, and synthesis of a macrophage stimulatory lipopeptide from Mycoplasma fermentans acting at picomolar concentration. *J. Exp. Med.* **1997**, *185*, 1951–1958. [CrossRef] [PubMed]
12. Takeuchi, O.; Kaufmann, A.; Grote, K.; Kawai, T.; Hoshino, K.; Morr, M.; Muhlradt, P.F.; Akira, S. Cutting edge: Preferentially the R-stereoisomer of the mycoplasmal lipopeptide macrophage-activating lipopeptide-2 activates immune cells through a toll-like receptor 2- and MyD88-dependent signaling pathway. *J. Immunol.* **2000**, *164*, 554–557. [CrossRef] [PubMed]
13. Takeuchi, O.; Kawai, T.; Muhlradt, P.F.; Morr, M.; Radolf, J.D.; Zychlinsky, A.; Takeda, K.; Akira, S. Discrimination of bacterial lipoproteins by Toll-like receptor 6. *Int. Immunol.* **2001**, *13*, 933–940. [CrossRef] [PubMed]
14. Grote, K.; Schuett, H.; Salguero, G.; Grothusen, C.; Jagielska, J.; Drexler, H.; Muhlradt, P.F.; Schieffer, B. Toll-like receptor 2/6 stimulation promotes angiogenesis via GM-CSF as a potential strategy for immune defense and tissue regeneration. *Blood* **2010**, *115*, 2543–2552. [CrossRef] [PubMed]
15. Grote, K.; Sonnenschein, K.; Kapopara, P.R.; Hillmer, A.; Grothusen, C.; Salguero, G.; Kotlarz, D.; Schuett, H.; Bavendiek, U.; Schieffer, B. Toll-like receptor 2/6 agonist macrophage-activating lipopeptide-2 promotes reendothelialization and inhibits neointima formation after vascular injury. *Arterioscler. Thromb. Vasc. Biol.* **2013**, *33*, 2097–2104. [CrossRef]
16. Grote, K.; Petri, M.; Liu, C.; Jehn, P.; Spalthoff, S.; Kokemuller, H.; Luchtefeld, M.; Tschernig, T.; Krettek, C.; Haasper, C.; et al. Toll-like receptor 2/6-dependent stimulation of mesenchymal stem cells promotes angiogenesis by paracrine factors. *Eur. Cell. Mater.* **2013**, *26*, 66–79. [CrossRef]
17. Limbourg, A.; Korff, T.; Napp, L.C.; Schaper, W.; Drexler, H.; Limbourg, F.P. Evaluation of postnatal arteriogenesis and angiogenesis in a mouse model of hind-limb ischemia. *Nat. Protoc.* **2009**, *4*, 1737–1746. [CrossRef]
18. Scholz, D.; Ito, W.; Fleming, I.; Deindl, E.; Sauer, A.; Wiesnet, M.; Busse, R.; Schaper, J.; Schaper, W. Ultrastructure and molecular histology of rabbit hind-limb collateral artery growth (arteriogenesis). *Virchows Arch.* **2000**, *436*, 257–270. [CrossRef]
19. Ito, W.D.; Arras, M.; Winkler, B.; Scholz, D.; Schaper, J.; Schaper, W. Monocyte chemotactic protein-1 increases collateral and peripheral conductance after femoral artery occlusion. *Circ. Res.* **1997**, *80*, 829–837. [CrossRef]
20. Buschmann, I.R.; Hoefer, I.E.; van Royen, N.; Katzer, E.; Braun-Dulleaus, R.; Heil, M.; Kostin, S.; Bode, C.; Schaper, W. GM-CSF: A strong arteriogenic factor acting by amplification of monocyte function. *Atherosclerosis* **2001**, *159*, 343–356. [CrossRef]
21. Das, S.; Goldstone, A.B.; Wang, H.; Farry, J.; D'Amato, G.; Paulsen, M.J.; Eskandari, A.; Hironaka, C.E.; Phansalkar, R.; Sharma, B.; et al. A Unique Collateral Artery Development Program Promotes Neonatal Heart Regeneration. *Cell* **2019**, *176*, 1128–1142. [CrossRef] [PubMed]

22. Chennupati, R.; Lamers, W.H.; Koehler, S.E.; De Mey, J.G. Endothelium-dependent hyperpolarization-related relaxations diminish with age in murine saphenous arteries of both sexes. *Br. J. Pharmacol.* **2013**, *169*, 1486–1499. [CrossRef]
23. Benjamin, E.J.; Muntner, P.; Alonso, A.; Bittencourt, M.S.; Callaway, C.W.; Carson, A.P.; Chamberlain, A.M.; Chang, A.R.; Cheng, S.; Das, S.R.; et al. American Heart Association Council on Epidemiology and Prevention Statistics Committee and Stroke Statistics Subcommittee. Heart Disease and Stroke Statistics-2019 Update: A Report From the American Heart Association. *Circulation* **2019**, *139*, e56–e528. [CrossRef] [PubMed]
24. Qadura, M.; Terenzi, D.C.; Verma, S.; Al-Omran, M.; Hess, D.A. Concise Review: Cell Therapy for Critical Limb Ischemia: An Integrated Review of Preclinical and Clinical Studies. *Stem Cells* **2018**, *36*, 161–171. [CrossRef] [PubMed]
25. Haghighat, L.; Ionescu, C.N.; Regan, C.J.; Altin, S.E.; Attaran, R.R.; Mena-Hurtado, C.I. Review of the Current Basic Science Strategies to Treat Critical Limb Ischemia. *Vasc. Endovascular Surg.* **2019**, *53*, 316–324. [CrossRef]
26. Seiler, C.; Pohl, T.; Wustmann, K.; Hutter, D.; Nicolet, P.A.; Windecker, S.; Eberli, F.R.; Meier, B. Promotion of collateral growth by granulocyte-macrophage colony-stimulating factor in patients with coronary artery disease: A randomized, double-blind, placebo-controlled study. *Circulation* **2001**, *104*, 2012–2017. [CrossRef]
27. Van Royen, N.; Schirmer, S.H.; Atasever, B.; Behrens, C.Y.; Ubbink, D.; Buschmann, E.E.; Voskuil, M.; Bot, P.; Hoefer, I.; Schlingemann, R.O.; et al. START Trial: A pilot study on STimulation of ARTeriogenesis using subcutaneous application of granulocyte-macrophage colony-stimulating factor as a new treatment for peripheral vascular disease. *Circulation* **2005**, *112*, 1040–1046. [CrossRef]
28. Van den Borne, S.W.; van de Schans, V.A.; Strzelecka, A.E.; Vervoort-Peters, H.T.; Lijnen, P.M.; Cleutjens, J.P.; Smits, J.F.; Daemen, M.J.; Janssen, B.J.; Blankesteijn, W.M. Mouse strain determines the outcome of wound healing after myocardial infarction. *Cardiovasc. Res.* **2009**, *84*, 273–282. [CrossRef]
29. Cho, M.L.; Ju, J.H.; Kim, H.R.; Oh, H.J.; Kang, C.M.; Jhun, J.Y.; Lee, S.Y.; Park, M.K.; Min, J.K.; Park, S.H.; et al. Toll-like receptor 2 ligand mediates the upregulation of angiogenic factor, vascular endothelial growth factor and interleukin-8/CXCL8 in human rheumatoid synovial fibroblasts. *Immunol. Lett.* **2007**, *108*, 121–128. [CrossRef]
30. Wang, W.; Xu, G.L.; Jia, W.D.; Ma, J.L.; Li, J.S.; Ge, Y.S.; Ren, W.H.; Yu, J.H.; Liu, W.B. Ligation of TLR2 by versican: A link between inflammation and metastasis. *Arch. Med. Res.* **2009**, *40*, 321–323. [CrossRef]
31. West, X.Z.; Malinin, N.L.; Merkulova, A.A.; Tischenko, M.; Kerr, B.A.; Borden, E.C.; Podrez, E.A.; Salomon, R.G.; Byzova, T.V. Oxidative stress induces angiogenesis by activating TLR2 with novel endogenous ligands. *Nature* **2010**, *467*, 972–976. [CrossRef] [PubMed]
32. Curtiss, L.K.; Black, A.S.; Bonnet, D.J.; Tobias, P.S. Atherosclerosis induced by endogenous and exogenous toll-like receptor (TLR)1 or TLR6 agonists. *J. Lipid Res.* **2012**, *53*, 2126–2132. [CrossRef] [PubMed]

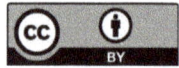

© 2020 by the authors. Licensee MDPI, Basel, Switzerland. This article is an open access article distributed under the terms and conditions of the Creative Commons Attribution (CC BY) license (http://creativecommons.org/licenses/by/4.0/).

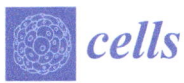

Article

Local Mast Cell Activation Promotes Neovascularization

Ilze Bot [1], Daniël van der Velden [1], Merel Bouwman [1,2,3], Mara J. Kröner [1], Johan Kuiper [1], Paul H. A. Quax [2,3] and Margreet R. de Vries [2,3,*]

1 Division of BioTherapeutics, Leiden Academic Centre for Drug Research, Leiden University, 2333CC Leiden, The Netherlands; i.bot@lacdr.leidenuniv.nl (I.B.); daniel.vandervelden@hu.nl (D.v.d.V.); merel_bouwman@hotmail.com (M.B.); marakroner@hotmail.com (M.J.K.); j.kuiper@lacdr.leidenuniv.nl (J.K.)
2 Department of Surgery, Leiden University Medical Center, 2300RC Leiden, The Netherlands; p.h.a.quax@lumc.nl
3 Einthoven Laboratory for Experimental Vascular Medicine, Leiden University Medical Center, 2300RC Leiden, The Netherlands
* Correspondence: m.r.de_vries@lumc.nl; Tel.: +31-715-265-147

Received: 18 December 2019; Accepted: 10 March 2020; Published: 12 March 2020

Abstract: Mast cells have been associated with arteriogenesis and collateral formation. In advanced human atherosclerotic plaques, mast cells have been shown to colocalize with plaque neovessels, and mast cells have also been associated with tumor vascularization. Based on these associations, we hypothesize that mast cells promote angiogenesis during ischemia. In human ischemic muscle tissue from patients with end-stage peripheral artery disease, we observed activated mast cells, predominantly located around capillaries. Also, in mouse ischemic muscles, mast cells were detected during the revascularization process and interestingly, mast cell activation status was enhanced up to 10 days after ischemia induction. To determine whether mast cells contribute to both arteriogenesis and angiogenesis, mast cells were locally activated immediately upon hind limb ischemia in C57Bl/6 mice. At day 9, we observed a 3-fold increase in activated mast cell numbers in the inguinal lymph nodes. This was accompanied by an increase in the amount of Ly6C^{high} inflammatory monocytes. Interestingly, local mast cell activation increased blood flow through the hind limb (46% at day 9) compared to that in non-activated control mice. Histological analysis of the muscle tissue revealed that mast cell activation did not affect the number of collaterals, but increased the collateral diameter, as well as the number of CD31$^+$ capillaries. Together, these data illustrate that locally activated mast cell contribute to arteriogenesis and angiogenesis.

Keywords: arteriogenesis; angiogenesis; innate immunity; mast cell

1. Introduction

The mast cell, part of the innate immune system, generally resides in tissues such as the lung and the skin to protect against pathogens like bacteria and parasites. Mast cells have also been described to participate in diseases such as asthma, allergies, and rheumatoid arthritis. Over the last decades, the mast cell has been implicated in cardiovascular diseases as well, for example in atherosclerosis [1,2], the underlying pathology of acute cardiovascular diseases including peripheral artery disease (PAD) [3,4]. Interestingly, mast cell numbers in advanced human atherosclerotic plaques obtained after endarterectomy surgery were seen to be of predictive value for the incidence of a secondary cardiovascular event [5]. In those plaques, mast cell density associated with the number of CD31$^+$ microvessels [5]. Mast cells have also been associated with arteriogenesis and collateral formation [6]. Mast cells can secrete growth factors and pro-inflammatory cytokines that can recruit immune cells such as neutrophils and monocytes to the site of inflammation, thus further enhancing a pro-inflammatory response [6–8]. Patients with systemic mastocytosis, a disease that is characterized by the excessive accumulation of mast cells in tissue or organs, experienced an increased prevalence of cardiovascular disease events, such as myocardial infarction, stroke, and importantly, peripheral artery disease, which is actually caused by the development of atherosclerosis in the arteries that supply oxygen to the extremities [9]. These associative data suggest that the mast cell may actively contribute to these underlying pathologies, and preclinical studies have been performed to elucidate underlying mast cell pathways that are causally related to vascular remodeling and the related disease outcome.

We speculate that mast cells may affect atherosclerotic plaque progression and PAD by increasing angiogenesis. Plaque angiogenesis has been shown to be related to atherosclerotic plaque progression and also, during tumor development, mast cells have been implicated in angiogenesis [10]. Mast cells have been shown to induce tumor endothelial proliferation by the release of Vascular Endothelial Growth Factor (VEGF) in response to the hypoxic environment in the tumor [10], which may be translatable to muscles in PAD patients, in which hypoxia occurs as well [11,12]. Although induction of neovascularization, in particular angiogenesis, maybe unfavorable for atherosclerosis progression, in PAD, the induction of neovascularization by mast cells, more precisely by inducing collateral formation and angiogenesis, may act as a repair pathway to resupply the ischemic limb tissue with oxygen. This neovascularization process requires a pro-inflammatory response, which is thus, on one hand, beneficial to resolve ischemia, but may on the other hand lead to enhanced progression of atherosclerosis. This two-faced process is also known as the Janus phenomenon [13]. Recently, the contribution of mast cells to arteriogenesis and collateral formation in a shear-stress induced mouse model of hind limb ischemia (HLI) has been described by Chillo and colleagues [6]. In that study, mast cells were systemically activated with the mast cell activator compound 48/80 upon ligation of the femoral artery, which resulted in increased hind limb perfusion. Treatment with the mast cell stabilizer cromolyn prevented the mast cell-induced effects on arteriogenesis and the investigators identified the neutrophil as a prominent effector cell involved in the mechanism behind mast cell-induced arteriogenesis. However, in that study, mast cell activation-dependent effects on angiogenesis in the ischemic muscles were not reported.

In this study, we aimed to investigate whether local induction of mast cell activation can stimulate blood flow recovery in a mouse hind limb ischemia model by inducing angiogenesis as well as arteriogenesis.

First, we analyzed the number and activation status of mast cells in human ischemic tissue, obtained after limb amputation. Next, we induced hind limb ischemia in mice by ligation of the femoral artery and at time of ligation, we activated mast cells in the hind limb by a skin sensitization/challenge protocol using a pluronic gel to apply the hapten DNP locally at the ligation site as described before [7,14], after which blood perfusion was measured using laser Doppler imaging. Mast cell activation increased reperfusion of the hind limb by not only increasing arteriogenesis, but also angiogenesis, which is at least partly induced by increasing the pro-inflammatory monocyte response.

2. Materials and Methods

2.1. Tissue Collection from Patients with End-Stage Peripheral Artery Disease

Sample collection of tissues from patients with end-stage peripheral artery disease undergoing limb amputation was approved by the Medical Ethics Committee of the Leiden University Medical Center (Protocol No. P12.265). Written informed consent was obtained from the participants. Inclusion criteria were a minimum age of 18 years and lower limb amputation, excluding ankle, foot, or toe amputations. Exclusion criteria were suspected or confirmed malignancy and inability to give informed consent. Gastrocnemius and soleus muscle samples obtained from 15 patients were formalin fixed, processed, paraffin embedded sectioned, and stained for mast cells. From these patients, $n = 1$ had type I diabetes and $n = 7$ suffered from type II diabetes.

2.2. Hind Limb Ischemia Model

This study was performed in accordance with the Directive 2010/63/EU of the European Parliament and Dutch government guidelines. All experiments were approved (reference number 14185) by the Leiden University and Leiden University Medical Center committee on animal welfare (Leiden, the Netherlands). Wild-type C57Bl/6J mice were bred in our in-house breeding facility. Male mice aged 8 to 12 weeks were housed in groups with free access to water and regular chow.

Before the unilateral hind limb ischemia, mice were anesthetized by i.p. injection of midazolam (8 mg/kg, Roche Diagnostics, Basel, Switzerland), medetomidine (0.4 mg/kg, Orion, Espoo, Finland), and fentanyl (0.08 mg/kg, Janssen Pharmaceuticals, Beerse, Belgium). Hind limb ischemia was induced by electrocoagulation on two locations of the left femoral artery; the first ligation proximal to the superficial epigastric artery and the second proximal to the bifurcation of the popliteal and saphenous artery [15,16]. After surgery, anesthesia was antagonized with with atipamezol (2.5 mg/kg, Orion, Espoo, Finland) and flumazenil (0.5 mg/kg, Fresenius Kabi, Bad Homburg vor der Höhe, Germany).and buprenorphine (0.1 mg/kg, MSD Animal Health, Keniworth, NJ, USA) was provided as a painkiller. For the time course, 5 mice per time point were used, whereas for both the long-term (t28) and short-term (t9) HLI experiments, 8–9 mice per group were used.

2.3. Local Mast Cell Activation with DPN treatment

Mice were skin-sensitized on the shaved abdomen and paws for 2 consecutive days with a dinitrofluorobenzene (DNFB (D1529) solution (0.5% v/v in acetone:olive oil (4:1), Sigma-Aldrich, St. Louis, MO, USA) as described previously to sensitize the mice for the hapten DNP [7,14]. In the control mice, a vehicle solution of acetone:olive oil (4:1) was applied. At the end of the hind limb ischemia procedure, which was scheduled one week after the skin-sensitization procedure, 50 µg dinitrophenyl hapten (DNP (D198501), Sigma-Aldrich, St. Louis, MO, USA) in a pluronic gel (25% w/v, Sigma-Aldrich, St. Louis, MO, USA) was applied around the ligated areas of the left hind limb to locally activate the mast cells. Empty pluronic gel was applied in the control mice. This model has been previously applied [7,14,17,18] and has been shown to specifically induce mast cells activation upon local hapten application.

2.4. Laser Doppler Perfusion Measurements

Before and directly after surgery and at 3, 7, 10, 14, 21, and 28 days after surgery, blood flow recovery to the ligated hind limb and the unligated control paw were measured using Laser Doppler Perfusion Imaging (LDPI) (Moor Instruments, Axminster, UK). Before the LDPI measurements, mice were anesthetized by i.p. injection of midazolam (8 mg/kg) and medetomidine (0.4 mg/kg,). Next, mice were placed in a double glazed pot, perfused with water at 37 °C for 5 min [19]. After LDPI, anesthesia was antagonized by subcutaneous injection of flumazenil (0.7 mg/kg). LDPI measurements in the ligated paw were normalized to measurements of the unligated paw, as an internal control. At sacrifice, after the last LDPI measurement, analgesic fentanyl (0.08 mg/kg) was administered, blood was drawn, and mice were sacrificed via cervical dislocation. The adductor and soleus muscles were harvested and fixed in 4% formaldehyde. For a second short experiment, animals were sacrificed at day 9, where blood was collected by orbital bleeding and the inguinal lymph nodes were isolated for further analyses. Again, the adductor and soleus muscles were harvested and fixed in 4% formaldehyde for histology analysis.

2.5. Immunohistochemistry

Mast cells were visualized by staining using a naphthol AS-D chloroacetate esterase staining kit (#91C, Sigma-Aldrich, St. Louis, MO, USA) and counted manually. A mast cell was considered resting when all granula were maintained inside the cell, while mast cells were assessed as activated when granula were deposited in the tissue surrounding the mast cell (examples are shown in Figure 1A).

Tissue size was quantified by the Leica image analysis system (Leica Ltd., Cambridge, UK). Paraffin embedded adductor and soleus muscle were stained with alpha smooth muscle actin (aSMA) (1A4, DAKO, Glostrup, Denmark) to visualize smooth muscle cell positive collaterals. Soleus muscles were stained for capillaries using CD31 (Sc-1506, Santa Cruz, Dallas, TX, USA) and macrophages using MAC3 (550292, BD-Pharmingen, Franklin Lakes, NJ, USA) together with aSMA and DAPI (Sigma, Santa Clara, CA, USA) as nuclear staining. For each antibody, negative controls were included using specific isotype-matched antibodies. The Pannoramic MIDI digital slide scanner (3DHistech, Budapest, Hungary) was used to create high-resolution images of the muscles. Snapshots (9 representative images per muscle) were taken using the caseviewer software (3DHistech) with a 40× magnification. aSMA positive collaterals were analyzed by counting the number of collaterals and measuring the diameters of each collateral with a visible lumen to determine arteriogenesis. CD31 positive capillaries and the number of MAC3 positive macrophages were quantified. All quantifications were performed using FIJI Image J image analysis software (ImageJ, Bethesda, MD, USA).

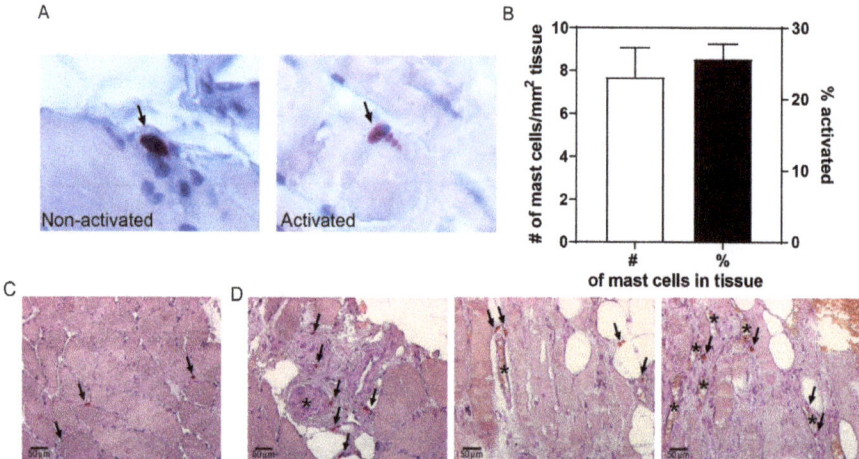

Figure 1. Mast cells in calf muscles of patients with peripheral artery disease. (**A**) Representative high-magnification image of a non-activated (left) and activated (right) mast cell, stained using a chloro-acetate esterase (CAE) staining and indicated by arrows. The non-activated mast cell shows the pink granula in the cytoplasm of the cell, whereas the pink granula are being released in the surroundings of the activated mast cell. (**B**) Quantification of the number of mast cells/mm^2 tissue, and the percentage of activated mast cells observed (n = 15). (**C**) Overview of a chloro-acetate esterase (CAE) staining of muscle tissue showing mast cells in pink (indicate by arrows) in between muscle fibers. (**D**) Representative overview images of mast cells surrounding microvessels (indicated by *) in human calf muscle tissue.

2.6. FACS Analysis

Blood was collected at sacrifice, after which red blood cells were lysed using an erythrocyte lysis buffer (0.1 mM EDTA, 10 mM NaHCO$_3$, 1 mM NH$_4$Cl, pH = 7.2). Subsequently, white blood cells were stained with the antibodies for flow cytometric analysis. Inguinal lymph nodes were harvested from all mice and processed through a 70 µm cell strainer to acquire single cell suspensions. Subsequently, the cell suspensions were stained for flow cytometry. In approximation, 200,000 cells per sample were stained with antibodies against extracellular proteins at a concentration of 0.1 µg/sample for 30 min as described previously [20,21]. All flow cytometry experiments were executed on a FACS Canto II (BDBiosciences, San Jose, CA, USA) and data were analyzed using FlowJo software (v10, BDBiosciences).

2.7. Statistical Analysis

Results are presented as mean ± standard error of the mean (SEM). A 2-tailed Student's t-test was used to compare individual groups. Non-Gaussian distributed data were analyzed using a 2-tailed Mann–Whitney U test. p-values < 0.05 were considered statistically significant and are indicated with *; p-values < 0.01 and < 0.001 are indicated by ** and ***, respectively.

3. Results

3.1. Mast Cells Localization in Calf Muscles of Peripheral Artery Disease Patients

To assess mast cell presence and its activation status in calf muscles of peripheral artery disease patients, we stained sections of ischemic muscle biopsies obtained after amputation surgery with a CAE staining and quantified the number of mast cells. On average, we detected 7.7 ± 1.4 mast cells/mm^2 tissue, of which 26 ± 2% was activated (Figure 1B). As shown in Figure 1C, mast cells, primarily non-activated, can be detected between the muscle fibers. Interestingly, mast cells, and in particular activated ones, generally appeared to colocalize with blood vessels in the muscle tissue (representative overview images in Figure 1D). The amount of mast cells in muscle tissue did not differ between patients that suffered from type I or II diabetes vs. patients that did not (7.5 ± 2.0 mast cells/mm^2 vs. 7.4 ± 2.1 mast cells/mm^2, respectively). Also, mast cell activation status in the muscle tissue was not affected by presence of diabetes (DM: 24.1 ± 2.3% vs. non-DM: 29.9 ± 3.1%).

3.2. Activation of Mast Cells upon Ischemia in a Murine Hindlimb Ischemia Model

To study whether mast cells accumulate in the murine muscle tissue upon hind limb ischemia, we quantified mast cell number and its activation status in adductor muscle tissue at 0, 7, 10, 21, and 28 days after the induction of hind limb ischemia. Similar to the human tissue, in murine muscles, mast cells were located in between muscle fibers and near blood vessels (Figure 2A). As the overall number of mast cells in this ischemic muscle tissue was relatively low, we included overview images of different locations in tissue to illustrate where mast cells reside (Figure 2A) Mast cell density, i.e., the number of mast cells per mm^2 tissue, did not change during the time-course of the experiment (Figure 2B), but mast cell activation status increased upon the induction of ischemia, in particular during the initial phase from day 0 up to day 10 (Figure 2C).

At day 7, a 33% increase in activated mast cells was observed compared to the percentage of activated mast cells at day 0, which further rose to a maximum of a 54% increase at 10 days after HLI. The number of activated mast cells then declined at 21 and 28 days to the level control (day 0; non-surgery) muscles (Figure 2B). Interestingly, most of these activated mast cells, as indicated by granules that reside outside the cell, were found in close proximity of capillaries in the muscle tissues (Figure 2A, lower panels) suggesting a direct relation between blood vessels and mast cells as we have shown previously in atherosclerosis [5].

3.3. Effect of Local Mast Cell Activation on Post Ischemic Blood Flow Recovery.

To study the effects of local mast cell activation on blood flow recovery, we applied the hapten DNP as part of our mast cell activation protocol on the gastrocnemius and adductor muscles directly after the hind limb ischemia procedure. We studied the subsequent blood flow recovery starting with eight mice per group, however between surgery and day 3, two mice in the DNP group and three mice in the control group had to be sacrificed because they reached humane end points. At day 10, a significant 44% increase in paw perfusion could be observed in the DNP treated group (left/right ratio of 0.70 ± 0.07) in comparison to the vehicle treated control group (left/right ratio of 0.49 ± 0.04). The enhanced increase in blood flow perfusion continued until the end of the experiment with significant differences between the groups at day 21 and day 28 (Figure 3A). We repeated the experiment, focusing on the early stage of blood flow recovery by sacrificing the mice at day 9 (short-term experiment). The experiment was started with nine mice per group; one mouse in the control and two mice in the DNP group reached the humane end point and were not included in the analysis. Similar to the t28 experiment, we observed an increase in paw perfusion in the DNP group at the day 9 time point of 46% (DNP: 0.66 ± 0.02 vs. control: 0.45 ± 0.05, Figure 3B).

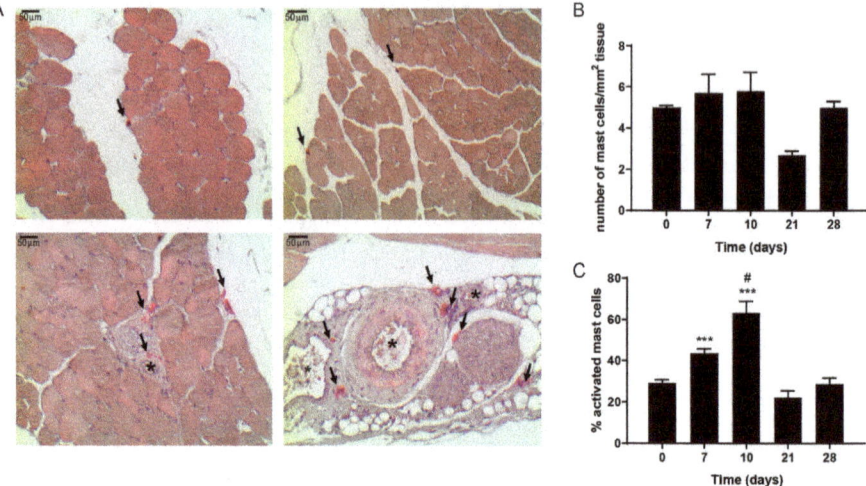

Figure 2. Mast cells in hind limb muscle tissue during ischemia in mice. (**A**) Representative images of mast cells in pink (CAE staining, indicated by arrows) in mouse ischemic muscle tissue (upper panels) and in close proximity to blood vessels (lower panels, indicated by *). (**B**) Mast cell density and (**C**) the percentage of activated mast cells in the hind limb muscle during recovery after ischemia. p-values of < 0.001 in comparison to t0 are indicated by *** p-value of < 0.05 in comparison to t7 is indicated by #.

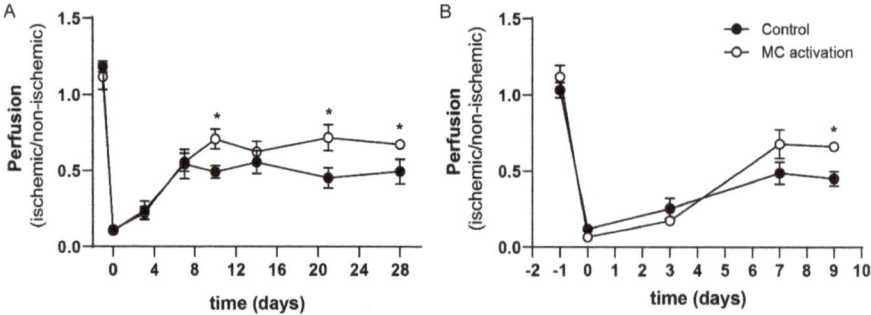

Figure 3. Perfusion of the ischemic hind limb in mast cell (MC) activated vs. control mice. Perfusion (ischemic/non-ischemic) as measured by Laser Doppler Perfusion Imaging (LDPI) from day 0 to day 28 in the long-term experiment (**A**) and in the short-term experiment from day 0 up to day 9 (**B**) after ligation of the femoral artery. * p-value of < 0.05 between the groups.

3.4. Local Mast Cell Activation Induced by DNP

We studied to what extent mast cell number and activation status were still affected after the single treatment with DNP of the ischemic hind limb. At nine days after ligation, the number of mast cell observed in the ligated and non-ligated adductor muscles were comparable (Figure 4A). In the ligated adductor muscles, the number of activated mast cells still tended to be increased at nine days after DNP treatment ($p = 0.11$), an effect that was lost at 28 days after ligation. In the soleus muscle of the DNP groups, both total mast cell numbers as well as the number of activated mast cells was still somewhat increased at nine days after ligation as compared to the controls (Figure 4B,C). Representative images of soleus muscle tissue are shown in Figure 4D.

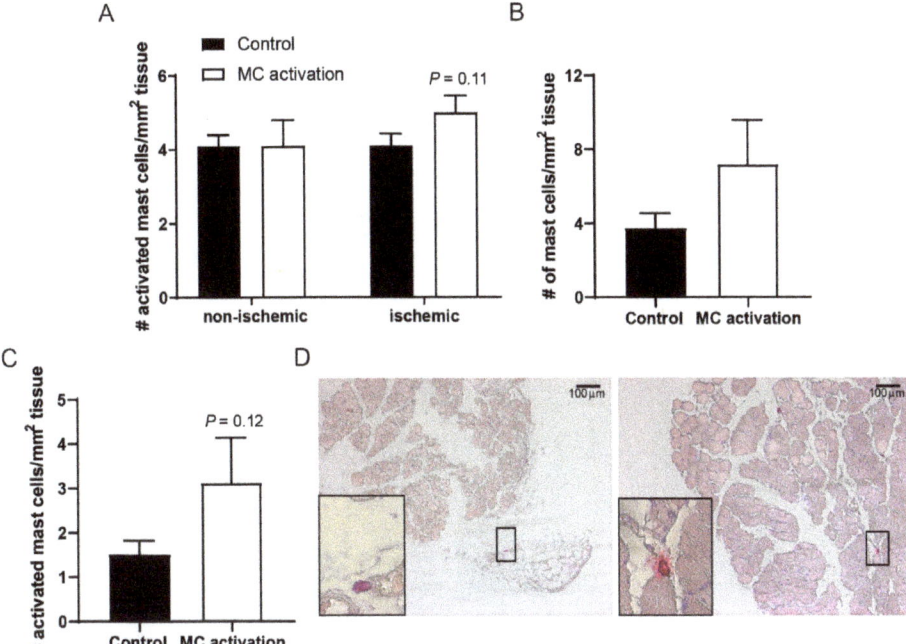

Figure 4. Activated mast cell numbers in muscle tissue of the ischemic hind limb. (**A**) The number of activated mast cells as measured by histology in the ischemic vs. non-ischemic adductor muscles of mice in which mast cells were activated compared to control mice at day 9 after the induction of ischemia. (**B**) Total mast cell numbers per mm^2 of ischemic soleus muscle tissue. (**C**) Number of activated mast cells per mm^2 of soleus muscle tissue at day 9 after ligation. (**D**) Representative overview images of the soleus muscles with a resting (control, left) and an activated mast cell (dinitrophenyl hapten, DNP, right) in high-magnification inserts.

Mast cell activation did not result in muscle hypertrophy, analyzed in both the ischemic and non-ischemic adductor muscles of the control and DNP-group at day 9 and day 28 after femoral artery ligation (data not shown).

3.5. Contribution of Arteriogenesis to the Increase in Blood Flow Recovery by Activated Mast Cells

Since restoration of blood flow recovery is a combination of shear stress induced arteriogenesis and ischemia induced angiogenesis [22], we studied these processes in the adductor muscle upstream of the ligation and in the soleus muscle, the ischemic region downstream of the ligation. Increased shear stress upstream of the ligation leads to arterialization of collaterals in the adductor muscle. At day 28, the number of collaterals did not differ between the ischemic and the non-ischemic adductor muscles in both the control and DNP treated group, nor did the number of collaterals differ between the control and DNP treated group (control: non-ischemic 32.7 ± 1.8, ischemic 28.7 ± 1.8, DNP: non-ischemic 34.6 ± 3.4, ischemic 32.2 ± 1.5). No differences in collateral numbers after ligation is frequently observed in hind limb ischemia studies since the pre-existing collaterals predominantly increase in size upon shear stress. Therefore, we also analyzed the surface area of the collaterals. The area of the collaterals in the ischemic muscles of the DNP treated mice was slightly increased compared to control mice (control: 318.4 ± 12.5 µm^2 vs. DNP: 381.2 ± 42.5 µm^2, $p = 0.205$) (Figure 5A). Also, the area of the collaterals in the non-ischemic vs. the ischemic hind limbs expressed as the ratio collateral area was somewhat increased between the control and DNP treated mice, but did not reach significance (control: 1.420±0.1 vs. DNP: 1.611 ± 0.2, $p = 0.509$).

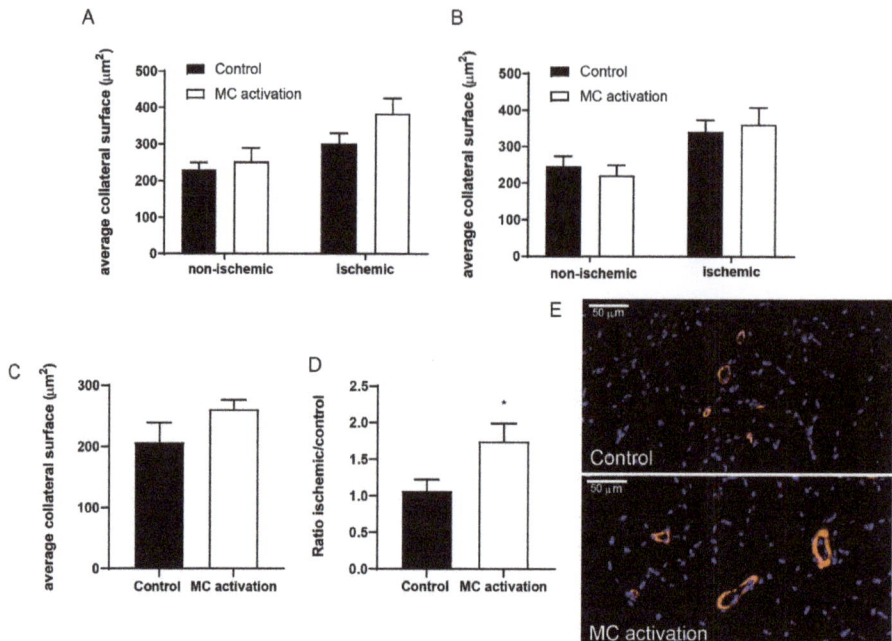

Figure 5. Arteriogenesis upon mast cell activation in the ischemic hind limb. The average collateral surface area in ischemic as compared to non-ischemic adductor muscles of mice in which mast cells were activated compared to controls at (**A**) 28 days after ligation and (**B**) 9 days after ligation. (**C**) The average collateral surface area in the soleus muscle of mice in which mast cells were activated compared to controls. (**D**) The collateral area ratio between ischemic and non-ischemic soleus muscles in mast cell activated compared to control mice at nine days after femoral artery ligation. (**E**). Representative pictures of smooth muscle cell actin positive collaterals in orange and nuclei in blue (DAPI) in both a control muscle and a muscle in which mast cells were activated. * $p < 0.05$.

In the short-term experiment with sacrifice at day 9, the number of collaterals also did not differ between the ischemic and the non-ischemic adductor muscles in both the control and DNP treated group, nor did the number of collaterals between the control and DNP treated group (control: Non-ischemic 27.3 ± 1.8, ischemic 30.7 ± 1.5, DNP: Non-ischemic 29.0 ± 1.8, ischemic 27.3 ± 1.8). Furthermore, no differences could be observed in collateral area in the ligated hind limbs between the control and DNP treated mice at day 9 (control 340.2 ± 29.2 μm^2 vs. DNP 362.1 ± 45.5 μm^2, $p = 0.680$) (Figure 5B) nor in the collateral area ratio (control 1.557 ± 0.3 vs. DNP 1.749 ± 0.3, $p = 0.633$).

In the downstream area of the ligation, the distal end of the collaterals in the soleus muscle are also exposed to increased shear stress. Comparable to the adductor muscle, the number of collaterals in the soleus muscle did not differ between the groups with or without ischemia at day 9 (control: Non-ischemic 23.8 ± 2.1, ischemic 26.3 ± 1.7, DNP: Non-ischemic 25.2 ± 2.0, ischemic 23.9 ± 1.9). A non-significant increase in soleus muscle collateral area could be observed in the ligated hind limbs of the DNP treated mice compared to the control mice (control 207.4 ± 31.7 μm^2 vs. DNP 261.7 ± 14.8 μm^2, $p = 0.163$) (Figure 5C). Interestingly, the collateral area ratio of the ischemic vs. the non-ischemic soleus of the individual mice was significantly increased in the DNP group vs. the control group (Control:

1.070 ± 0.2 vs. DNP: 1.751 ± 0.2, $p = 0.026$) (Figure 5D), suggesting that local mast cell activation does increase collateral diameter downstream of the ligation.

3.6. Effects of Mast Cell Activation on Angiogenesis

As a measure for the angiogenic response, CD31 positive capillaries were quantified in the right non-ischemic and the left ischemic soleus muscles. Local mast cell activation resulted in an increased number of angiogenic capillaries in the ischemic soleus muscles (Figure 6A). Quantification revealed a 66% significant increase in the number of capillaries (control: 211 ± 31 vs. DNP: 351 ± 55 µm^2, $p = 0.039$, Figure 6B), whereas in the control non-ischemic muscles, no significant difference in the number of capillaries were observed (control 176 ± 15 vs. DNP 196 ± 40 µm^2).

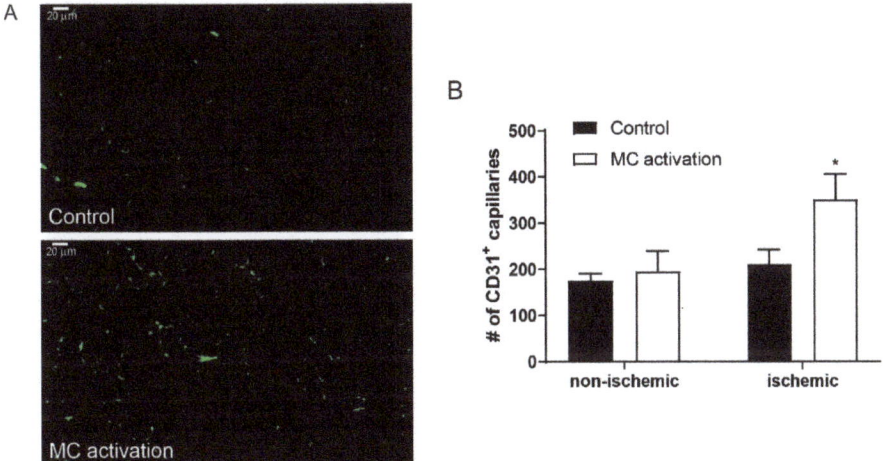

Figure 6. Activated mast cells induce angiogenesis in the ischemic hind limb. (**A**) CD31 staining of the ischemic soleus muscles shows the presence of CD31$^+$ capillaries in control mice and in mice in which mast cells were activated. (**B**) Quantification of the number of CD31$^+$ capillaries in non-ischemic and ischemic soleus muscle with (white bars) or without local (black bars) mast cell activation, measured at nine days after femoral artery ligation. *$p < 0.05$.

3.7. Local Mast Cell Activation Induces a Pro-Inflammatory Monocyte Response

To determine whether local mast cell activation induced a pro-inflammatory response in the hind limb, we analyzed the inguinal lymph nodes draining from the hind limbs in which mast cells were activated at day 9 after ligation. To do so, we measured the number of CD117$^+$FcεR$^+$ cells and analyzed CD63 as a common mast cell activation marker. Interestingly, mast cells numbers were highly increased in the DNP group (Figure 7A), similarly to the number of activated mast cells (Figure 7B), which suggests that mast cells have drained from the muscle tissue to the lymph nodes. The number of CD11b$^+$Ly6G^{high} neutrophils in the lymph nodes did not differ between the groups (Figure 7C), nor did the amount of T- and B-cells (data not shown). The number of CD11b$^+$Ly6G^{low} monocytes in the draining lymph nodes was significantly increased upon mast cell activation (Figure 7D), which was due to an increase in both the Ly6C$^{low/mid}$ and the Ly6C^{high} monocytes (Figure 7E,F). In the circulation, neutrophil and total monocyte numbers were not affected (Figure 7G,H), however within the monocyte population, the relative amount of inflammatory Ly6C^{high} monocytes was significantly increased (Figure 7I). We also measured plasma IL-6 and CCL2 levels as markers of a systemic inflammatory response at 9 days after ligation but were unable to detect any differences between the control mice and those in which mast cells were locally activated (data not shown). To further investigate the local effect of mast cell activation on the pro-inflammatory response in the ischemic tissue, we used a MAC3 staining to quantify the number of macrophages present. Here, in contrast to the number of inflammatory monocytes in the draining lymph nodes, no effect on the macrophage numbers in the ischemic soleus muscles was observed at day 9 (control: 14.1 ± 3.2 vs. DNP 8.1 ± 1.8, $p = 0.141$, Figure 7J,K).

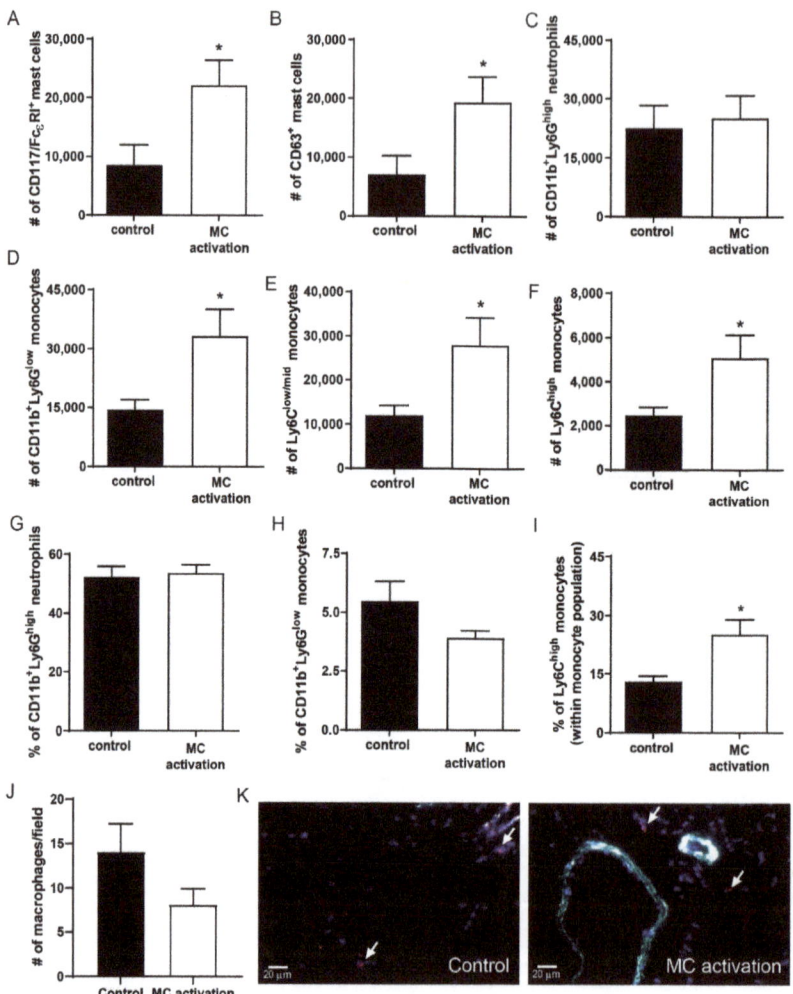

Figure 7. Inflammatory cell analysis in the ischemic hind limb at nine days after ischemia induction. (**A**) Total CD117$^+$FcεRI$^+$ mast cell numbers and (**B**) the number of CD63$^+$ activated mast cells were measured in the inguinal lymph node (iLN) draining from the ischemic hind limb of mice in the DNP-group and the controls using flow cytometry. (**C**) The number of CD11b$^+$Ly6C^{high} neutrophils in the iLN. (**D**) The number of CD11b$^+$Ly6G^{low} monocytes of which, (**E**) Ly6C$^{low/mid}$ and (**F**) Ly6C^{high} monocytes. (**G**) Percentage of neutrophils, (**H**) percentage of total monocytes, and (**I**) percentage of inflammatory monocytes within the total monocyte population were measured in the circulation of control mice vs. mice in which mast cells were activated. (**J**) The number of macrophages per microscopic field in the ischemic soleus muscles of mice in which mast cells were activated vs. controls at nine days after ligation. (**K**) Representative micrographs of macrophages in red (indicated by arrows) and aSMA$^+$ collaterals in cyan and nuclei (DAPI) in blue. * $p < 0.05$.

4. Discussion

In this study, we aimed to determine the contribution of mast cell activation to angiogenesis in hind limb ischemia. First, we demonstrated the presence of mast cells in human ischemic limb tissue, and both non-activated and activated mast cells were observed. Interestingly, activated mast cells were predominantly present around the capillaries in the ischemic limb, similarly as that described previously in the atherosclerotic plaque, where mast cells were seen to colocalize with microvessels [5]. In addition, mast cells have previously been associated with microvessel density in the brain [23]. Although mast cells have been associated with obesity and diabetes in experimental models of disease [24], the presence of diabetes did not affect mast cell numbers in the human ischemic tissue, which is in line with previous human studies in which intraplaque mast cells numbers did not differ between cardiovascular patients with and without diabetes mellitus [5].

In ischemic mouse hind limbs, the mast cells that colocalized with capillaries were mostly activated early in the revascularization process. Apparently, the ischemic environment in the hind limb causes the mast cells to degranulate. However, the mechanisms via which mast cells are activated upon ischemia remain largely unknown. In ischemia/reperfusion studies, reactive oxygen species, but also alarmins/DAMPS, have been suggested to activate mast cells [24]. The composition of the mast cell secretome completely depends on the specific stimuli and receptors involved, which indicates that the ischemic microenvironment can influence how mast cells are activated and which mediators these cells secrete. In this study, we aimed to determine whether local mast cell activation using a sensitization and challenge protocol in the ischemic hind limb would improve limb perfusion by inducing neovascularization. Similarly as described previously [6], we have established that mast cell activation promotes limb perfusion as indicated by enhanced blood flow to the lower limbs. Previously, it was suggested that neutrophils were the culprit immune effector cells during the neovascularization process in the ischemic hind limb [6]. In our study, we actually show that mast cell activation induced a pro-inflammatory monocyte response, while not affecting neutrophil numbers, either systemically or locally in the draining lymph nodes. The difference in observed immune response between the studies may be explained by the fact that we analyzed these monocyte responses at nine days after the induction of ischemia, whereas neutrophils are usually early responders and act in the first few days after injury. Furthermore, the difference in mast cell activation methods used may have affected the composition of the releasate, resulting in a difference in immune responses in the two studies. The increased immune response in the draining lymph nodes from the ischemic hind limb was not reflected by a difference in macrophage count in the muscle tissue itself at nine days after ligation. Again, this may be due to the timeframe of the study or to local secretion of pro-inflammatory mediators.

To further elucidate the underlying mechanisms that have caused the increased limb perfusion, both angiogenesis and arteriogenesis processes in the ischemic hind limbs were analyzed. In the adductor muscle, we were unable to detect any significant differences in either the number or the surface area of the collaterals, both at 9 and 28 days after femoral artery ligation. In the soleus muscle downstream of the ischemia, however, at day 9 we did observe an increase in the collateral surface area ratio in the mice in which mast cells were activated, suggesting that mast cells increase limb perfusion by expansion of pre-existing collaterals, as arteriogenesis is defined. At the same time point, we observed that the number of CD31 positive capillaries in the soleus muscle was significantly increased upon mast cell activation, and as this did not occur in the non-ischemic muscles, we can conclude that this is a specific local effect of mast cell activation. Together, these effects early in the revascularization process can explain the increase in paw perfusion induced in our model and that both arteriogenesis and angiogenesis in the ischemic muscles are responsible for the increased perfusion. To further elucidate the underlying mechanisms, it would be of interest to study arteriogenesis and angiogenesis processes in mast cell deficient mouse models. However, in our hands, survival of mast cell deficient Kit$^{W-sh/W-sh}$ mice upon hind limb ischemia was too limited to study these processes (unpublished data), and we therefore decided to apply a more therapeutics mast cell activation protocol, which made use of a local delayed type hypersensitivity approach. Previously, we have established that this method induces a specific mast cell activation response [7], however it would also be of interest to study other local mast cell activation approaches to determine which method induces the best neovascularization response without side effects.

As our data imply that mast cell activation improves limb perfusion after an ischemic episode, it is of great interest to determine how we can use these data for therapeutic application. As mentioned earlier, excessive mast cell activation can have detrimental effects on atherosclerotic plaque stability, the lungs, and other tissues in which mast cells reside. Also, an enhanced systemic inflammatory response induced by activated mast cells may be beneficial upon ischemia, but may also negatively affect other sources of inflammation, the so-called Janus phenomenon [13]. Local mast cell activation in the ischemic area may be a more suitable option. Furthermore, the identification of ischemia-specific mast cell activation pathways may provide novel therapeutic strategies to specifically target mast cell activation in the ischemic area. Further research may shed more light on the therapeutic opportunities for intervention.

In conclusion, in this study, we show that mast cells colocalize with capillaries in human ischemic tissue and in ischemic mouse limbs, where mast cells are activated in the early phase after the induction of ischemia. Locally induced mast cell activation in the hind limb leads to an increase in recovery of paw perfusion, which was associated with increased arterio- and angiogenesis, and with an increased inflammatory response, suggesting that mast cells actively contribute to tissue neovascularization.

Author Contributions: Conceptualization, I.B. and M.R.d.V.; formal analysis, I.B., D.v.d.V., M.B. and M.R.d.V.; investigation, I.B., D.v.d.V., M.B., M.J.K. and M.R.d.V.; resources, I.B., J.K., P.H.A.Q. and M.R.d.V.; supervision, I.B and M.R.d.V.; visualization, I.B and M.R.d.V.; writing—original draft, I.B. and M.R.d.V.; writing—review and editing, I.B., J.K., P.H.A.Q. and M.R.d.V. All authors have read and agreed to the published version of the manuscript.

Funding: This research received no external funding.

Conflicts of Interest: The authors declare no conflict of interest.

References

1. Kaartinen, M.; Penttila, A.; Kovanen, P.T. Accumulation of activated mast cells in the shoulder region of human coronary atheroma, the predilection site of atheromatous rupture. *Circulation* **1994**, *90*, 1669–1678. [CrossRef] [PubMed]
2. Kovanen, P.T.; Kaartinen, M.; Paavonen, T. Infiltrates of activated mast cells at the site of coronary atheromatous erosion or rupture in myocardial infarction. *Circulation* **1995**, *92*, 1084–1088. [CrossRef] [PubMed]
3. Bot, I.; Shi, G.P.; Kovanen, P.T. Mast cells as effectors in atherosclerosis. *Arter. Thromb. Vasc. Biol.* **2015**, *35*, 265–271. [CrossRef] [PubMed]
4. Shi, G.P.; Bot, I.; Kovanen, P.T. Mast cells in human and experimental cardiometabolic diseases. *Nat. Rev. Cardiol.* **2015**, *12*, 643–658. [CrossRef]
5. Willems, S.; Vink, A.; Bot, I.; Quax, P.H.; de Borst, G.J.; de Vries, J.P.; van de Weg, S.M.; Moll, F.L.; Kuiper, J.; Kovanen, P.T.; et al. Mast cells in human carotid atherosclerotic plaques are associated with intraplaque microvessel density and the occurrence of future cardiovascular events. *Eur. Heart J.* **2013**, *34*, 3699–3706. [CrossRef]
6. Chillo, O.; Kleinert, E.C.; Lautz, T.; Lasch, M.; Pagel, J.I.; Heun, Y.; Troidl, K.; Fischer, S.; Caballero-Martinez, A.; Mauer, A.; et al. Perivascular Mast Cells Govern Shear Stress-Induced Arteriogenesis by Orchestrating Leukocyte Function. *Cell Rep.* **2016**, *16*, 2197–2207. [CrossRef]
7. Bot, I.; de Jager, S.C.; Zernecke, A.; Lindstedt, K.A.; van Berkel, T.J.; Weber, C.; Biessen, E.A. Perivascular mast cells promote atherogenesis and induce plaque destabilization in apolipoprotein E-deficient mice. *Circulation* **2007**, *115*, 2516–2525. [CrossRef]
8. Sun, J.; Sukhova, G.K.; Wolters, P.J.; Yang, M.; Kitamoto, S.; Libby, P.; MacFarlane, L.A.; Mallen-St, C.J.; Shi, G.P. Mast cells promote atherosclerosis by releasing proinflammatory cytokines. *Nat. Med.* **2007**, *13*, 719–724. [CrossRef]

9. Indhirajanti, S.; van Daele, P.L.A.; Bos, S.; Mulder, M.T.; Bot, I.; Roeters van Lennep, J.E. Systemic mastocytosis associates with cardiovascular events despite lower plasma lipid levels. *Atherosclerosis* **2018**, *268*, 152–156. [CrossRef]
10. Albini, A.; Bruno, A.; Noonan, D.M.; Mortara, L. Contribution to Tumor Angiogenesis From Innate Immune Cells Within the Tumor Microenvironment: Implications for Immunotherapy. *Front. Immunol.* **2018**, *9*, 527. [CrossRef]
11. van Weel, V.; Seghers, L.; de Vries, M.R.; Kuiper, E.J.; Schlingemann, R.O.; Bajema, I.M.; Lindeman, J.H.; Delis-van Diemen, P.M.; van Hinsbergh, V.W.; van Bockel, J.H.; et al. Expression of vascular endothelial growth factor, stromal cell-derived factor-1, and CXCR4 in human limb muscle with acute and chronic ischemia. *Arter. Thromb. Vasc. Biol.* **2007**, *27*, 1426–1432. [CrossRef] [PubMed]
12. Campia, U.; Gerhard-Herman, M.; Piazza, G.; Goldhaber, S.Z. Peripheral Artery Disease: Past, Present, and Future. *Am. J. Med.* **2019**, *132*, 1133–1141. [CrossRef] [PubMed]
13. Epstein, S.E.; Stabile, E.; Kinnaird, T.; Lee, C.W.; Clavijo, L.; Burnett, M.S. Janus phenomenon: The interrelated tradeoffs inherent in therapies designed to enhance collateral formation and those designed to inhibit atherogenesis. *Circulation* **2004**, *109*, 2826–2831. [CrossRef] [PubMed]
14. de Vries, M.R.; Wezel, A.; Schepers, A.; van Santbrink, P.J.; Woodruff, T.M.; Niessen, H.W.; Hamming, J.F.; Kuiper, J.; Bot, I.; Quax, P.H. Complement factor C5a as mast cell activator mediates vascular remodelling in vein graft disease. *Cardiovasc. Res.* **2013**, *97*, 311–320. [CrossRef]
15. de Vries, M.R.; Seghers, L.; van, B.J.; Peters, H.A.; de Jong, R.C.; Hamming, J.F.; Toes, R.E.; van Hinsbergh, V.W.; Quax, P.H. C57BL/6 NK cell gene complex is crucially involved in vascular remodeling. *J. Mol. Cell Cardiol.* **2013**, *64*, 51–58. [CrossRef]
16. Simons, K.H.; Aref, Z.; Peters, H.A.B.; Welten, S.P.; Nossent, A.Y.; Jukema, J.W.; Hamming, J.F.; Arens, R.; de Vries, M.R.; Quax, P.H.A. The role of CD27-CD70-mediated T cell co-stimulation in vasculogenesis, arteriogenesis and angiogenesis. *Int. J. Cardiol.* **2018**, *260*, 184–190. [CrossRef]
17. Kraneveld, A.D.; Buckley, T.L.; van Heuven-Nolsen, D.; van, S.Y.; Koster, A.S.; Nijkamp, F.P. Delayed-type hypersensitivity-induced increase in vascular permeability in the mouse small intestine: Inhibition by depletion of sensory neuropeptides and NK1 receptor blockade. *Br. J. Pharm.* **1995**, *114*, 1483–1489. [CrossRef]
18. den Dekker, W.K.; Tempel, D.; Bot, I.; Biessen, E.A.; Joosten, L.A.; Netea, M.G.; van der Meer, J.W.; Cheng, C.; Duckers, H.J. Mast cells induce vascular smooth muscle cell apoptosis via a toll-like receptor 4 activation pathway. *Arterioscler. Thromb. Vasc. Biol.* **2012**, *32*, 1960–1969. [CrossRef]
19. Aref, Z.; de Vries, M.R.; Quax, P.H.A. Variations in Surgical Procedures for Inducing Hind Limb Ischemia in Mice and the Impact of These Variations on Neovascularization Assessment. *Int J. Mol. Sci* **2019**, *20*, 3704. [CrossRef]
20. Kritikou, E.; van der Heijden, T.; Swart, M.; van Duijn, J.; Slutter, B.; Wezel, A.; Smeets, H.J.; Maffia, P.; Kuiper, J.; Bot, I. Hypercholesterolemia Induces a Mast Cell-CD4(+) T Cell Interaction in Atherosclerosis. *J. Immunol.* **2019**, *202*, 1531–1539. [CrossRef]
21. Wezel, A.; Lagraauw, H.M.; van der Velden, D.; de Jager, S.C.; Quax, P.H.; Kuiper, J.; Bot, I. Mast cells mediate neutrophil recruitment during atherosclerotic plaque progression. *Atherosclerosis* **2015**, *241*, 289–296. [CrossRef] [PubMed]
22. Nowak-Sliwinska, P.; Alitalo, K.; Allen, E.; Anisimov, A.; Aplin, A.C.; Auerbach, R.; Augustin, H.G.; Bates, D.O.; van Beijnum, J.R.; Bender, R.H.F.; et al. Consensus guidelines for the use and interpretation of angiogenesis assays. *Angiogenesis* **2018**, *21*, 425–532. [CrossRef] [PubMed]
23. Ollikainen, E.; Tulamo, R.; Frosen, J.; Lehti, S.; Honkanen, P.; Hernesniemi, J.; Niemela, M.; Kovanen, P.T. Mast cells, neovascularization, and microhemorrhages are associated with saccular intracranial artery aneurysm wall remodeling. *J. Neuropathol Exp. Neurol.* **2014**, *73*, 855–864. [CrossRef] [PubMed]
24. He, Z.; Ma, C.; Yu, T.; Song, J.; Leng, J.; Gu, X.; Li, J. Activation mechanisms and multifaceted effects of mast cells in ischemia reperfusion injury. *Exp. Cell Res.* **2019**, *376*, 227–235. [CrossRef] [PubMed]

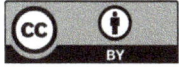

© 2020 by the authors. Licensee MDPI, Basel, Switzerland. This article is an open access article distributed under the terms and conditions of the Creative Commons Attribution (CC BY) license (http://creativecommons.org/licenses/by/4.0/).

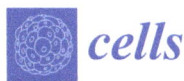

Article

Isoform-Specific Roles of ERK1 and ERK2 in Arteriogenesis

Nicolas Ricard [1], Jiasheng Zhang [1], Zhen W. Zhuang [1] and Michael Simons [1,2,*]

[1] Yale Cardiovascular Research Center, Department of Internal Medicine, Yale University School of Medicine, New Haven, CT 06511, USA; nic.ricard@gmail.com (N.R.); jiasheng.zhang@yale.edu (J.Z.); zhen.zhuang@yale.edu (Z.W.Z.)
[2] Department of Cell Biology, Yale University School of Medicine, New Haven, CT 06511, USA
* Correspondence: michael.simons@yale.edu; Tel.: +203-737-4643

Received: 5 November 2019; Accepted: 18 December 2019; Published: 21 December 2019

Abstract: Despite the clinical importance of arteriogenesis, this biological process is poorly understood. ERK1 and ERK2 are key components of a major intracellular signaling pathway activated by vascular endothelial growth (VEGF) and FGF2, growth factors critical to arteriogenesis. To investigate the specific role of each ERK isoform in arteriogenesis, we used mice with a global *Erk1* knockout as well as *Erk1* and *Erk2* floxed mice to delete *Erk1* or *Erk2* in endothelial cells, macrophages, and smooth muscle cells. We found that ERK1 controls macrophage infiltration following an ischemic event. Loss of ERK1 in endothelial cells and macrophages induced an excessive macrophage infiltration leading to an increased but poorly functional arteriogenesis. Loss of ERK2 in endothelial cells leads to a decreased arteriogenesis due to decreased endothelial cell proliferation and a reduced eNOS expression. These findings show for the first time that isoform-specific roles of ERK1 and ERK2 in the control of arteriogenesis.

Keywords: angiogenesis; arteriogenesis; ERK; VEGF; endothelial cells; inflammation; macrophages

---

1. Introduction

Blood vessel development and growth encompasses three distinct biological processes—vasculogenesis, angiogenesis, and arteriogenesis [1]. The term vasculogenesis denotes the formation of the primitive vascular plexus from progenitor cells in embryo and this mode of blood vessel formation is limited to embryonic development. Angiogenesis encompasses the process of new capillary formation from pre-existing capillary beds that involves proliferation, sprouting and, migration of endothelial cells. Finally, arteriogenesis refers to the growth of new arteries and arterioles either de novo or from pre-existing arterial collaterals [2]. Arteriogenesis, the process of new arterial vasculature growth, is critical to the restoration of tissue perfusion following the development of a functionally significant decrease of arterial inflow. It is important to note that compromised arterial inflow results in two distinct events: distal tissue ischemia that leads to local angiogenesis (e.g., angiogenesis along the myocardial infarction border zone) and arteriogenesis that occurs in close proximity to the site of arterial trunk occlusion, a territory that is typically not ischemic [3,4].

While molecular controls of angiogenesis are well understood, events triggering and regulating arteriogenesis are still a matter of intense study and controversy. Vascular endothelial growth factor (VEGF) is the main factor driving angiogenesis in response to tissue hypoxia [5], yet VEGF is equally critical to arteriogenesis [6]. Indeed, disruption of VEGF signaling and, in particular, a reduction in VEGF-induced endothelial ERK1/2 signaling, has been shown to result in decreased arteriogenesis [7].

While angiogenesis involves simple proliferation and sprouting of capillary endothelial cells, arteriogenesis requires a coordinated response that involves multiple cell types that, in addition to endothelial and vascular smooth muscle cells, include a panoply of inflammatory cells including lymphocytes [8,9], natural killer cells [10], macrophages [11], and mast cells [12]. The presence of inflammatory cells (and a local inflammatory response at an arteriogenic site) is critical as these cells serve as the major source of VEGF in the absence of tissue ischemia [13–17].

Endothelial response to VEGF stimulation encompasses a complex series of events that include activation of various intracellular signaling cascades [18]. Of these, activation of ERK1/2 has been directly linked to the extent of arteriogenesis [7]. Remarkably, little is known about the individual contribution of ERK isoforms to this process. Global deletion of *Erk2* is embryonic lethal [19] whereas a global deletion of *Erk1* has no apparent vascular phenotype [20]. Furthermore, endothelial-specific deletion of *Erk2* on the *Erk1* global knockout background is lethal early on in embryonic development due to impaired vascular development [21]. Another key role played by the two ERKs in the adult endothelium is the regulation of vascular normalcy and integrity [22].

In this paper, we focused on the role of ERK1/2 isoforms in adult arteriogenesis. Induction of acute hindlimb ischemia resulted in excessive but poorly functional arteriogenesis in mice with a global deletion of *Erk1* whereas mice with endothelial-specific deletion of *Erk2* exhibited a decreased arteriogenesis. Since arteriogenesis involves a number of cell types, we generated a floxed *Erk1* mouse line and conditionally deleted the gene in macrophages, endothelial, and smooth muscle cells. While endothelial or macrophage deletions of *Erk1* failed to recapitulate the phenotype of the *Erk1*$^{-/-}$ mice, combined deletion of *Erk1* in endothelial cells and macrophages came close to the phenotype in global *Erk1* null mice. Altogether, these results show that endothelial and macrophage *Erk1* is critical to endothelial/macrophage crosstalk and effective adult arteriogenesis.

2. Methods

2.1. Mice

Mapk3$^{-/-}$ mice (denominated *Erk1*$^{-/-}$), *Mapk1*^{tm1Gela}/J mice (denominated *Erk2*$^{Fl/Fl}$), and B6.129P2-Lyz2tm1(cre)Ifo/J mice (denominated LysMCre) were purchased from the Jackson Laboratory. *Cdh5CreER*^{T2} mice were a generous gift from Ralf Adams. *Myh11CreER*^{T2} mice were a generous gift from Dan Greif. All mice, including the wild type (WT) mice, are *Mus musculus* on a pure C57Bl6 genetic background. *Erk1*$^{Fl/Fl}$ mice were realized by inserting 2 loxP sequences in introns between exons 2 and 3 and exons 8 and 9 of the Erk1 gene. Tamoxifen injections to induce deletion by the Cdh5Cre or Myc11Cre were done with 5 injections of 1.5 mg of tamoxifen on 5 consecutive days. Control mice received the same quantity of tamoxifen. For retinal angiogenesis, 100 µg of tamoxifen were administrated by IP injections starting at P1 to P4. BrdU was injected 2 h prior to euthanasia. Animals were housed and used in accordance with protocols and policies approved by the Yale Institutional Animal Care and Use Committee.

2.2. Endothelial Cells, Macrophages, and Aortic Smooth Muscle Cell Isolations and Quantitative PCR

Endothelial cells were isolated from mouse livers and lungs. Briefly, livers and lungs were collected and digested in a solution of collagenase and dispase (Roche/Sigma Aldrich, St Louis, MO, USA). The suspensions were then washed and filtered. Endothelial cells were isolated using magnetic beads anti-Rat IgG (Invitrogen, Camarillo, CA, USA) previously coated with rat anti-mouse CD31 antibody (BD). After extensive washing, cells were lysed and RNA was isolated using PicoPure RNa isolation kit (ThermoFisher, Waltham, MA, USA) or cultured.

Macrophages were isolated from the peritoneal cavity as previously described [23]. Macrophages were selected using magnetic beads anti-Rat IgG (Invitrogen) previously coated with rat anti-mouse F4/80 antibody (Invitrogen). After extensive washing, cells were lysed, and RNA was isolated using PicoPure RNa isolation kit (ThermoFisher).

Smooth muscle cells were isolated from the aorta. Aortas were collected and digested in 175 U/mL collagenase (Worthington), 1.25 U/mL elastase (Worthington, Lakewood, NJ, USA), and HBSS for 25 to 30 min at 37 °C. Adventitia layer was then pulled out. Media and endothelium were cut and digested in 175 U/mL collagenase and 2.5 U/mL elastase in HBSS for 1 h at 37 °C. Endothelial cells were bound toon beads previously coated with rat anti-mouse CD31 antibody were used and discarded. The remaining smooth muscle cells were lysed and RNA was isolated using PicoPure RNa isolation kit (ThermoFisher).

cDNAs were synthetized with iScript Reverse Transcription Supermix (Bio-Rad, Hercules, CA, USA) and qPCRs were performed using SsoAdvanced Universal SYBR Green Supermix (Bio-Rad).

2.3. shRNA Infection

shRNA targeting ERK1 and ERK2 (Sigma-Aldrich, St Louis, MO, USA) were encapsulated into lentivirus that were then. Lentivirus were produced in 293T cells using second generation lentiviral system (Invitrogen).

2.4. Hindlimb Ischemia Model

This was done as previously described by our lab [6]. Laser Doppler flow-imaging was carried out using a Moor Infrared Laser Doppler Imager (LDI; Moor Instruments Ltd., Wilmington, DE, USA) under ketamine and xylazine anesthesia.

2.5. Micro-CT Imaging

Microcomputed tomography (micro-CT) of the hindlimb vasculature was done by injecting 0.7 mL bismuth contrast solution in the descending aorta and the vasculature was imaged and quantified as previously described [6].

2.6. Western Blot

Cells were lysed in RIPA buffer (Boston BioProducts, Ashland, MA, USA). Proteins were titrated using Bio-Rad Protein Assay Dye Reagent (Bio-Rad). A total of 20 ng of proteins were loaded on a 4–12% acrylamide gel (Bio-Rad) and then transferred on a PVDF membrane (Millipore). Primary antibodies used were: F4/80 (Invitrogen), ERK (Cell Signaling, Danvers, MA, USA), and β-actin (Sigma-Aldrich).

2.7. Immunofluorescent Staining

Frozen sections were treated with ice cold acetone. Permeabilization was done in triton 0.1%. Primary antibodies were: F4/80 (Invitrogen) and IsolectinB4 (Invitrogen). Pictures were taken using an SP5 confocal microscope (Leica, Allendale, NJ, USA).

2.8. xCELLigence Real-Time Cell Analysis (RTCA)

Endothelial cell proliferation was measured by using an xCELLigence RTCA instrument (Roche Diagnostics) and E-plate 16 (a modified 16-well plate, Roche Diagnostics). The E-plate 16 was coated with 0.1% gelatin, loaded with 100 µL cell-free medium, and left in a tissue culture hood for 30 min to reach equilibrium. The E-plate 16 was placed into the RTCA instrument to measure the background impedance. Thereafter, 100 µL cell suspensions with fewer than 3500 cells were added into each well of the E-plate 16, which was then placed in a tissue culture incubator for 30 min to allow cells to settle down before being measured by the RTCA device. The impedance value of E-plate 16 was automatically monitored every 15 min. FGF2 was added at 100 ng/mL.

2.9. Endothelial Migration

HUVEC migration was measured in a wound-healing assay, which used ibidi Culture-Inserts (ibidi) to generate the wound. An ibidi Culture-Insert has dimensions of 9 mm × 9 mm × 5 mm (width × length × height) and is composed of two wells. One or two inserts were placed into one well of a six-well plate. After being coated with 0.1% gelatin, both wells of inserts were loaded with 100 µL cell suspension. FGF2 and VEGF were used at 100 ng/mL.

2.10. Statistical Analyses

Statistical tests were performed using the software GraphPad Prism 8.

3. Results

3.1. Erk1 KO Mice Exhibit Excessive but Poorly Functional Arteriogenesis

To assess the role of ERK1 in arteriogenesis, we ligated the common femoral artery (CFA) of $Erk1^{-/-}$ mice and assessed blood flow recovery over time using laser Doppler imaging while the anatomical extent of arteriogenesis was studied using micro-CT. While blood flow recovery was reduced in $Erk1^{-/-}$ mice compared to wild type (WT) controls (Figure 1A,B), the micro-CT-determined extent of arteriogenesis was dramatically increased (Figure 1C,D). Since macrophages are the critical source of VEGF in this model and since the extent of arteriogenesis generally correlates with the amount of VEGF-A present [24], we used immunocytochemistry to assess the extent of macrophage accumulation in the arteriogenic zone. Staining with an F4/80 antibody of the thigh muscles around the area of CFA, ligation was carried out three and seven days following hindlimb ischemia. There was a marked increase in macrophage tissue infiltration in $Erk1^{-/-}$ mice compared to WT mice (Figure 1E). To confirm these findings, we carried out Western blotting using total thigh muscle lysates. In agreement with immunocytochemical findings, we observed a massive increase in F4/80 signal (Figure 1F).

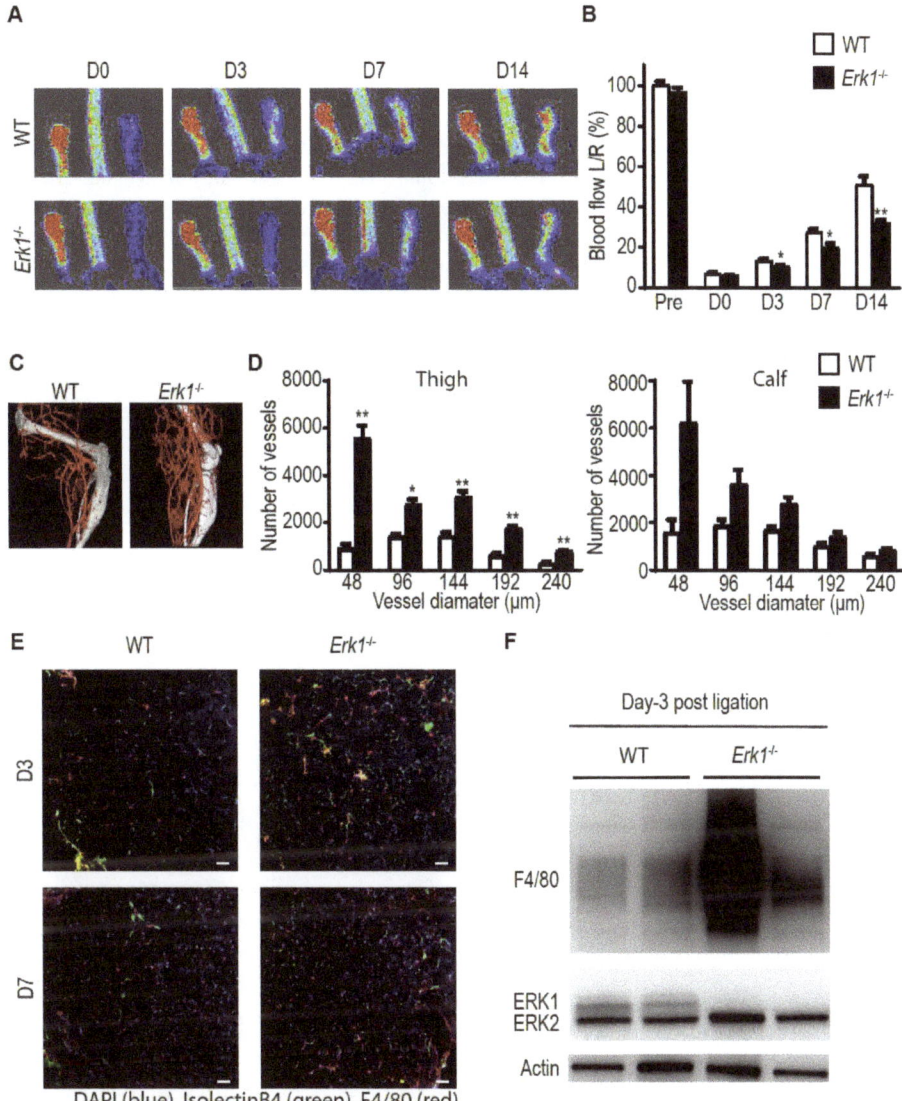

Figure 1. *Erk1*−/− mice exhibit excessive but dysfunctional arteriogenesis. (**A,B**) Blood flow recovery after ligation of the CFA in *Erk1*−/− mice assessed by laser-Doppler right after the surgery and 3, 7, and 14 days thereafter. Bar graph represents mean with SEM ($n = 10$ mice) * $p < 0.05$, ** $p < 0.005$ using two-way ANOVA followed by Sidak's multiple comparison test. (**C,D**) Quantification of the hindlimb vasculature by micro-CT three weeks after femoral artery ligation. Bar graph represents mean with SEM ($n = 4$ mice) * $p < 0.05$, ** $p < 0.005$ using two-way ANOVA followed by Sidak's multiple comparison test. (**E,F**) Macrophage infiltration in the thigh from *Erk1*−/− mice assessed by staining or Western blotting. Scale bar, 50 μm. Bar graph represents mean with SEM ($n = 3$ mice) * $p < 0.05$ using t-test.

3.2. Erk1 Deletions in Endothelial Cells, Macrophages, or Smooth Muscle Cells Do Not Affect Arteriogenesis

To identify the cell type(s) involved in the defective arteriogenic phenotype seen in $Erk1^{-/-}$ mice, we created mice with two intronic loxP sites in the $Erk1$ (*Mapk3*) gene (hereafter denominated as $Erk1^{Fl/Fl}$ (Figure 2A)). Since endothelial cells are critical to arteriogenesis [6], these mice were crossed with a strain carrying an inducible Cre recombinase under the control of the VE-cadherin promotor (Cdh5CreER^{T2}) [25] generating a Cdh5CreER^{T2};Erk1$^{f/f}$ line ($Erk1^{iEC-/-}$). Administration of tamoxifen to eight-week-old $Erk1^{Fl/Fl}$ mice resulted in a high efficiency deletion of endothelial *ERK1* (Figure 2B). One week after tamoxifen treatment, common femoral arteries (CFA) of $Erk1^{iEC-/-}$ and control mice were ligated. Surprisingly, laser-Doppler assessment of blood flow recovery in $Erk1^{iEC-/-}$ mice showed that it was similar to that of WT control mice (Figure 2C,D). We next turned our attention to macrophages. Similarly to Cdh5 CreER^{T2}, LysM Cre [26] was very effective in deleting *Erk1* (Figure 2E). Blood flow recovery after CFA ligation was not impaired compared to WT mice after either *Erk1* gene deletion (Figure 2F,G). We next deleted the *Erk1* gene in smooth muscle cells (SMC) using the Myh11CreER^{T2} driver line [27]. *Erk1* gene was efficiently deleted in SMC (Figure 2H) and this deletion had no effect on the blood flow recovery after CFA (Figure 2I,J).

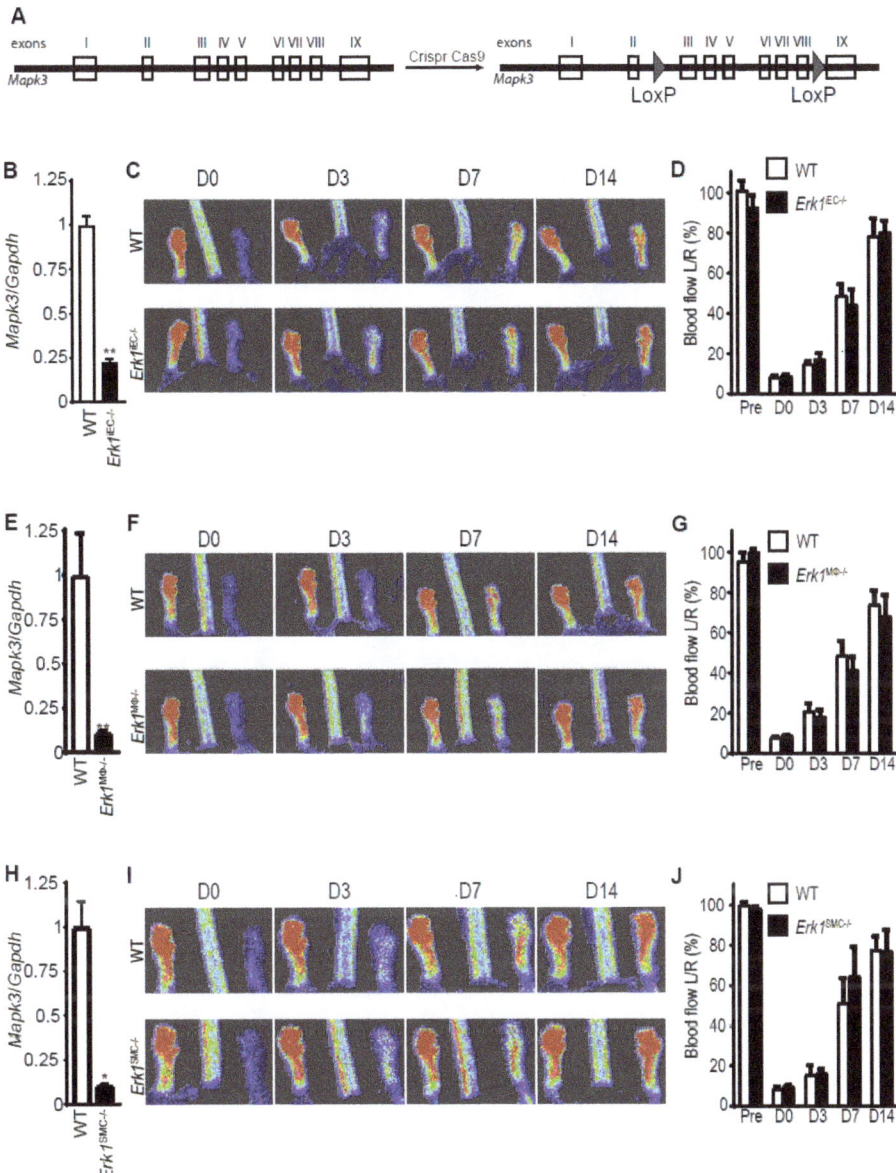

Figure 2. *Erk1* deletions in endothelial cells, macrophages, or smooth muscle cells do not affect arteriogenesis. (**A**) Generation of *Erk1* floxed mice by insertion of LoxP sites between exons 2 and 3 and exons 8 and 9. (**B**) Efficiency of *Erk1* deletion in endothelial cells was assessed by Q-PCR of endothelial cells isolated from mouse livers. Bar graph represents mean with SEM ($n = 4$ mice) ** $p <$ 0.005 using Mann–Whitney test. (**C,D**) Blood flow recovery after ligation of the CFA in $Erk1^{iEC-/-}$ mice assessed by laser Doppler right after the surgery and 3, 7, and 14 days after the surgery. Bar graph represents mean with SEM ($n = 8$ mice). (**E**) Efficiency of *Erk1* deletion in macrophages was assessed by Q-PCR of peritoneal macrophages. Bar graph represents mean with SEM ($n = 4$ mice) ** $p < 0.005$ using Mann–Whitney test. (**F,G**) Blood flow recovery after ligation of the CFA in $Erk1^{M\Phi-/-}$ mice assessed by laser-Doppler right after the surgery and 3, 7, and 14 days thereafter. Bar graph represents mean with

SEM (*n* = 6 mice). (**H**) Efficiency of *Erk1* deletion in smooth muscle cells was assessed by Q-PCR of smooth muscle cells isolated from the mouse aortas. Bar graph represents mean with SEM (*n* = 4 mice) * $p < 0.05$ using Mann–Whitney test. (**I,J**) Blood flow recovery after ligation of the CFA in $Erk1^{SMC-/-}$ mice assessed by laser-Doppler right after the surgery and 3, 7, and 14 days after the surgery. Bar graph represents mean with SEM (*n* = 5 mice).

3.3. Erk1 Deletions in Endothelial Cells and Macrophages Leads to an Excessive but Poorly Functional Arteriogenesis

Finally, we bred mice with macrophage- ($Erk1^{M\phi KO}$) and endothelial ($Erk1^{iECKO}$)-specific deletions to generate double knockout mice with ERK1 expression disrupted in both cell types ($Erk1^{iECKO/M\phi KO}$). Induction of hindlimb ischemia in these mice led to impaired blood flow recovery that was similar to that observed in the *Erk1* global null mice (Figure 3A,B) and the anatomical extent of arteriogenesis was increased (Figure 3C,D). We carried out Western blotting using total thigh muscle lysates and we observed a massive increase in F4/80 signal (Figure 3E).

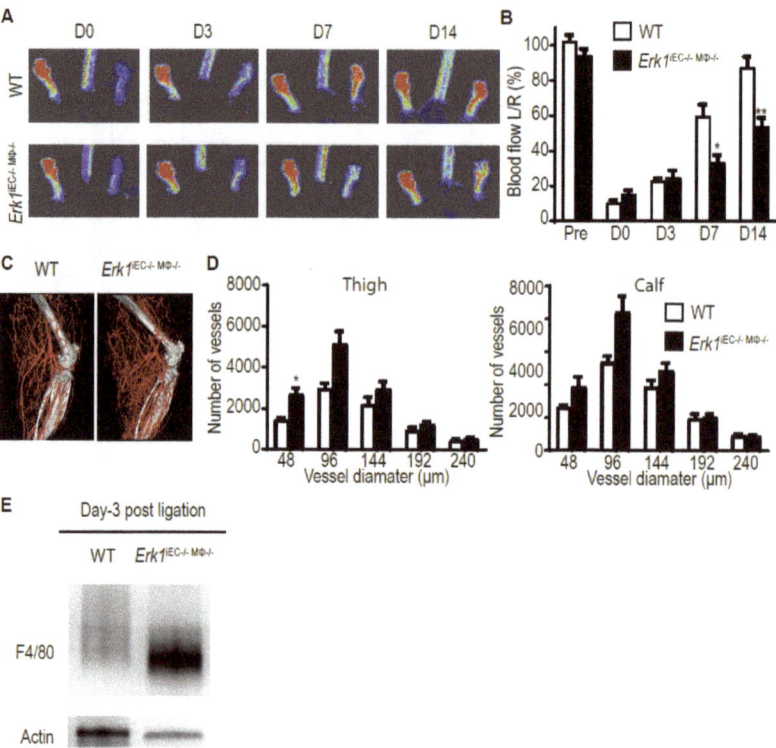

Figure 3. *Erk1* deletion in macrophages and endothelial cells leads to an excessive but poorly functional arteriogenesis. (**A,B**) Blood flow recovery after ligation of the femoral artery in $Erk1^{iEC-/-M\phi-/-}$ mice assessed by laser-Doppler right after the surgery and 3, 7, and 14 days thereafter. Bar graph represents mean with SEM (*n* = 6 mice) * $p < 0.05$, ** $p < 0.005$ using two-way ANOVA followed by Sidak's multiple comparison test. (**C,D**) Quantification of the hindlimb vasculature by micro-CT three weeks after femoral artery ligation. Bar graph represents mean with SEM (*n* = 6 mice) * $p < 0.05$ using two-way ANOVA followed by Sidak's multiple comparison test. (**E**) Macrophage infiltration in the thigh from $Erk1^{iEC-/-M\phi-/-}$ KO mice assessed by Western blotting. Bar graph represents mean with SEM (*n* = 3 mice) * $p < 0.05$ using *t*-test.

3.4. Erk2 Deletions in Endothelial, but Not Other Cell Types, Decreases Arteriogenesis

We next deleted endothelial *Erk2* (*Mapk1*) using the same Cdh5CreER^{T2} line. As in the case of *Erk1*, the administration of tamoxifen to eight-week-old *Erk2*$^{Fl/Fl}$ mice resulted in high efficiency deletion of the endothelial *Erk2* (Figure 4A). However, unlike the *Erk1*$^{iEC-/-}$ mice, the deletion of endothelial *Erk2* resulted in reduced flow recovery in *Erk2*$^{iEC-/-}$ compared to WT mice (Figure 4B,C). Surprisingly, there was no difference in the anatomical extent of arteriogenesis as determined by micro-CT imaging (Figure 4D,E). Endothelial nitric oxide synthase (eNOS) is a key enzyme producing the vasodilator NO and its activity is critical to arteriogenesis [28]. We found a decreased eNOS expression in *Erk2* KO endothelial cells compared to endothelial cells from WT mice (Figure 4F). We next focused on macrophages. LysM Cre was very effective in deleting *Erk2* in mice (Figure 4G). However, blood flow recovery after CFA ligation was not impaired compared to WT mice after *Erk2* gene deletion (Figure 4H,I). We next deleted the *Erk2* gene in smooth muscle cells using Myh11CreER^{T2} driver line (Figure 4J). *Erk2* deletion had no effect on the blood flow recovery (Figure 4K,L).

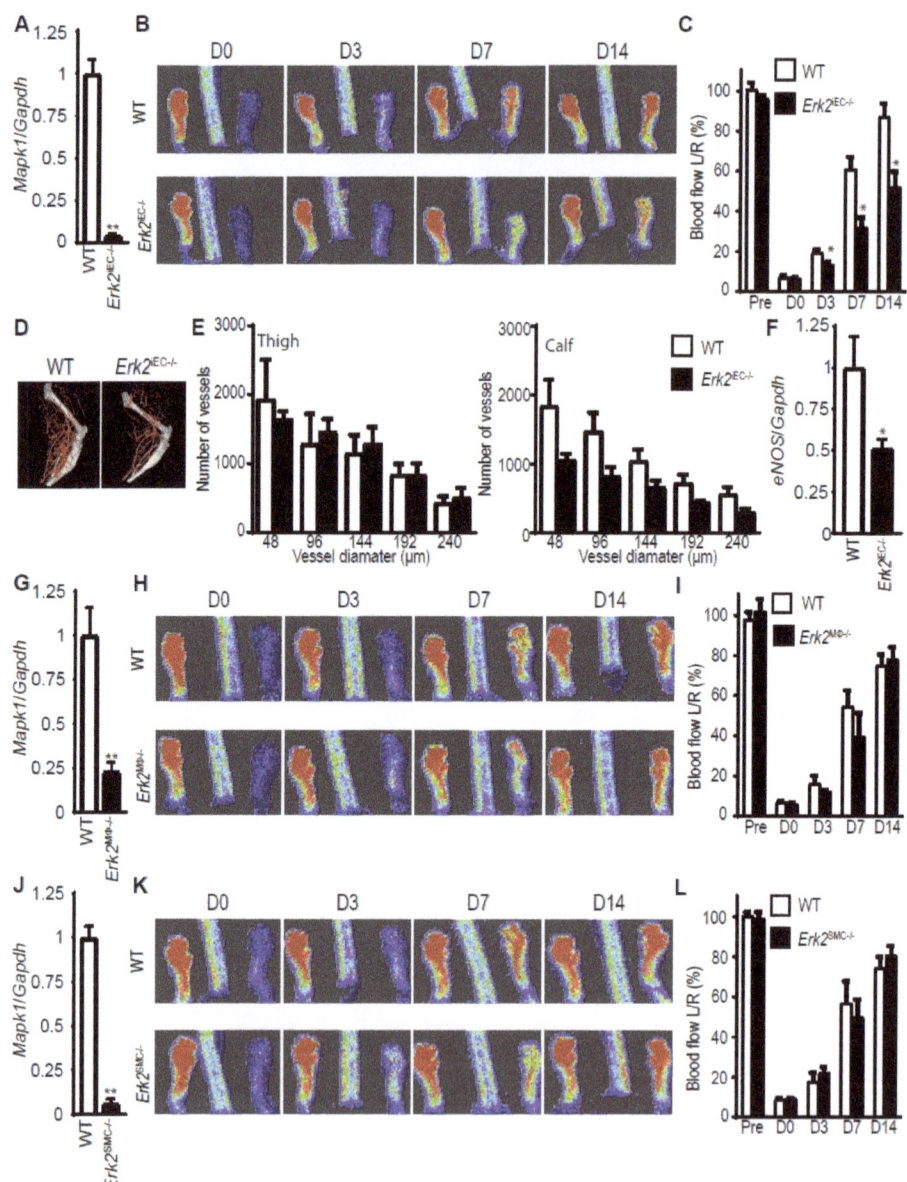

Figure 4. *Erk2* deletion in endothelial cells, but not in other cell types, decreases arteriogenesis. (**A**) Efficiency of *Erk2* deletion in endothelial cells was assessed by Q-PCR of endothelial cells isolated from mouse livers. Bar graph represents mean with SEM (n = 4 mice) ** $p < 0.005$ using Mann–Whitney test. (**B,C**) Blood flow recovery after ligation of the CFA in $Erk2^{iEC-/-}$ mice assessed by laser-Doppler right after the surgery and 3, 7, and 14 days thereafter. Bar graph represents mean with SEM (n = 5 mice) * $p < 0.05$ using two-way ANOVA followed by Sidak's multiple comparison test. (**D,E**) Quantification of the hindlimb vasculature by micro-CT three weeks after femoral artery ligation. Bar graph represents mean with SEM (n = 3 mice). (**F**) eNOS expression in endothelial cells isolated from livers from $Erk2^{iEC-/-}$ mice. * $p < 0.05$ using Mann–Whitney test. (**G**) Efficiency of *Erk2* deletion in macrophages was assessed by Q-PCR on macrophages from the peritoneal cavity. Bar graph represents mean with

Erk2 deletion in endothelial cells, but not in other cell types, decreases arteriogenesis. (**A**) Efficiency of *Erk2* deletion in endothelial cells was assessed by Q-PCR of endothelial cells isolated from mouse livers. Bar graph represents mean with SEM ($n = 4$ mice) ** $p < 0.005$ using Mann–Whitney test. (**B,C**) Blood flow recovery after ligation of the CFA in *Erk2*$^{iEC-/-}$ mice assessed by laser-Doppler right after the surgery and 3, 7, and 14 days thereafter. Bar graph represents mean with SEM ($n = 5$ mice) * $p < 0.05$ using two-way ANOVA followed by Sidak's multiple comparison test. (**D,E**) Quantification of the hindlimb vasculature by micro-CT three weeks after femoral artery ligation. Bar graph represents mean with SEM ($n = 3$ mice). (**F**) eNOS expression in endothelial cells isolated from livers from *Erk2*$^{iEC-/-}$ mice. * $p < 0.05$ using Mann–Whitney test. (**G**) Efficiency of *Erk2* deletion in macrophages was assessed by Q-PCR on macrophages from the peritoneal cavity. Bar graph represents mean with SEM ($n = 4$ mice) ** $p < 0.005$ using Mann–Whitney test. (**H,I**) Blood flow recovery after ligation of the femoral artery in *Erk2*$^{MΦ-/-}$ mice assessed by laser-Doppler right after the surgery and 3, 7, and 14 days thereafter. Bar graph represents mean with SEM ($n = 4$ mice). (**J**) Efficiency of *Erk2* deletion in smooth muscle cells was assessed by Q-PCR of smooth muscle cells isolated from mouse aortas. Bar graph represents mean with SEM ($n = 4$ mice) ** $p < 0.005$ using Mann–Whitney test. (**K,L**) Blood flow recovery after ligation of the femoral artery in *Erk2*$^{SMC-/-}$ mice assessed by laser-Doppler right after the surgery and 3, 7, and 14 days thereafter. Bar graph represents mean with SEM ($n = 6$ mice).

3.5. ERK Isoform Effect on Endothelial Cell Proliferation and Migration

To gain an insight into differences in ERK1- vs. ERk2-specific effects in the endothelium, we examined the effect of either isoform deletion on endothelial cell proliferation and migration. Administration of BrdU to P6 *Erk1*$^{-/-}$ mice showed no differences in the extent of endothelial cell proliferation in the retinal vasculature vs. WT controls (Figure 5A,B). In contrast, BrdU labeling in *Erk2*^{iECKO} mice showed a ~50% reduction in endothelial proliferation. A combination of EC-specific *Erk2* and global *Erk1* knockouts (*Erk2*^{iECKO}; *Erk1*$^{-/-}$ mice) did not result in a further decline in endothelial proliferation demonstrating that *Erk2* is the primary driver of this process. These findings were confirmed in vitro: *Erk2* but not *Erk1* knockdown resulted in decreased EC proliferation in an FGF2 growth assay (Figure 5C). In contrast, both ERKs were involved in EC migration response to VEGF-A or FGF2 stimulation in in vitro cell wounding assays (Figure 5D).

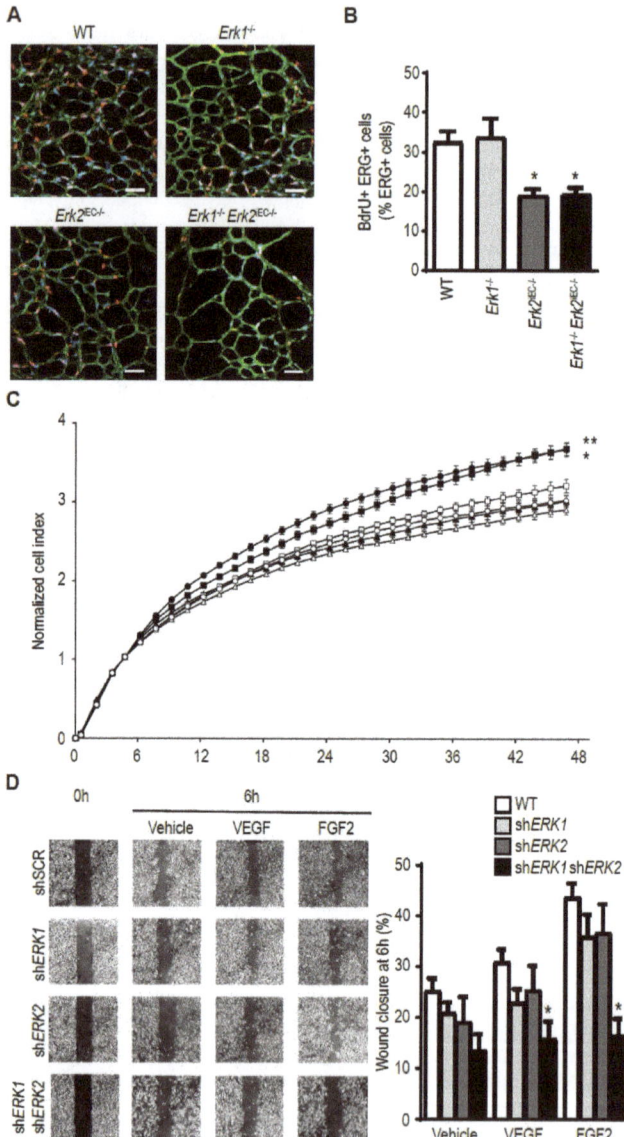

Figure 5. ERK isoform effect on endothelial cell proliferation and migration. (**A**,**B**) Assessment of endothelial cells proliferation in the retina of six-day-old pups by BrdU quantification. * $p < 0.05$ compared to WT using Kruskel–Wallis test with Dunn's multiple comparison test. Scale bar, 50 µm. Bar graph represents mean with SEM ($n = 5$ mice). (**C**) Assessment of proliferation of pulmonary endothelial cells from WT mice (circle), $Erk1^{-/-}$ mice (square), or $Erk2^{iECKO}$ mice (triangle). White symbols are cells treated with vehicle, and black symbols cells treated with FGF2. Bar graph represents mean with SEM ($n = 6$ wells) * $p < 0.05$, ** $p < 0.005$ compared to WT treated with vehicle using Kruskel–Wallis test with Dunn's multiple comparison test. (**D**) Assessment of migration of HUVEC treated with shRNA scrambled, or against *ERK1*, or against *ERK2* and stimulated with (VEGFA$_{165}$ or FGF2. Bar graph represents mean with SEM ($n = 4$ wells) * $p < 0.05$ compared to siSCR of each condition using Kruskel–Wallis test with Dunn's multiple comparison test.

4. Discussion

The results of this study show that ERK isoforms have a differential effect on arteriogenesis. While a global *Erk1* knockout impaired blood flow recovery due to inefficient arteriogenesis, it took a combination of endothelial- and macrophage-specific knockout of this isoform to match the global deletion phenotype. The principal driver of response appeared to be a large increase in tissue macrophage levels that likely resulted in abnormally high VEGF levels and exuberant, albeit inefficient, arteriogenesis. In contrast, endothelial-specific deletion of the *Erk2* isoform resulted in reduced blood flow recovery even though the anatomical extent of arteriogenesis appeared normal. The culprit in this case was a dramatic reduction in endothelial eNOS expression that led to vasoconstriction. Neither ERK isoform deletion by itself in smooth muscle cells affected either blood flow recovery or arteriogenesis per se, while deletion of both genes resulted in a transient decrease of blood flow recovery.

Arteriogenesis is a process leading to the formation of arteries and arterioles. It can proceed either by remodeling of pre-existing collateral arteries or by expansion and arterialization of the capillary bed [2,5,29]. Arteriogenesis is distinct from angiogenesis, a process defined as sprouting and proliferation of the existing capillary bed [2]. Importantly, the two processes are regulated by distinctly different sets of factors. While hypoxia is the primary driver of angiogenesis, arteriogenesis is induced by a combination of shear stress and other mechanical factors [2,5,30]. At the same time, VEGF, and its subsequent induction of endothelial ERK activation, are crucial to both angiogenesis and arteriogenesis [31–35]. One important distinction, however, is the source of VEGF: while, in angiogenesis, VEGF is produced locally due to tissue ischemia, in arteriogenic settings macrophages are the key source of the growth factor [24].

While the importance of the VEGF/VEGFR2/ERK signaling cascade in both angiogenesis and arteriogenesis has been clearly recognized, how this signaling cascade promotes the two distinct means of vascular growth has been unclear. ERK activation is thought to be involved in the proliferation and migration of endothelial cells. Interestingly, our data indicate that endothelial proliferation is largely controlled by ERK2 while migration is the additive function of both isoforms. These results are in agreement with the study of Lefloch et al. who found that ERK2 controls cell proliferation in NIH 3T3 cells [36]. Other isoforms-specific effects of ERK signaling are regulation of macrophage accumulation by ERK1 and regulation of eNOS expression by ERK2.

Both global and a combination of macrophage- and/endothelial-specific *Erk1* knockouts led to markedly increased macrophage accumulation at the site of arteriogenesis after the common femoral artery ligation that was coupled with exuberant but ineffective arteriogenesis. The critical role macrophages play in arteriogenesis is well established. While the M2 subset (macrophages involved in wounds healing and vascular growth) have been described as a principle source of VEGF [37,38], other cell population, including blood-derived inflammatory cells, and mechanical factors can also contribute [13,39]. The observed increase in tissue macrophage levels in these mutant strains is likely derived from circulating monocytes [11] although a proliferation of resident M2 macrophages cannot be ruled out [39,40]. Endothelial cells play a crucial role in monocyte recruitment by increasing expression of the Notch ligand Dll1 [11], as has been observed in this study. Activation of Notch signaling in recruited monocytes polarizes them to an arteriogenic M2 phenotype [11]. Similarly, haploinsufficiency of *Phd2*, encoding the PHD2 oxygen sensor, leads to an expansion of tissue-resident M2-like macrophages, an increased release in arteriogenic factors, and an improved vascular reperfusion in the hindlimb ischemia model [37]. Here, we found that ERK1 controls endothelial-macrophage crosstalk, and that exacerbated macrophage infiltration increases arteriogenesis extent but decreases arteriogenesis functionality. However, a combination of the macrophage- and endothelial-specific *Erk1* knockout phenotype is not as severe as in the *Erk1* global knockout mice, suggesting that other cell types are also may be involved in the phenotype found in the *Erk1* global knockout mice.

In addition to the Dll1 signaling, endothelial cells also regulate macrophage infiltration via MAPK pathways. There are four distinct MAPK pathways: ERK1/2, ERK5, p38, and JNK. While we show that ERK1 controls macrophage recruitment, p38 MAPK pathway has also been shown to be involved in this process [41]. Indeed, a p38 downstream effector MAP-kinase-activated protein kinase 2 (MK2) induces MCP-1 expression in endothelial cells, which promotes monocyte chemoattraction. Thus, at least two different MAPK pathways are involved in the promotion of macrophage infiltration.

Effective blood flow recovery requires not only expansion of the arterial bed thereby ensuring adequate blood supply, but also effective organization and function of this newly formed vasculature. Interestingly, these processes appear to be differentially regulated. We and others have previously reported a dissociation between the extent of anatomical arteriogenesis and effective blood flow. Thus, a mouse strain with an endothelial loss of NF-kB signaling due to deletion of *Rela* showed increased and disorganized arteriogenesis and decreased tissue perfusion after CFA ligation [42]. This was driven by decreased expression of Dll4 that is NF-kB dependent. Delta-like 4 (Dll4) promotes arterial differentiation and restricts vessel branching by direct endothelial cell–cell signaling. Indeed, a similar phenotype was observed in adult $Dll4^{+/-}$ mice. These animals also show reduced blood flow recovery after femoral artery occlusion despite exuberant arteriogenesis [43]. Finally, mice with an endothelial-specific deletion of HIF2α also display increased arteriogenesis abut impaired blood flow recovery in the same hindlimb model [44]. Our description of excessive arteriogenesis yet impaired perfusion in ERK1 null mice adds to this growing body of literature.

In contrast to *Erk1*, *Erk2* knockout in endothelial cells resulted in impaired blood flow recovery despite the normal anatomical extent of arteriogenesis. This is likely due to a decrease in endothelial proliferation combined with decreased expression of eNOS and a corresponding fall in NO production that is critical to the maintenance of arterial tone. Indeed, these observations match a similar decrease in blood flow recovery in endothelial eNOS knockout mice.

ERK1 and ERK2 isoforms share 84% of their amino-acid sequences. ERK1 is larger than ERK2 due to an extension of 17 amino-acids at its N-terminal and two amino-acids at its C-terminal. It has been long a matter of debate whether ERK1 and ERK2 have isoform-specific functions or are totally redundant [45]. ERK2 is expressed at higher levels than ERK1 in most mammalian tissues [46,47]. This difference in expression level may account for the difference in phenotype of the global knockout. Indeed, $Erk1^{-/-}$ mice are viable and fertile [20], whereas $Erk2^{-/-}$ mice die at an early stage in development [19]. Several studies support the functional redundancy of ERK1 and ERK2. Indeed, deletion of *Erk2* but not *Erk1* affected NIH 3T3 cell proliferation in vitro while overexpression of *Erk1* in *Erk2*-deficient NIH 3T3 cells rescued this proliferation defect [36]. ERK1 can also rescue the loss of ERK2 in vivo. Indeed, overexpression of *Erk1* in $Erk2^{-/-}$ mice, generating mice expressing only the ERK1 isoform, fully rescue the developmental defects associated with the loss of ERK2 [47]. We recently published that loss of endothelial *Erk2* in a global $Erk1^{-/-}$ background in adult mice is lethal, whereas loss of one of the two isoforms in the endothelium of adult mice has no vascular phenotype [22]. Interestingly, deletion of *Erk2* by a ubiquitously expressed Cre in adult $Erk1^{-/-}$ mice is lethal in less than three weeks due to multiple organ failure [48]. However, adult mice with only one allele of ERK regardless of the isoform survive [48]. These results suggest redundant roles between ERK1 and ERK2. On the other hand, other studies suggest isoform-specific functions (review in [45]). Notably, in a model of myocardial ischemia/reperfusion injury, myocardial infarction extent was found to be similar in $Erk1^{-/-}$ mice and WT mice [49]. However, mice lacking one *Erk2* allele ($Erk2^{+/-}$), developed increased infarct areas compared with WT mice.

In summary, our data demonstrate specific roles of ERK isoforms in endothelial cells. While ERK1 controls macrophage infiltration following an ischemic event, ERK2 primarily controls endothelial cell proliferation and eNOS expression. Both isoforms are involved in regulation of migration.

Author Contributions: N.R. and M.S. designed experiments. J.Z. and Z.W.Z. carried out animal studies. N.R. and M.S. wrote the manuscript. M.S. supervised the study. All authors have read and agreed to the published version of the manuscript.

Funding: Funded in part by NIH grant 2PO1 HL107205.

Conflicts of Interest: The authors declare no conflict of interest.

References

1. Rizzi, A.; Benagiano, V.; Ribatti, D. Angiogenesis versus arteriogenesis. *Rom. J. Morphol. Embryol.* **2017**, *58*, 15–19. [PubMed]
2. Faber, J.E.; Chilian, W.M.; Deindl, E.; Van Royen, N.; Simons, M. A brief etymology of the collateral circulation. *Arterioscler. Thromb. Vasc. Biol.* **2014**, *34*, 1854–1859. [CrossRef] [PubMed]
3. Lee, C.W.; Stabile, E.; Kinnaird, T.; Shou, M.; Devaney, J.M.; Epstein, S.E.; Burnett, M.S. Temporal patterns of gene expression after acute hindlimb ischemia in mice: Insights into the genomic program for collateral vessel development. *J. Am. Coll. Cardiol.* **2004**, *43*, 474–482. [CrossRef] [PubMed]
4. Scholz, D.; Ziegelhoeffer, T.; Helisch, A.; Wagner, S.; Friedrich, C.; Podzuweit, T.; Schaper, W. Contribution of arteriogenesis and angiogenesis to postocclusive hindlimb perfusion in mice. *J. Mol. Cell. Cardiol.* **2002**, *34*, 775–787. [CrossRef] [PubMed]
5. Simons, M.; Eichmann, A. Molecular controls of arterial morphogenesis. *Circ. Res.* **2015**, *116*, 1712–1724. [CrossRef] [PubMed]
6. Moraes, F.; Paye, J.; Mac Gabhann, F.; Zhuang, Z.W.; Zhang, J.; Lanahan, A.A.; Simons, M. Endothelial cell-dependent regulation of arteriogenesis. *Circ. Res.* **2013**, *113*, 1076–1086. [CrossRef]
7. Lanahan, A.A.; Lech, D.; Dubrac, A.; Zhang, J.; Zhuang, Z.W.; Eichmann, A.; Simons, M. Ptp1b is a physiologic regulator of vascular endothelial growth factor signaling in endothelial cells. *Circulation* **2014**, *130*, 902–909. [CrossRef]
8. Stabile, E.; Burnett, M.S.; Watkins, C.; Kinnaird, T.; Bachis, A.; La Sala, A.; Miller, J.M.; Shou, M.; Epstein, S.E.; Fuchs, S. Impaired arteriogenic response to acute hindlimb ischemia in cd4-knockout mice. *Circulation* **2003**, *108*, 205–210. [CrossRef]
9. Stabile, E.; Kinnaird, T.; La Sala, A.; Hanson, S.K.; Watkins, C.; Campia, U.; Shou, M.; Zbinden, S.; Fuchs, S.; Kornfeld, H.; et al. Cd8+ t lymphocytes regulate the arteriogenic response to ischemia by infiltrating the site of collateral vessel development and recruiting cd4+ mononuclear cells through the expression of interleukin-16. *Circulation* **2006**, *113*, 118–124. [CrossRef]
10. Van Weel, V.; Toes, R.E.; Seghers, L.; Deckers, M.M.; De Vries, M.R.; Eilers, P.H.; Sipkens, J.; Schepers, A.; Eefting, D.; Van Hinsbergh, V.W.; et al. Natural killer cells and cd4+ t-cells modulate collateral artery development. *Arterioscler. Thromb. Vasc. Biol.* **2007**, *27*, 2310–2318. [CrossRef]
11. Krishnasamy, K.; Limbourg, A.; Kapanadze, T.; Gamrekelashvili, J.; Beger, C.; Hager, C.; Lozanovski, V.J.; Falk, C.S.; Napp, L.C.; Bauersachs, J.; et al. Blood vessel control of macrophage maturation promotes arteriogenesis in ischemia. *Nat. Commun.* **2017**, *8*, 952. [CrossRef] [PubMed]
12. Ribatti, D. A new role of mast cells in arteriogenesis. *Microvasc. Res.* **2018**, *118*, 57–60. [CrossRef] [PubMed]
13. Li, J.; Hampton, T.; Morgan, J.P.; Simons, M. Stretch-induced vegf expression in the heart. *J. Clin. Investig.* **1997**, *100*, 18–24. [CrossRef] [PubMed]
14. Pipp, F.; Heil, M.; Issbrucker, K.; Ziegelhoeffer, T.; Martin, S.; Van Den Heuvel, J.; Weich, H.; Fernandez, B.; Golomb, G.; Carmeliet, P.; et al. Vegfr-1-selective vegf homologue plgf is arteriogenic: Evidence for a monocyte-mediated mechanism. *Circ. Res.* **2003**, *92*, 378–385. [CrossRef] [PubMed]
15. Morrison, A.R.; Yarovinsky, T.O.; Young, B.D.; Moraes, F.; Ross, T.D.; Ceneri, N.; Zhang, J.; Zhuang, Z.W.; Sinusas, A.J.; Pardi, R.; et al. Chemokine-coupled beta2 integrin-induced macrophage rac2-myosin iia interaction regulates vegf-a mrna stability and arteriogenesis. *J. Exp. Med.* **2014**, *211*, 1957–1968. [CrossRef] [PubMed]
16. Ahn, G.O.; Seita, J.; Hong, B.J.; Kim, Y.E.; Bok, S.; Lee, C.J.; Kim, K.S.; Lee, J.C.; Leeper, N.J.; Cooke, J.P.; et al. Transcriptional activation of hypoxia-inducible factor-1 (hif-1) in myeloid cells promotes angiogenesis through vegf and s100a8. *Proc. Natl. Acad. Sci. USA* **2014**, *111*, 2698–2703. [CrossRef] [PubMed]
17. Heil, M.; Ziegelhoeffer, T.; Pipp, F.; Kostin, S.; Martin, S.; Clauss, M.; Schaper, W. Blood monocyte concentration is critical for enhancement of collateral artery growth. *Am. J. Physiol. Heart Circ. Physiol.* **2002**, *283*, H2411–H2419. [CrossRef]
18. Simons, M.; Gordon, E.; Claesson-Welsh, L. Mechanisms and regulation of endothelial vegf receptor signalling. *Nat. Rev. Mol. Cell. Biol.* **2016**, *17*, 611–625. [CrossRef]
19. Hatano, N.; Mori, Y.; Oh-hora, M.; Kosugi, A.; Fujikawa, T.; Nakai, N.; Niwa, H.; Miyazaki, J.; Hamaoka, T.; Ogata, M. Essential role for erk2 mitogen-activated protein kinase in placental development. *Genes. Cells* **2003**, *8*, 847–856. [CrossRef]

20. Pages, G.; Guerin, S.; Grall, D.; Bonino, F.; Smith, A.; Anjuere, F.; Auberger, P.; Pouyssegur, J. Defective thymocyte maturation in p44 map kinase (erk 1) knockout mice. *Science* **1999**, *286*, 1374–1377.
21. Srinivasan, R.; Zabuawala, T.; Huang, H.; Zhang, J.; Gulati, P.; Fernandez, S.; Karlo, J.C.; Landreth, G.E.; Leone, G.; Ostrowski, M.C. Erk1 and erk2 regulate endothelial cell proliferation and migration during mouse embryonic angiogenesis. *PLoS ONE* **2009**, *4*, e8283. [CrossRef] [PubMed]
22. Ricard, N.; Scott, R.P.; Booth, C.J.; Velazquez, H.; Cilfone, N.A.; Baylon, J.L.; Gulcher, J.R.; Quaggin, S.E.; Chittenden, T.W.; Simons, M. Endothelial erk1/2 signaling maintains integrity of the quiescent endothelium. *J. Exp. Med.* **2019**, *216*, 1874–1890. [CrossRef] [PubMed]
23. Ray, A.; Dittel, B.N. Isolation of mouse peritoneal cavity cells. *J. Vis. Exp.* **2010**. [CrossRef] [PubMed]
24. Ziegelhoeffer, T.; Fernandez, B.; Kostin, S.; Heil, M.; Voswinckel, R.; Helisch, A.; Schaper, W. Bone marrow-derived cells do not incorporate into the adult growing vasculature. *Circ. Res.* **2004**, *94*, 230–238. [CrossRef]
25. Sorensen, I.; Adams, R.H.; Gossler, A. Dll1-mediated notch activation regulates endothelial identity in mouse fetal arteries. *Blood* **2009**, *113*, 5680–5688. [CrossRef]
26. Clausen, B.E.; Burkhardt, C.; Reith, W.; Renkawitz, R.; Forster, I. Conditional gene targeting in macrophages and granulocytes using lysmcre mice. *Transgenic Res.* **1999**, *8*, 265–277. [CrossRef]
27. Wirth, A.; Benyo, Z.; Lukasova, M.; Leutgeb, B.; Wettschureck, N.; Gorbey, S.; Orsy, P.; Horvath, B.; Maser-Gluth, C.; Greiner, E.; et al. G12-g13-larg-mediated signaling in vascular smooth muscle is required for salt-induced hypertension. *Nat. Med.* **2008**, *14*, 64–68. [CrossRef]
28. Lee, M.Y.; Gamez-Mendez, A.; Zhang, J.; Zhuang, Z.; Vinyard, D.J.; Kraehling, J.; Velazquez, H.; Brudvig, G.W.; Kyriakides, T.R.; Simons, M.; et al. Endothelial cell autonomous role of akt1: Regulation of vascular tone and ischemia-induced arteriogenesis. *Arterioscler. Thromb. Vasc. Biol.* **2018**, *38*, 870–879. [CrossRef]
29. Mac Gabhann, F.; Peirce, S.M. Collateral capillary arterialization following arteriolar ligation in murine skeletal muscle. *Microcirculation* **2010**, *17*, 333–347. [CrossRef]
30. Heil, M.; Schaper, W. Influence of mechanical, cellular, and molecular factors on collateral artery growth (arteriogenesis). *Circ. Res.* **2004**, *95*, 449–458. [CrossRef]
31. Shin, M.; Beane, T.J.; Quillien, A.; Male, I.; Zhu, L.J.; Lawson, N.D. Vegfa signals through erk to promote angiogenesis, but not artery differentiation. *Development* **2016**, *143*, 3796–3805. [CrossRef] [PubMed]
32. Kofler, N.M.; Simons, M. Angiogenesis versus arteriogenesis: Neuropilin 1 modulation of vegf signaling. *F1000Prime Rep.* **2015**, *7*, 26. [CrossRef] [PubMed]
33. Lucitti, J.L.; Mackey, J.K.; Morrison, J.C.; Haigh, J.J.; Adams, R.H.; Faber, J.E. Formation of the collateral circulation is regulated by vascular endothelial growth factor-a and a disintegrin and metalloprotease family members 10 and 17. *Circ. Res.* **2012**, *111*, 1539–1550. [CrossRef] [PubMed]
34. Hong, C.C.; Peterson, Q.P.; Hong, J.Y.; Peterson, R.T. Artery/vein specification is governed by opposing phosphatidylinositol-3 kinase and map kinase/erk signaling. *Curr. Biol.* **2006**, *16*, 1366–1372. [CrossRef] [PubMed]
35. Ren, B.; Deng, Y.; Mukhopadhyay, A.; Lanahan, A.A.; Zhuang, Z.W.; Moodie, K.L.; Mulligan-Kehoe, M.J.; Byzova, T.V.; Peterson, R.T.; Simons, M. Erk1/2-akt1 crosstalk regulates arteriogenesis in mice and zebrafish. *J. Clin. Investig.* **2010**, *120*, 1217–1228. [CrossRef]
36. Lefloch, R.; Pouyssegur, J.; Lenormand, P. Single and combined silencing of erk1 and erk2 reveals their positive contribution to growth signaling depending on their expression levels. *Mol. Cell. Biol.* **2008**, *28*, 511–527. [CrossRef]
37. Takeda, Y.; Costa, S.; Delamarre, E.; Roncal, C.; De Oliveira, R.L.; Squadrito, M.L.; Finisguerra, V.; Deschoemaeker, S.; Bruyere, F.; Wenes, M.; et al. Macrophage skewing by phd2 haplodeficiency prevents ischaemia by inducing arteriogenesis. *Nature* **2011**, *479*, 122–126. [CrossRef]
38. Troidl, C.; Jung, G.; Troidl, K.; Hoffmann, J.; Mollmann, H.; Nef, H.; Schaper, W.; Hamm, C.W.; Schmitz-Rixen, T. The temporal and spatial distribution of macrophage subpopulations during arteriogenesis. *Curr. Vasc. Pharmacol.* **2013**, *11*, 5–12. [CrossRef]
39. Li, J.; Brown, L.F.; Hibberd, M.G.; Grossman, J.D.; Morgan, J.P.; Simons, M. VEGF, flk-1, and flt-1 expression in a rat myocardial infarction model of angiogenesis. *Am. J. Physiol.* **1996**, *270*, H1803–H1811. [CrossRef]
40. Jenkins, S.J.; Ruckerl, D.; Cook, P.C.; Jones, L.H.; Finkelman, F.D.; Van Rooijen, N.; MacDonald, A.S.; Allen, J.E. Local macrophage proliferation, rather than recruitment from the blood, is a signature of th2 inflammation. *Science* **2011**, *332*, 1284–1288. [CrossRef]

41. Limbourg, A.; Von Felden, J.; Jagavelu, K.; Krishnasamy, K.; Napp, L.C.; Kapopara, P.R.; Gaestel, M.; Schieffer, B.; Bauersachs, J.; Limbourg, F.P.; et al. Map-kinase activated protein kinase 2 links endothelial activation and monocyte/macrophage recruitment in arteriogenesis. *PLoS ONE* **2015**, *10*, e0138542. [CrossRef] [PubMed]
42. Tirziu, D.; Jaba, I.M.; Yu, P.; Larrivee, B.; Coon, B.G.; Cristofaro, B.; Zhuang, Z.W.; Lanahan, A.A.; Schwartz, M.A.; Eichmann, A.; et al. Endothelial nuclear factor-kappab-dependent regulation of arteriogenesis and branching. *Circulation* **2012**, *126*, 2589–2600. [CrossRef] [PubMed]
43. Cristofaro, B.; Shi, Y.; Faria, M.; Suchting, S.; Leroyer, A.S.; Trindade, A.; Duarte, A.; Zovein, A.C.; Iruela-Arispe, M.L.; Nih, L.R.; et al. Dll4-notch signaling determines the formation of native arterial collateral networks and arterial function in mouse ischemia models. *Development* **2013**, *140*, 1720–1729. [CrossRef] [PubMed]
44. Skuli, N.; Majmundar, A.J.; Krock, B.L.; Mesquita, R.C.; Mathew, L.K.; Quinn, Z.L.; Runge, A.; Liu, L.; Kim, M.N.; Liang, J.; et al. Endothelial hif-2alpha regulates murine pathological angiogenesis and revascularization processes. *J. Clin. Investig.* **2012**, *122*, 1427–1443. [CrossRef]
45. Busca, R.; Pouyssegur, J.; Lenormand, P. Erk1 and erk2 map kinases: Specific roles or functional redundancy? *Front. Cell Dev. Biol.* **2016**, *4*, 53. [CrossRef]
46. Busca, R.; Christen, R.; Lovern, M.; Clifford, A.M.; Yue, J.X.; Goss, G.G.; Pouyssegur, J.; Lenormand, P. Erk1 and erk2 present functional redundancy in tetrapods despite higher evolution rate of erk1. *BMC Evol. Biol.* **2015**, *15*, 179. [CrossRef]
47. Fremin, C.; Saba-El-Leil, M.K.; Levesque, K.; Ang, S.L.; Meloche, S. Functional redundancy of erk1 and erk2 map kinases during development. *Cell. Rep.* **2015**, *12*, 913–921. [CrossRef]
48. Blasco, R.B.; Francoz, S.; Santamaria, D.; Canamero, M.; Dubus, P.; Charron, J.; Baccarini, M.; Barbacid, M. C-Raf, but not B-Raf, is essential for development of K-Ras oncogene-driven non-small cell lung carcinoma. *Cancer Cell* **2011**, *19*, 652–663. [CrossRef]
49. Lips, D.J.; Bueno, O.F.; Wilkins, B.J.; Purcell, N.H.; Kaiser, R.A.; Lorenz, J.N.; Voisin, L.; Saba-El-Leil, M.K.; Meloche, S.; Pouysségur, J.; et al. MEK1-ERK2 signaling pathway protects myocardium from ischemic injury in vivo. *Circulation* **2004**, *109*, 1938–1941. [CrossRef]

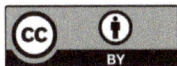

© 2019 by the authors. Licensee MDPI, Basel, Switzerland. This article is an open access article distributed under the terms and conditions of the Creative Commons Attribution (CC BY) license (http://creativecommons.org/licenses/by/4.0/).

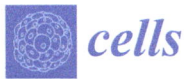

Article

Contribution of the Potassium Channels $K_V1.3$ and $K_{Ca}3.1$ to Smooth Muscle Cell Proliferation in Growing Collateral Arteries

Manuel Lasch [1,2], Amelia Caballero Martinez [1], Konda Kumaraswami [1], Hellen Ishikawa-Ankerhold [1,3], Sarah Meister [4] and Elisabeth Deindl [1,*]

1. Walter-Brendel-Centre of Experimental Medicine, University Hospital, LMU Munich, 80539 Munich, Germany; Manuel.Lasch@med.uni-muenchen.de (M.L.); a_caballeromartinez@hotmail.com (A.C.M.); Kumaraswami.Konda@med.uni-muenchen.de (K.K.); Hellen.Ishikawa-Ankerhold@med.uni-muenchen.de (H.I.-A.)
2. Department of Otorhinolaryngology, Head and Neck Surgery, University Hospital, LMU Munich, 80539 Munich, Germany
3. Department of Internal Medicine I, Faculty of Medicine, University Hospital, LMU Munich, 80539 Munich, Germany
4. Department of Obstetrics and Gynaecology, University Hospital, LMU Munich, 80539 Munich, Germany; Sarah.Meister@med.uni-muenchen.de
* Correspondence: Elisabeth.Deindl@med.uni-muenchen.de; Tel.: +49-2180-76504

Received: 19 February 2020; Accepted: 3 April 2020; Published: 8 April 2020

Abstract: Collateral artery growth (arteriogenesis) involves the proliferation of vascular endothelial cells (ECs) and smooth muscle cells (SMCs). Whereas the proliferation of ECs is directly related to shear stress, the driving force for arteriogenesis, little is known about the mechanisms of SMC proliferation. Here we investigated the functional relevance of the potassium channels $K_V1.3$ and $K_{Ca}3.1$ for SMC proliferation in arteriogenesis. Employing a murine hindlimb model of arteriogenesis, we found that blocking $K_V1.3$ with PAP-1 or $K_{Ca}3.1$. with TRAM-34, both interfered with reperfusion recovery after femoral artery ligation as shown by Laser-Doppler Imaging. However, only treatment with PAP-1 resulted in a reduced SMC proliferation. qRT-PCR results revealed an impaired downregulation of α smooth muscle-actin (αSM-actin) and a repressed expression of fibroblast growth factor receptor 1 (*Fgfr1*) and platelet derived growth factor receptor b (*Pdgfrb*) in growing collaterals in vivo and in primary murine arterial SMCs in vitro under $K_V1.3$. blockade, but not when $K_{Ca}3.1$ was blocked. Moreover, treatment with PAP-1 impaired the mRNA expression of the cell cycle regulator early growth response-1 (*Egr1*) in vivo and in vitro. Together, these data indicate that $K_V1.3$ but not $K_{Ca}3.1$ contributes to SMC proliferation in arteriogenesis.

Keywords: arteriogenesis; collateral artery growth; SMC proliferation; potassium channel; $K_V1.3$; $K_{Ca}3.1$; FGFR-1; Egr-1; PDFG-R; αSM-actin

1. Introduction

Arteriogenesis, which is defined as the growth of pre-existing arteriolar connections into functional arteries compensating for the loss of an artery due to occlusion [1], particularly involves the proliferation of vascular endothelial cells (ECs) and smooth muscle cells (SMCs). The driving force for arteriogenesis is increased fluid shear stress [2,3]. This mechanical force, which can be sensed directly by ECs, has recently been shown to be linked to local activation of collateral ECs. By mediating the release of extracellular RNA (eRNA) from ECs, eRNA promotes the binding of vascular endothelial growth factor A (VEGFA) to VEGF receptor 2 (VEGFR2) [4], thereby promoting local vascular EC proliferation as well as activation of a mechanosensory complex, consisting of VEGFR2, platelet endothelial cell adhesion molecule 1 (PECAM-1), and vascular endothelial cell cadherin (VE-cadherin) [5], triggering collateral artery growth.

SMCs, located at the abluminal side, are not able to sense shear stress, and relatively little is known about the mechanisms triggering SMC proliferation in arteriogenesis. Growth factors, such as fibroblast growth factor 2 (FGF-2) and platelet-derived growth factor BB (PDGF-BB) have been shown to be important for SMC proliferation in arteriogenesis [6,7] (and own unpublished results of M. Lasch). This might in particular be related to their function to induce the expression of early growth response 1 (*Egr1*) [8], a transcriptional regulator, which has been shown to control cell cycle progression in arteriogenesis [9]. Interestingly, it has been demonstrated that the receptor for FGF-2, namely FGFR-1, which is expressed on collateral SMCs but not on ECs, is increased expressed only during a short time frame after induction of arteriogenesis [10]. These data indicate that the point in time of FGF-2 application is critical and might explain the outcome of clinical studies in which FGF-2 treatment showed limited effects in patients with vascular occlusive diseases [11,12].

The proliferation of vascular SMCs in arteriogenesis is characterized by the transition from the contractile to the synthetic (proliferating) SMC type. This process is associated with reduced mRNA and protein levels of contractile genes such as α-smooth muscle actin (αSM-actin) and paralleled by an increased expression of *Egr1*. [9,13,14]. The opposed gene expression of contractile genes and *Egr1*, which is tightly regulated by the transcriptional co-activators myocardin and myocardin-related transcription factors (MRTFs) and the ternary complex factor ETS like protein Elk-1, which compete for the binding to the transcription factor serum response factor (SRF) [15–17], has been demonstrated for the process of arteriogenesis by our group [9].

The potassium channels $K_V1.3$ and $K_{Ca}3.1$ have been shown to be involved in cell cycle regulation by activating intracellular signaling pathways [18,19], and to play a role in modulating vascular SMC proliferation [20,21]. Since the mechanisms triggering vascular SMC proliferation in arteriogenesis are still not very well described, we decided to investigate the functional contribution of $K_V1.3$ and $K_{Ca}3.1$ to the proliferation of vascular SMCs in collateral artery growth. The mode of action of these potassium channels in terms of proliferation is still under debate and several mechanisms, either ion flux dependent or independent, have been proposed [18,19]. Both potassium channels, $K_V1.3$ and $K_{Ca}3.1$, have been demonstrated to be upregulated in proliferating SMCs, whereby their specific blockade interfered with cell cycle progression. Increased expression levels of $K_V1.3$ have been detected in vitro in proliferating SMCs isolated from murine femoral arteries or from human donors [21,22] as well as under pathological situations such as neointima hyperplasia in vivo [22,23]. Moreover, it has been shown that blockade of $K_V1.3$ with selective blockers such as 5-(4-phenoxybutoxy)psoralen (PAP-1) inhibited migration and proliferation of SMCs in vitro [22,23] and in vivo [23,24]. Similar to $K_V1.3$, $K_{Ca}3.1$ has been found to be upregulated upon stimulation with PDGF-BB in proliferating SMCs in vitro [20] and in models of hyperplasia in vivo [25,26]. Blocking $K_{Ca}3.1$ with the selective blocker TRAM-34 in contrast interfered with SMC proliferation both, in vitro and in vivo [20,25,27,28]. Besides its effect on SMC proliferation, $K_{Ca}3.1$ plays a major role in endothelium-derived hyperpolarizing factor (EDHF)-mediated vasodilation as shown in $K_{Ca}3.1$ deficient mice [29].

In the present study we investigated the relevance of the potassium channels $K_V1.3$ and $K_{Ca}3.1$ for SMC proliferation in growing collateral arteries by performing blocking studies employing the selective channel blockers PAP-1 and TRAM-34, respectively. From our results we conclude that $K_V1.3$ contributes to SMC proliferation in arteriogenesis, whereas $K_{Ca}3.1$ is more likely to be involved in vasodilation.

2. Materials and Methods

2.1. Animal Protocol and Treatments

Male C57BL6/J mice, purchased from Charles River, were housed in cages and kept under 12 h day/night cycle with food and water ad libitum. All experiments were approved by the Bavarian Animal Care and Use Committee (ethical approval code ROB-55.2-1-54-2532-73-12 and

ROB-55.2Vet-2532.Vet_02-17-99) and carried out according to the guidelines of the German law for protection of animal life. Mice at the age of 6 to 10 weeks were anesthetized with a combination of 0.5 mg/kg medetomidine (Pfister Pharma), 5 mg/kg midazolam (Ratiopharm GmbH), and 0.05 mg/kg fentanyl (CuraMED Pharma). Arteriogenesis was induced by right femoral artery ligation (FAL, occlusion (occ)), whereas the left femoral artery was sham operated (Figure 1) as previously described in [30].

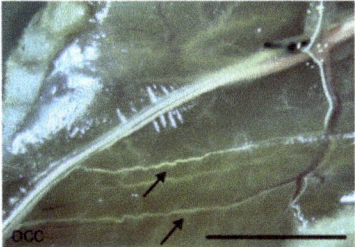 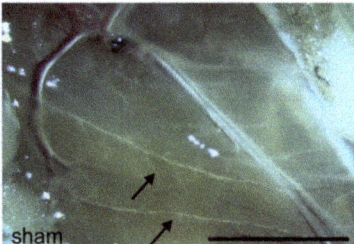

Figure 1. Photographs of superficial collateral arteries in mouse adductor muscles. Photographs were taken 7 days after induction of arteriogenesis by femoral artery ligation (left picture) or sham operation (right picture). Mice were perfused with latex to better visualize collateral arteries. Pre-existing collaterals appear very fine and straight (arrows, right picture). Seven days after induction of arteriogenesis, grown collateral arteries show a typical corkscrew formation with increased vascular caliber size (arrows, left picture). Scale bar 5 mm

To block potassium channels, mice were treated either with the selective $K_V1.3$ channel blocker (5-(4-phenoxybutoxy)psoralen (PAP-1, 40 mg/kg/d, intraperitoneally (i.p), Sigma-Aldrich) [31], or the selective $K_{Ca}3.1$ channel blocker TRAM-34 (120 mg/kg/d, i.p., Alomone Labs) [27], dissolved in peanut oil, at doses previously described [27,31]. The treatments started 4 h before the surgical procedure. Moreover, to uphold constant blood levels of the blockers, mice received two doses per day, one in the morning and one in the afternoon. When mice were treated with BrdU (Sigma-Aldrich), they received a single dose (1.25 mg/d dissolved in phosphate buffered saline (PBS), i.p.) starting directly after the surgical procedure.

2.2. Laser Doppler Perfusion Measurements and Tissue Sampling

The laser Doppler perfusion measurements were performed as described in [4]. In brief, hindlimb perfusion was measured using the laser Doppler imaging technique (Moor LDI2-IR, LDI 5061 and Moor Software 3.01, Moor Instruments) under temperature-controlled conditions (37 °C), and perfusion was calculated by right to left (occlusion (occ) to sham) flux ratios.

Prior to tissue sampling for (immuno-) histology, mice were perfused with an adenosine buffer (1% adenosine, 5% bovine serum albumin (BSA), both from Sigma-Aldrich dissolved in PBS, PAN Biotech, pH 7.4) for maximal vasodilation followed by perfusion with 3% paraformaldehyde (PFA, Merck) dissolved in PBS, pH 7.4, for cryoconservation, or 4% PFA for paraffin embedding [2]. For qRT-PCR analyses, mice were perfused with latex flexible compound (Chicago Latex) to visualize superficial collateral arteries (see also Figure 1) for dissection. After isolation, superficial collateral arteries were snap frozen on dry ice and stored at −80 °C until further investigations [9].

2.3. Cell Culture

Mouse primary artery smooth muscle cells (catalog number C57-6081, CellBiologics) were cultured in a SMC growth medium (SMCGM, CellBiologics) containing insulin and the growth factors fibroblast growth factor 2 (FGF-2) and epidermal growth factor (EGF) together with 20% fetal calf serum (FCS, PAN). For serum starvation, cells were cultured in Dulbecco's modified Eagle's medium (DMEM, Thermo Fisher Scientific) with 1% FCS for 24 h. Thereafter, negative controls were stimulated with medium containing 2% FCS, positive controls with 10% FCS.

2.4. Histology, Immunohistology, Proliferation Assay, and Immunocytochemistry

Giemsa staining on paraffin fixed tissue samples was performed according to standard procedures, and slices were analyzed using an Axioskop 40 microscope (Carl Zeiss AG). BrdU staining of paraffin fixed tissue sections was performed with a BrdU detection kit (BD Pharmingen) according to the manufacturer´s procedure using the same microscope for evaluating the tissue sections.

To investigate the proliferation of mouse primary artery SMCs, a BrdU proliferation assay kit (Roche) was used according to the manufacturer´s instructions. In brief, mouse primary artery SMCs were seeded in a 96-well plate overnight, and after serum starvation in DMEM containing 1% FCS for 24 h, the mouse primary artery SMCs were cultured in DMEM with 10% FCS and treated with or without PAP-1 or TRAM-34, respectively, together with 10 mM BrdU. Cell proliferation was assessed by colorimetry with an Infinite F200 ELISA reader (TECAN).

For immunofluorescence staining, cryofixed tissue sections (10 µm) were stained with a rabbit anti-$K_V1.3$ (catalog number APC-101) or a rabbit anti-$K_{Ca}3.1$ (catalog number APC-064) antibody (both from Alomone Labs) followed by a goat anti-rabbit IgG Alexa fluor 488-conjugated antibody (catalog number 711-545-153, Jackson ImmunoResearch) together with a Cy3-conjugated mouse anti-αSM-actin antibody (catalog number C6198, Sigma-Aldrich) and an Alexa fluor 647-conjugated rat anti-CD31 antibody (catalog number 102515, BioLegend), followed by DAPI counter staining (catalog number 62248, Thermo Fisher Scientific). Images were taken with an Axio Imager 2 fluorescence microscope equipped with and an Axion ICc 5 camera and Axiovert software (Carl Zeiss) or using a LSM 880 confocal laser scanning microscope equipped with an Airycan module (Carl Zeiss) with ZEN black software for imaging acquisition. Imaging analysis of $K_V1.3$ or $K_{Ca}3.1$ expression in αSM-actin positive SMCs or CD31 positive ECs was performed using the ZEN blue software. For the colocalization anaylsis, the ZEN colocalization tool was used (Carl Zeiss AG). The three-dimensional (3D) projection surface reconstruction of the images where done by using the Imaris software (Bitplane).

2.5. RNA Isolation, cDNA Synthesis, and qRT-PCR

The total RNA was isolated from the mouse primary artery SMCs or collateral arteries with Trizol (Life Technologies) and the residual DNA was removed by digestion with RQ1 RNase-Free DNase (Promega). Thereafter, RNA was purified with RNeasy MinElute columns (Qiagen) and reverse transcribed to cDNA using the QuantiTect® Reverse Transcription Kit (Qiagen) according to the manufacturer´s procedure. The qRT-PCR was performed as previously described [32] using the Power SYBR Green Kit (Life Technologies) and a StepOnePlus cycler (Life Technologies) and the following primers: 18S rRNA forward 5′-GGACAGGATTGACAGATTGATAG-3′, reverse 5′-CTCGTTCGTTATCGGAATTAAC-3′, αSM-actin forward 5′-GAGCATCCGACACTGCTG-3′, reverse 5′-GTACGTCCAGAGGCATAG-3′, fibroblast growth factor receptor-1 (*Fgfr1*) forward 5′-CTTGCCGTATGTCCAGATCC-3′, reverse 5′-TCCGTAGATGAAGCACCTCC-3′, platelet derived growth factor b (*Pdgfrb*) forward 5′-AGGACAACCGTACCTTGGGTGACT-3′, reverse 5′-CAGTTCTGACACGTACCGGGTCTC-3′, early growth response 1 (*Egr1*) forward 5′-CGAACAACCCTATGAGCACCTG-3′, and reverse 5′-CAGAGGAAGACGATGAAGCAGC-3′. To control specific amplification, melt curve analyses and agarose gels were performed. Data were analyzed using the ∆∆Ct method [33] and results were normalized to the expression level of the 18S rRNA.

2.6. Statistical Analyses

Statistical analyses were performed using the GraphPad software PRISM6. All data are stated as means ± SEM. Results were tested for normality and statistical analyses were performed as specified in the figure legends. Results were considered to be statistically significant at $p \leq 0.05$.

3. Results

3.1. $K_V1.3$ and $K_{Ca}3.1$ are Localized in Collateral Arteries

Employing a murine hindlimb model of arteriogenesis, we investigated whether the potassium channel $K_V1.3$ or $K_{Ca}3.1$, respectively, were expressed in adductor collateral arteries.

Immunofluorescence imaging revealed that $K_V1.3$ and $K_{Ca}3.1$ labelling strongly colocalized with αSM-actin, a marker for SMCs, but weakly with CD 31, which is a marker for ECs (Figures 2 and 3).

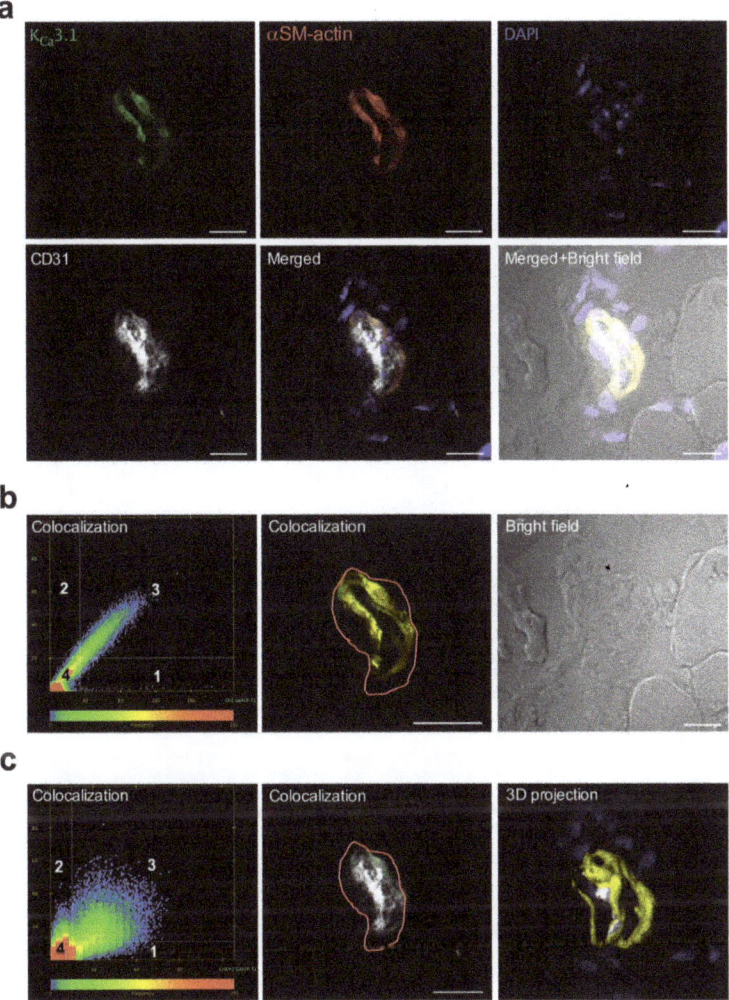

Figure 2. Localization of $K_{Ca}3.1$ in ECs and SMCs of murine collateral arteries. (**a**) Representative confocal immunofluorescence images of transversal sections of collateral arteries isolated 3 h after induction of arteriogenesis. Tissue sections were stained with an antibody against $K_{Ca}3.1$ (green), together with the SMC marker αSM-actin (red), the EC marker CD31 (grey), and DAPI (blue); (**b**,**c**) Scatterplots showing the colocalization analysis, (left lower panel) represents pixels that have low intensity levels in both channels, green and red (**b**), or green and gray (**c**). Quadrant 4 (lower left bottom) represents pixels that are referred to as background and are not taken into consideration for colocalization analysis. Quadrant 1 represents pixels that have high green intensities and low red intensities and Quadrant 2 represents pixels that have high red intensities and low green intensities. Quadrant 3 represents pixels with high intensity levels in both green and red (b) or green and gray (c). These pixels are considered to be colocalized. Bright field image is also displayed. (**c**) 3D projection surface rendering is showing the localization of the $K_{Ca}3.1$ with the labelling CD 31 and αSM-actin display on the panel (c) right lower position. Scale bar 20 μm.

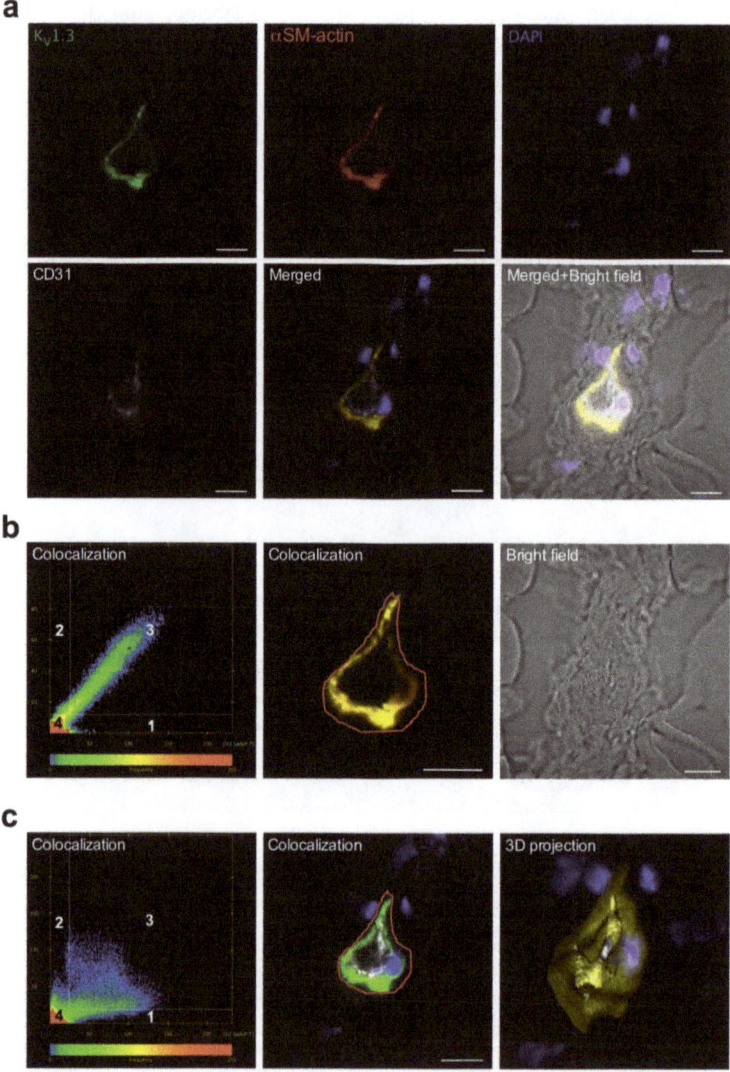

Figure 3. Localization of $K_V1.3$ in ECs and SMCs of murine collateral arteries. (**a**) Representative confocal immunofluorescence images of transversal sections of collateral arteries isolated 3 h after induction of arteriogenesis. Tissue sections were stained with an antibody against $K_V1.3$ (green), together with the SMC marker αSM-actin (red), the EC marker CD31 (grey), and DAPI (blue); (**b**,**c**) Scatterplots showing the colocalization analysis. Quadrant 4 (left lower left panel) represents pixels that have low intensity levels in both channels, green and red (**b**) or green and grey (**c**), and these pixels are referred to as background and are not taken into consideration for colocalization analysis. Quadrant 1 represent pixels that have high green intensities and low red intensities and Quadrant 2 represents pixels that have high red intensities and low green intensities. Quadrant 3 represents pixels with high intensity levels in both green and red in (**b**) and green and grey in (**c**). These pixels are considered to be colocalized. Scale bar 20 µm. Bright field image is also displayed. (**c**) 3D projection surface rendering is showing the localization of the $K_V1.3$ with the labelling CD 31 and αSM-actin on the panel (**c**) right lower position.

3.2. Blockade of $K_V1.3$ But Not of $K_{Ca}3.1$ Impaired Arteriogenesis by Inhibiting Collateral SMC Proliferation

To investigate the functional relevance of the potassium channels for arteriogenesis, the $K_V1.3$ channel was blocked with PAP-1, and the $K_{Ca}3.1$ channel with TRAM-34. The laser Doppler perfusion measurements revealed that both treatments significantly interfered with reperfusion recovery after femoral artery ligation (Figure 4).

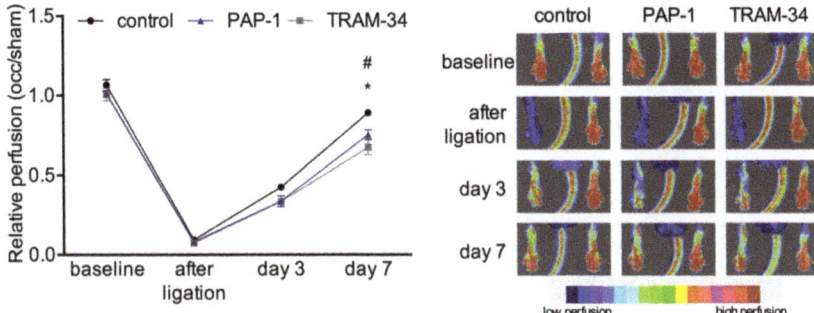

Figure 4. Laser Doppler perfusion measurements. Line plot (left panel) along with corresponding flux images (right panel) of laser Doppler perfusion measurements. Mice were treated with solvent (control), PAP-1, or TRAM-34, respectively, and the perfusion was calculated by right to left (occlusion (occ) to sham) ratio before, immediately after, and at day 3 and 7 after the surgical procedure (left panel). Data are means ± SEM, n = 6 per group. * $p < 0.05$ (PAP-1 vs. control) and # $p < 0.05$ (TRAM-34 vs. control) from two-way ANOVA with Bonferroni's multiple comparison test. The right panel shows representative flux images of murine paws with the tail in the center. Cold colors (blue, green) indicate low perfusion, whereas warm colors (yellow, red) indicate high perfusion (see scale).

To quantify the effects of channel blockade on vascular cell proliferation, we performed immunohistochemical analyses of the proliferation marker BrdU in transversal sections of collateral arteries at day 7 after induction of arteriogenesis. The results showed that both treatment with the $K_V1.3$ blocker PAP-1 and with $K_{Ca}3.1$ blocker TRAM-34 did not interfered with EC proliferation in growing collaterals. However, the PAP-1 treatment significantly reduced SMC proliferation, an effect that was not observed when mice were treated with TRAM-34 (Figure 5a–c).

During the transition from the synthetic to the proliferative phase, the mRNA expression level of αSM-actin has been shown to be downregulated 12h after induction of arteriogenesis [9], and confirmed in the present study by qRT-PCR analyses (Figure 5d). Interestingly, in TRAM-34 treated mice, the expression level of αSM-actin was comparable to that of the control mice at 12 h after induction of arteriogenesis, however, it was significantly increased in PAP-1 treated mice at the same point in time (Figure 5e).

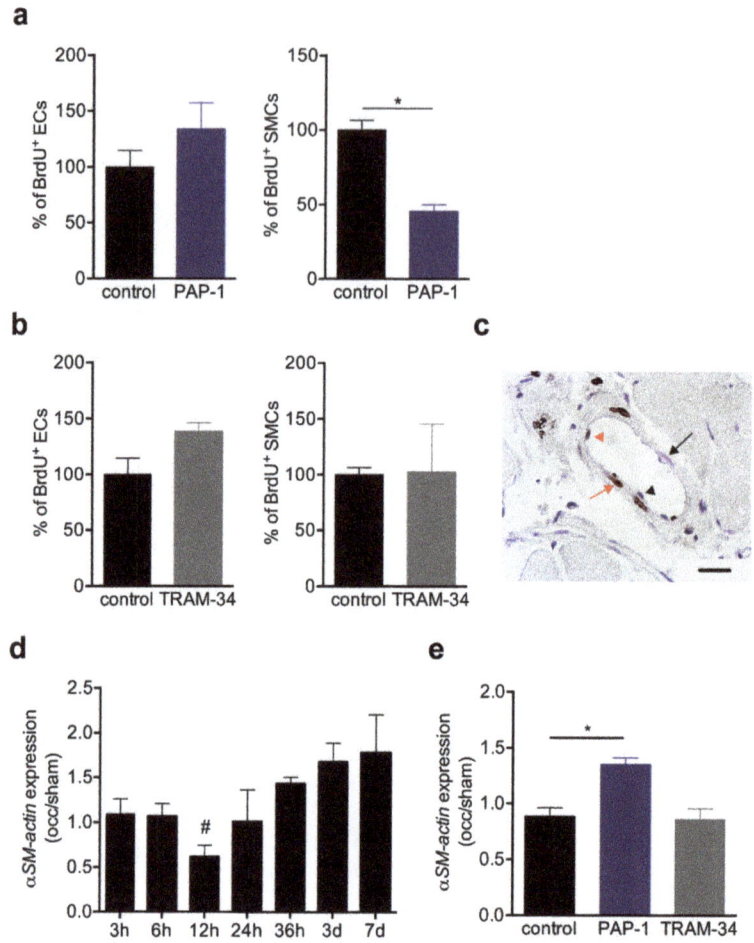

Figure 5. BrdU incorporation and αSM-actin expression in collaterals. (**a,b**) Bar graphs represent the results of quantitative analyses of BrdU$^+$ ECs (left panels) and SMCs (right panels) in solvent (control), (**a**) PAP-1 or (**b**) TRAM-34-treated mice at day 7 after induction of arteriogenesis. Data are means ± SEM, $n = 3$ mice per group. * $p < 0.05$ from unpaired student´s t-test. The numbers of BrdU$^+$ cells in control collaterals were defined as 100%; (**c**) Representative picture of a BrdU stained collateral at day 7 after induction of arteriogenesis. Scale bar 20 µm; (**d,e**) The bar graphs represent the expression levels of αSM-actin (occlusion/sham (occ/sham)) in collateral arteries (**d**) at different time points after induction of arteriogenesis or (**e**) at 12 h after induction of arteriogenesis in control, PAP-1, or TRAM-34 treated mice. The qRT-PCR results were normalized to the expression level of the 18SrRNA. Data are means ± SEM, n > 3 per group. * $p < 0.05$ from unpaired student's t-test and refers in (**d**) to occ vs. sham.

3.3. $K_V1.3$ and $K_{Ca}3.1$ Blockade Inhibits Mouse Primary Artery SMCs Proliferation In Vitro

To gain further insights into the role of the potassium channels on SMC proliferation, we performed in vitro investigations on mouse primary artery SMCs. Immunocytological analyses showed that $K_V1.3$, as well as $K_{Ca}3.1$, are localized perinuclear in mouse primary artery SMCs. Somehow, weaker signals were seen in the cytoplasm and at the cytoplasmic membrane (Figure 6).

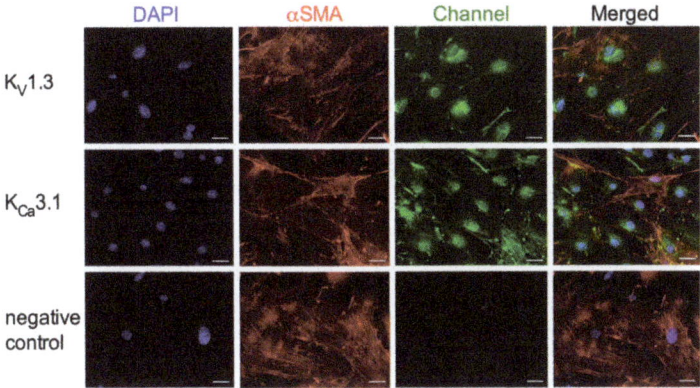

Figure 6. Immunocytological analyses on $K_V1.3$ and $K_{Ca}3.1$ localization in mouse primary artery SMCs. Cells were stained with antibodies against the $K_V1.3$ (upper panels, green) or the $K_{Ca}3.1$ channel (middle panels, green) together with an antibody against the SMC marker αSM-actin (red) and counterstained with DAPI (blue) to show the nuclei. For negative control (lower panels) the primary antibody was omitted. Scale bar 40 µm.

To analyze the effects of $K_V1.3$ and $K_{Ca}3.1$ blockade on SMC proliferation in in vitro mouse, primary artery SMCs were treated with different concentrations of PAP-1 (0.1, 1, and 5 µM) or TRAM-34 (10, 100, and 500 µM), respectively. Interestingly, in in vitro, both PAP-1 and TRAM-34 treatments interfered with SMC proliferation, as shown by the BrdU incorporation assay (Figure 7).

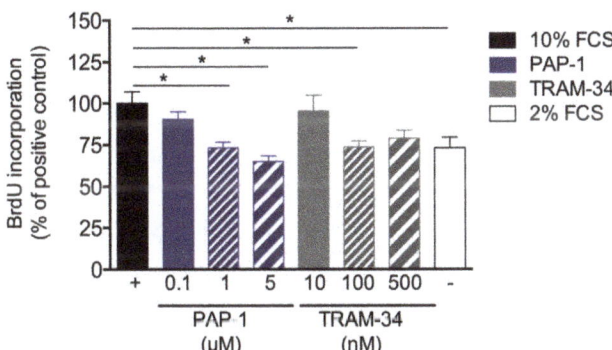

Figure 7. Proliferation assay of mouse primary artery SMCs. Mouse primary artery SMCs were cultured with 10% FCS with or without treatment of different concentrations of the $K_V1.3$ blocker PAP-1 or the $K_{Ca}3.1$ blocker TRAM-34. Cell proliferation was investigated by means of BrdU incorporation. Values are expressed as percentages of the positive control (+), i.e., mouse primary artery SMCs stimulated with 10% FCS. For the negative control (−), mouse primary artery SMCs cultured with 2% FCS. Data are means ± SEM, $n > 6$ per group. * $p < 0.05$ from one-way ANOVA with Bonferroni's multiple comparison test.

3.4. $K_V1.3$ Blockade Repressed the Expression of FGFR-1, PDGFR-ß, and Egr1 in Mouse Primary Artery SMCs In Vitro and During Arteriogenesis In Vivo

Receptor tyrosine kinases such as FGFR-1 and PDGFR-ß are well described for their relevance in SMC proliferation. Our qRT-PCR results on the expression level of *Fgfr1* and *Pdgfrb* provided evidence that treatment of mouse primary artery SMCs with the $K_V1.3$ channel blocker PAP-1 significantly interfered with the expression of both growth factor receptors, whereas the treatment with the $K_{Ca}3.1$

channel blocker TRAM-34 showed no significant influence (Figure 8a). Moreover, in collateral arteries 12 h after induction of arteriogenesis, a significant downregulation was evident for both *Fgfr1* and *Pdgfrb* when $K_V1.3$ was blocked with PAP-1, while treatment with the $K_{Ca}3.1$ blocker TRAM-34 showed no significant effect (Figure 8b). To further investigate the relevance of the $K_V1.3$ potassium channel for SMC proliferation in vitro and during arteriogenesis in vivo, qRT-PCR analyses were performed on the cell cycle regulator Egr1. Our results evidenced that blocking $K_V1.3$ with PAP-1 in vitro, as well during arteriogenesis in vivo, significantly interfered with the mRNA expression of *Egr1* (Figure 8c,d).

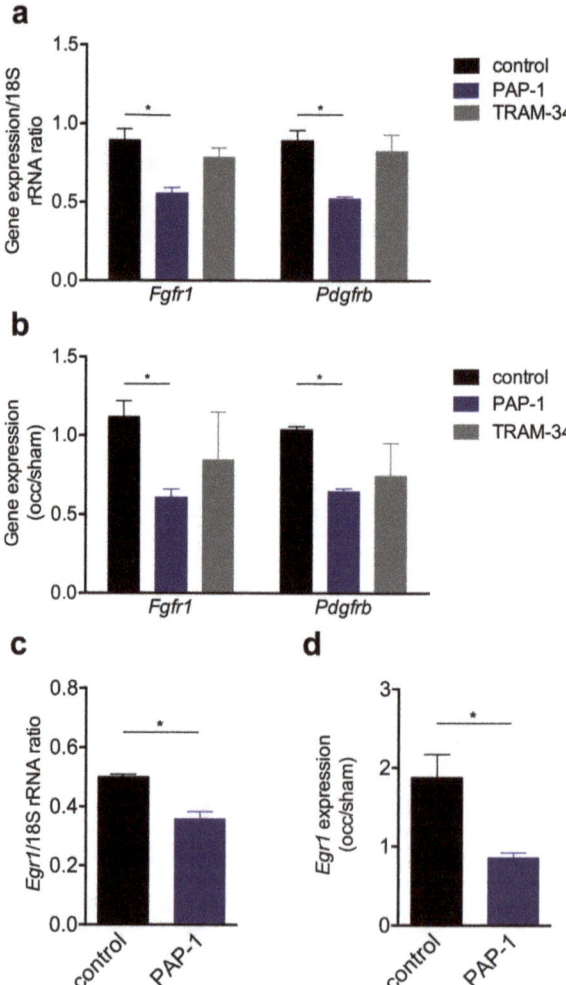

Figure 8. The qRT-PCR results of the expression levels of *Fgfr1*, *Pdgfrb*, and *Egr1* in vitro and during arteriogenesis in vivo. (**a,c**) Bar graphs represent the mRNA expression levels of Fgfr1, Pdgfrb, or Egr1 in vitro and (**b,d**) in vivo. In vitro mouse primary artery SMCs were cultured without (control) or with 1 µM PAP-1 or 100 nM TRAM-34, respectively. In vivo the expression level of *Fgfr1*, *Pdgfrb*, and *Egr1* were investigated 12 h after induction of arteriogenesis in collateral arteries and are expressed as occlusion (occ) to sham ratio. All qRT-PCR results were normalized to the expression level of the corresponding 18S rRNA. Data are means ± SEM, n = 3 per group. * $p < 0.05$ from one-way ANOVA with Bonferroni's multiple comparison test.

4. Discussion

The process of arteriogenesis mainly involves the proliferation of ECs and SMCs. Whereas the mechanisms relevant for EC proliferation are relatively well defined, little is known about the mechanism involved in SMC proliferation. Using a murine hindlimb model of arteriogenesis, here, we report that the voltage-gated potassium channel $K_V1.3$, but not the Ca^{2+}-gated potassium channel $K_{Ca}3.1$, is of importance for SMC proliferation in collateral arteries. Selectively blocking $K_V1.3$ with PAP-1 resulted in a reduced perfusion recovery (Figure 4), which was associated with reduced numbers of proliferating SMCs (Figure 5). More in-depth in vivo and in vitro studies demonstrated a role for $K_V1.3$ in the expression of the tyrosine kinase receptors *Fgfr1* and *Pdgfrb*, as well as of the transcriptional regulator *Egr1* (Figure 8), all relevant for proper SMC proliferation in arteriogenesis.

Elevated shear stress is the driving force for arteriogenesis [2,3]. This mechanical stress can be sensed by ECs but not by SMCs. The mechanisms how this mechanical force is translated into biochemical signals resulting in endothelial proliferation have been described in [4]. However, little is known about the mechanisms triggering SMC proliferation in arteriogenesis. To address this point, we decided to study the relevance of the potassium channels $K_V1.3$ and $K_{Ca}3.1$, which have been shown to play a role in smooth muscle proliferation in other experimental settings and processes [20,21]. Our immunohistological investigations demonstrated that both $K_V1.3$ and $K_{Ca}3.1$ are mainly localized in SMCs of collateral arteries of murine hindlimbs (Figures 2 and 3).

To investigate the relevance of $K_V1.3$ for arteriogenesis, we performed blocking studies employing PAP-1, described as a selective $K_V1.3$ blocker [31]. The laser Doppler perfusion measurements evidenced a significant reduction in perfusion recovery when mice were treated with PAP-1 (Figure 4). Moreover, our histological results showed a significant reduction of proliferating SMCs but not ECs in growing collateral arteries (Figure 5).

Proliferating SMCs are characterized by a reduced expression of the contractile marker αSM-actin a [34], which has been demonstrated by our group for the process of arteriogenesis [9] and confirmed in the present study (Figure 5). Blocking $K_V1.3$ during collateral artery growth, however, interfered with the downregulation of αSM-actin (Figure 5). To investigate whether the reduced proliferation rate of SMCs in arteriogenesis was directly related to $K_V1.3$ blockade in SMCs, but not in other cells such as leukocytes, which also play an important role in arteriogenesis [18,35,36], we analyzed the proliferative behavior of primary murine SMCs under $K_V1.3$ blockade in vitro. Our results revealed a correlation between the concentration of PAP-1 in culture medium and the inhibition of mouse primary artery SMC proliferation (Figure 7), attributing $K_V1.3$ with a role in SMC proliferation. Together, our data suggest a direct correlation between the blockade of the potassium channel $K_V1.3$ and the inhibition of SMC proliferation during the process of arteriogenesis. Our data are in line with results from Cidad et al., who demonstrated an inhibition of femoral artery SMC proliferation when $K_V1.3$ was blocked pharmacologically with PAP-1 or with Margatoxin or when $K_V1.3$ was knocked down by siRNA treatment [22].

Previous results have shown that SMC proliferation in arteriogenesis is dependent on the activation of FGFR-1. Already in 2003, we had demonstrated that FGFR-1, which was expressed in SMCs but not in ECs, was upregulated in the early phase of arteriogenesis, i.e., within the first 24 h after induction of collateral artery growth by femoral artery ligation, and that blocking this tyrosine kinase receptor with polyanetholsulfonic acid (PAS) interfered with the process of arteriogenesis [10]. A parallel study showed that a combined treatment of rodents with the cognate ligand of FGFR-1, namely FGF-2, and the cognate ligand of PDGFR-β, namely PDGF-BB, significantly promoted the process of arteriogenesis [6]. In that study, an upregulation of PDGF receptors by FGF-2 was suggested and was later confirmed by Zhang et al. [37]. PDGF-BB has been described as a potent inducer of the synthetic phenotype of a SMC and has been shown to act synergistically with FGF-2 to induce the downregulation of contractile genes such as αSM-actin during vascular SMC proliferation [38]. In particular, it has been demonstrated that PDGF-BB activates FGFR-1 via engaging PDGFR-β, thereby mediating the downregulation of αSM-actin and smooth muscle 22α (SM22-α) expression. The PDGFR-β/PDGF-BB and FGFR-1/FGF-2 signaling pathways have also been effectively described to promote the upregulation of the transcription factor Egr1 [8], the expression of which was regulated in opposition to that of contractile genes, and which we have found to mediate cell cycle progression in arteriogenesis [9]. In the present study, we found that treatment of mice with the $K_V1.3$ blocker PAP-1 during the process of arteriogenesis resulted in a downregulation of *Fgfr1*, *Pdgfrb*, and *Egr1* (Figure 8), whereas αSM-actin was upregulated (Figure 5). Accordingly, all genes are regulated in the opposite way as described for proper arteriogenesis [9,10]. Although one could speculate that the impaired expression of *Fgfr1* and/or *Pdgfrb* could be responsible for the impaired expression of their downstream genes, i.e., *Egr1* and αSM-actin, this is somehow unlikely as all genes show a hampered expression at the same point of time. Therefore, we wondered if another factor could be involved in $K_V1.3$ mediated gene expression. Interestingly, in silico analyses (data not shown) revealed several binding sites for the transcription factor specificity protein 1 (Sp1) in the promoter regions of *Fgfr1*, *Pdgfrb*, and *Egr1*. However, whether Sp1 is indeed involved in potassium channel $K_V1.3$ mediated gene expression remains to be determined by further studies. Our data indicate that $K_V1.3$ plays a major role in SMC proliferation, especially in the process of arteriogenesis, by influencing signal transduction cascades associated with the expression of the growth factor receptors *Fgfr1* and *Pdgfrb* and their downstream genes being involved in phenotype switch and cell cycle regulation.

In contrast to our findings regarding PAP-1 administration, treatment of mice with the $K_{Ca}3.1$ selective blocker TRAM-34 did not influence vascular SMC proliferation or differential gene expression in growing collaterals in vivo (Figures 5 and 8). The laser Doppler perfusion measurements, however, evidenced a reduced perfusion recovery after femoral artery ligation (Figure 4). Interestingly, $K_{Ca}3.1$ has been shown to be upregulated by fluid shear stress [39], the driving force for arteriogenesis [2,3]. Moreover, it has been demonstrated by blocking studies employing TRAM-34 in vivo, that $K_{Ca}3.1$ plays a role in EC proliferation during angiogenesis (Grigic, Eichler 2005) and in SMC proliferation, e.g., during atherogenesis [27]. Our study, however, revealed that $K_{Ca}3.1$ is not involved in EC or in SMC proliferation in collateral artery growth (Figure 5). Of course, one could argue that the dose of TRAM-34 used in the present study was not high enough to block $K_{Ca}3.1$ in vivo, but identical dosages were shown to be effective in hampering vascular cell proliferation in a model of intima hyperplasia [25] and atherosclerotic lesions in mice [27]. Together, these data indicate that the mechanisms of SMC proliferation in the different pathophysiological situations are diverging. Indeed, it has been shown by Bi et al. in vitro [20] that $K_{Ca}3.1$ mediated SMC proliferation blocked by TRAM-34 was not associated with any change in expression of *Pdgfrb*, supporting the data of the present investigations (Figure 8). As our laser Doppler perfusion measurements revealed a reduced perfusion recovery upon femoral artery ligation (Figure 4), which was not associated with a reduced collateral artery cell proliferation (Figure 5), we hypothesize that $K_{Ca}3.1$ could overtake a function in EDHF-mediated collateral vasodilation, a well described function of this potassium channel [29,40]. However, further studies are necessary to prove this hypothesis. A similar effect on reduced perfusion recovery upon femoral artery ligation has been described for nitric oxide synthase 3 (NOS3)-deficient mice, also attributing nitric oxide a role in vasodilation during arteriogenesis [41]. In terms of $K_{Ca}3.1$, it could be interesting to know that the Ca^{2+}-channel transient receptor potential cation channel, subfamily V, member 4 (TRPV4) has previously been shown to play a role in arteriogenesis by promoting vascular cell proliferation [42]. TRPV4 is described as shear stress sensitive channel which plays an important role in the regulation of vascular tone by modulating intracellular Ca^{2+} levels [43]. However, TRPV4 has also been shown to promote collateral artery growth in several animal models [42,44,45]. It has been suggested that upon activation of this receptor, a first increase in intracellular Ca^{2+} levels could result in EDHF-mediated vasodilation, whilst a prolonged raise could activate transcription factors causing vascular cell proliferation [42,45]. It is tempting to speculate that $K_{Ca}3.1$ is involved in this EDHF mediated vasodilation, but further studies are necessary to investigate this assumption.

5. Conclusions

From our investigations, we conclude that the potassium channel $K_V 1.3$, but not $K_{Ca} 3.1$, contributes to SMC proliferation in arteriogenesis by controlling the expression of growth factor receptors, as well as their downstream genes relevant for phenotype switch and cell cycle progression.

Author Contributions: M.L. wrote and prepared the manuscript; A.C.M., K.K., H.I.-A., and S.M. the experiments; E.D. conducted the scientific direction and wrote the manuscript. All authors have read and agreed to the published version of the manuscript.

Funding: This research received no external funding.

Acknowledgments: We thank Anna Kluever for proofreading the manuscript.

Conflicts of Interest: The authors declare no conflict of interest.

References

1. Faber, J.E.; Chilian, W.M.; Deindl, E.; van Royen, N.; Simons, M. A brief etymology of the collateral circulation. *Arter. Thromb. Vasc. Biol.* **2014**, *34*, 1854–1859. [CrossRef]
2. Lasch, M.; Nekolla, K.; Klemm, A.H.; Buchheim, J.I.; Pohl, U.; Dietzel, S.; Deindl, E. Estimating hemodynamic shear stress in murine peripheral collateral arteries by two-photon line scanning. *Mol. Cell Biochem.* **2019**, *453*, 41–51. [CrossRef]
3. Pipp, F.; Boehm, S.; Cai, W.J.; Adili, F.; Ziegler, B.; Karanovic, G.; Ritter, R.; Balzer, J.; Scheler, C.; Schaper, W.; et al. Elevated fluid shear stress enhances postocclusive collateral artery growth and gene expression in the pig hind limb. *Arter. Thromb. Vasc. Biol.* **2004**, *24*, 1664–1668. [CrossRef]
4. Lasch, M.; Kleinert, E.C.; Meister, S.; Kumaraswami, K.; Buchheim, J.I.; Grantzow, T.; Lautz, T.; Salpisti, S.; Fischer, S.; Troidl, K.; et al. Extracellular RNA released due to shear stress controls natural bypass growth by mediating mechanotransduction in mice. *Blood* **2019**, *134*, 1469–1479. [CrossRef]
5. Tzima, E.; Irani-Tehrani, M.; Kiosses, W.B.; Dejana, E.; Schultz, D.A.; Engelhardt, B.; Cao, G.; DeLisser, H.; Schwartz, M.A. A mechanosensory complex that mediates the endothelial cell response to fluid shear stress. *Nature* **2005**, *437*, 426–431. [CrossRef] [PubMed]
6. Cao, R.; Bråkenhielm, E.; Pawliuk, R.; Wariaro, D.; Post, M.J.; Wahlberg, E.; Leboulch, P.; Cao, Y. Angiogenic synergism, vascular stability and improvement of hind-limb ischemia by a combination of PDGF-BB and FGF-2. *Nat. Med.* **2003**, *9*, 604–613. [CrossRef] [PubMed]
7. De Paula, E.V.; Flores-Nascimento, M.C.; Arruda, V.R.; Garcia, R.A.; Ramos, C.D.; Guillaumon, A.T.; Annichino-Bizzacchi, J.M. Dual gene transfer of fibroblast growth factor-2 and platelet derived growth factor-BB using plasmid deoxyribonucleic acid promotes effective angiogenesis and arteriogenesis in a rodent model of hindlimb ischemia. *Transl. Res.* **2009**, *153*, 232–239. [CrossRef] [PubMed]
8. Vogel, S.; Kubin, T.; Brancik, M.; Deindl, E.; von der Ahe, D.; Zimmermann, R. Signal transduction pathways in smooth muscle cells. In *Arteriogenesis*; Schaper, W., Schaper, J., Eds., Kluwer Academic Publishers: Boston, MA, USA; Dordrecht, The Netherlands; London, UK, 2004.
9. Pagel, J.I.; Ziegelhoeffer, T.; Heil, M.; Fischer, S.; Fernandez, B.; Schaper, W.; Preissner, K.T.; Deindl, E. Role of early growth response 1 in arteriogenesis: Impact on vascular cell proliferation and leukocyte recruitment in vivo. *Thromb. Haemost.* **2012**, *107*, 562–574. [CrossRef]
10. Deindl, E.; Hoefer, I.E.; Fernandez, B.; Barancik, M.; Heil, M.; Strniskova, M.; Schaper, W. Involvement of the fibroblast growth factor system in adaptive and chemokine-induced arteriogenesis. *Circ. Res.* **2003**, *92*, 561–568. [CrossRef]
11. Lederman, R.J.; Mendelsohn, F.O.; Anderson, R.D.; Saucedo, J.F.; Tenaglia, A.N.; Hermiller, J.B.; Hillegass, W.B.; Rocha-Singh, K.; Moon, T.E.; Whitehouse, M.J.; et al. Therapeutic angiogenesis with recombinant fibroblast growth factor-2 for intermittent claudication (the TRAFFIC study): A randomised trial. *Lancet* **2002**, *359*, 2053–2058.

12. Simons, M.; Annex, B.H.; Laham, R.J.; Kleiman, N.; Henry, T.; Dauerman, H.; Udelson, J.E.; Gervino, E.V.; Pike, M.; Whitehouse, M.J.; et al. Pharmacological treatment of coronary artery disease with recombinant fibroblast growth factor-2: Double-blind, randomized, controlled clinical trial. *Circulation* **2002**, *105*, 788–793.
13. Scholz, D.; Ito, W.; Fleming, I.; Deindl, E.; Sauer, A.; Wiesnet, M.; Busse, R.; Schaper, J.; Schaper, W. Ultrastructure and molecular histology of rabbit hindlimb collateral artery growth (arteriogenesis). *Virchows Arch.* **2000**, *436*, 257–270. [CrossRef]
14. Wolf, C.; Cai, J.W.; Vosschulte, R.; Koltai, S.; Mousavipour, D.; Scholz, D.; Afsah-Hedjri, A.; Schaper, W.; Schaper, J. Vascular remodeling and altered protein expression during growth of coronary collateral arteries. *J. Mol. Cell Cardiol.* **1998**, *30*, 2291–2305. [CrossRef] [PubMed]
15. Pagel, J.I.; Deindl, E. Early growth response 1–a transcription factor in the crossfire of signal transduction cascades. *Indian. J. Biochem. Biophys.* **2011**, *48*, 226–235. [PubMed]
16. Wang, D.Z.; Olson, E.N. Control of smooth muscle development by the myocardin family of transcriptional coactivators. *Curr. Opin. Genet. Dev.* **2004**, *14*, 558–566. [CrossRef] [PubMed]
17. Wang, Z.; Wang, D.Z.; Hockemeyer, D.; McAnally, J.; Nordheim, A.; Olson, E.N. Myocardin and ternary complex factors compete for SRF to control smooth muscle gene expression. *Nature* **2004**, *428*, 185–189. [CrossRef]
18. Pérez-García, M.T.; Cidad, P.; López-López, J.R. The secret life of ion channels: Kv1.3 potassium channels and proliferation. *Am. J. Physio.l Cell Physiol.* **2018**, *314*, C27–C42. [CrossRef]
19. Urrego, D.; Tomczak, A.P.; Zahed, F.; Stühmer, W.; Pardo, L.A. Potassium channels in cell cycle and cell proliferation. *Philos Trans. R Soc. Lond. B Biol. Sci.* **2014**, *369*, 20130094. [CrossRef]
20. Bi, D.; Toyama, K.; Lemaitre, V.; Takai, J.; Fan, F.; Jenkins, D.P.; Wulff, H.; Gutterman, D.D.; Park, F.; Miura, H. The intermediate conductance calcium-activated potassium channel KCa3.1 regulates vascular smooth muscle cell proliferation via controlling calcium-dependent signaling. *J. Biol. Chem.* **2013**, *288*, 15843–15853. [CrossRef]
21. Cidad, P.; Miguel-Velado, E.; Ruiz-McDavitt, C.; Alonso, E.; Jiménez-Pérez, L.; Asuaje, A.; Carmona, Y.; García-Arribas, D.; López, J.; Marroquín, Y.; et al. Kv1.3 channels modulate human vascular smooth muscle cells proliferation independently of mTOR signaling pathway. *Pflug. Arch.* **2015**, *467*, 1711–1722. [CrossRef]
22. Cidad, P.; Moreno-Domínguez, A.; Roqué, M.; Novensá, L.; Barquín, L.; Heras, M.; Pérez-García, M.T.; López-López, J.R. Characterization of ion channels involved in the proliferative response of femoral artery smooth muscle cells. *Arter. Thromb. Vasc. Biol.* **2010**, *30*, 1203–1211. [CrossRef]
23. Cheong, A.; Li, J.; Sukumar, P.; Kumar, B.; Zeng, F.; Riches, K.; Munsch, C.; Wood, I.C.; Porter, K.E.; Beech, D.J. Potent suppression of vascular smooth muscle cell migration and human neointimal hyperplasia by KV1.3 channel blockers. *Cardiovasc. Res.* **2011**, *89*, 282–289. [CrossRef]
24. Cidad, P.; Novensa, L.; Garabito, M.; Batlle, M.; Dantas, A.P.; Heras, M.; Lopez-Lopez, J.R.; Perez-Garcia, M.T.; Roque, M. K+ channels expression in hypertension after arterial injury, and effect of selective Kv1.3 blockade with PAP-1 on intimal hyperplasia formation. *Cardiovasc. Drugs Ther.* **2014**, *28*, 501–511. [CrossRef] [PubMed]
25. Kohler, R.; Wulff, H.; Eichler, I.; Kneifel, M.; Neumann, D.; Knorr, A.; Grgic, I.; Kampfe, D.; Si, H.; Wibawa, J.; et al. Blockade of the intermediate-conductance calcium-activated potassium channel as a new therapeutic strategy for restenosis. *Circulation* **2003**, *108*, 1119–1125. [CrossRef] [PubMed]
26. Tharp, D.L.; Wamhoff, B.R.; Wulff, H.; Raman, G.; Cheong, A.; Bowles, D.K. Local delivery of the KCa3.1 blocker, TRAM-34, prevents acute angioplasty-induced coronary smooth muscle phenotypic modulation and limits stenosis. *Arter. Thromb. Vasc. Biol.* **2008**, *28*, 1084–1089. [CrossRef]
27. Toyama, K.; Wulff, H.; Chandy, K.G.; Azam, P.; Raman, G.; Saito, T.; Fujiwara, Y.; Mattson, D.L.; Das, S.; Melvin, J.E.; et al. The intermediate-conductance calcium-activated potassium channel KCa3.1 contributes to atherogenesis in mice and humans. *J. Clin. Investig.* **2008**, *118*, 3025–3037. [CrossRef] [PubMed]
28. Wulff, H.; Miller, M.J.; Hansel, W.; Grissmer, S.; Cahalan, M.D.; Chandy, K.G. Design of a potent and selective inhibitor of the intermediate-conductance Ca2+-activated K+ channel, IKCa1: A potential immunosuppressant. *Proc. Natl. Acad. Sci. USA* **2000**, *97*, 8151–8156. [CrossRef] [PubMed]
29. Si, H.; Heyken, W.T.; Wolfle, S.E.; Tysiac, M.; Schubert, R.; Grgic, I.; Vilianovich, L.; Giebing, G.; Maier, T.; Gross, V.; et al. Impaired endothelium-derived hyperpolarizing factor-mediated dilations and increased blood pressure in mice deficient of the intermediate-conductance Ca2+-activated K+ channel. *Circ. Res.* **2006**, *99*, 537–544. [CrossRef]

30. Limbourg, A.; Korff, T.; Napp, L.C.; Schaper, W.; Drexler, H.; Limbourg, F.P. Evaluation of postnatal arteriogenesis and angiogenesis in a mouse model of hind-limb ischemia. *Nat. Protoc.* **2009**, *4*, 1737–1746. [CrossRef]
31. Schmitz, A.; Sankaranarayanan, A.; Azam, P.; Schmidt-Lassen, K.; Homerick, D.; Hansel, W.; Wulff, H. Design of PAP-1, a selective small molecule Kv1.3 blocker, for the suppression of effector memory T cells in autoimmune diseases. *Mol. Pharmacol.* **2005**, *68*, 1254–1270. [CrossRef]
32. Lasch, M.; Caballero-Martinez, A.; Troidl, K.; Schloegl, I.; Lautz, T.; Deindl, E. Arginase inhibition attenuates arteriogenesis and interferes with M2 macrophage accumulation. *Lab. Investig.* **2016**, *96*, 830–838. [CrossRef]
33. Pfaffl, M.W. A new mathematical model for relative quantification in real-time RT-PCR. *Nucleic Acids Res.* **2001**, *29*, e45. [CrossRef]
34. Mack, C.P. Signaling mechanisms that regulate smooth muscle cell differentiation. *Arterioscler. Thromb. Vasc. Biol.* **2011**, *31*, 1495–1505. [CrossRef] [PubMed]
35. Simons, K.H.; Aref, Z.; Peters, H.A.B.; Welten, S.P.; Nossent, A.Y.; Jukema, J.W.; Hamming, J.F.; Arens, R.; de Vries, M.R.; Quax, P.H.A. The role of CD27-CD70-mediated T cell co-stimulation in vasculogenesis, arteriogenesis and angiogenesis. *Int. J. Cardiol.* **2018**, *260*, 184–190. [CrossRef] [PubMed]
36. Van Weel, V.; Toes, R.E.; Seghers, L.; Deckers, M.M.; de Vries, M.R.; Eilers, P.; Sipkens, J.; Schepers, A.; Eefting, D.; van Hinsbergh, V.W.; et al. Natural killer cells and CD4+ T-cells modulate collateral artery development. *Arter. Thromb. Vasc. Biol.* **2007**, *27*, 2310–2318. [CrossRef] [PubMed]
37. Zhang, J.; Cao, R.; Zhang, Y.; Jia, T.; Cao, Y.; Wahlberg, E. Differential roles of PDGFR-alpha and PDGFR-beta in angiogenesis and vessel stability. *FASEB J.* **2009**, *23*, 153–163. [CrossRef] [PubMed]
38. Chen, P.Y.; Simons, M.; Friesel, R. FRS2 via fibroblast growth factor receptor 1 is required for platelet-derived growth factor receptor beta-mediated regulation of vascular smooth muscle marker gene expression. *J. Biol. Chem.* **2009**, *284*, 15980–15992. [CrossRef] [PubMed]
39. Brakemeier, S.; Kersten, A.; Eichler, I.; Grgic, I.; Zakrzewicz, A.; Hopp, H.; Kohler, R.; Hoyer, J. Shear stress-induced up-regulation of the intermediate-conductance Ca(2+)-activated K(+) channel in human endothelium. *Cardiovasc. Res.* **2003**, *60*, 488–496. [CrossRef]
40. Eichler, I.; Wibawa, J.; Grgic, I.; Knorr, A.; Brakemeier, S.; Pries, A.R.; Hoyer, J.; Kohler, R. Selective blockade of endothelial Ca2+-activated small- and intermediate-conductance K+-channels suppresses EDHF-mediated vasodilation. *Br. J. Pharmacol.* **2003**, *138*, 594–601. [CrossRef]
41. Mees, B.; Wagner, S.; Ninci, E.; Tribulova, S.; Martin, S.; van Haperen, R.; Kostin, S.; Heil, M.; de Crom, R.; Schaper, W. Endothelial nitric oxide synthase activity is essential for vasodilation during blood flow recovery but not for arteriogenesis. *Arter. Thromb. Vasc. Biol.* **2007**, *27*, 1926–1933. [CrossRef]
42. Troidl, C.; Troidl, K.; Schierling, W.; Cai, W.-J.; Nef, H.; Möllmann, H.; Kostin, S.; Schimanski, S.; Hammer, L.; Elsässer, A.; et al. Trpv4 induces collateral vessel growth during regeneration of the arterial circulation. *J. Cell Mol. Med.* **2009**, *13*, 2613–2621. [CrossRef]
43. Nilius, B.; Droogmans, G.; Wondergem, R. Transient receptor potential channels in endothelium: Solving the calcium entry puzzle? *Endothelium* **2003**, *10*, 5–15. [CrossRef]
44. Schierling, W.; Troidl, K.; Apfelbeck, H.; Troidl, C.; Kasprzak, P.M.; Schaper, W.; Schmitz-Rixen, T. Cerebral arteriogenesis is enhanced by pharmacological as well as fluid-shear-stress activation of the Trpv4 calcium channel. *Eur. J. Vasc. Endovasc. Surg.* **2011**, *41*, 589–596. [CrossRef] [PubMed]
45. Troidl, C.; Nef, H.; Voss, S.; Schilp, A.; Kostin, S.; Troidl, K.; Szardien, S.; Rolf, A.; Schmitz-Rixen, T.; Schaper, W.; et al. Calcium-dependent signalling is essential during collateral growth in the pig hind limb-ischemia model. *J. Mol. Cell. Cardiol.* **2010**, *49*, 142–151. [CrossRef] [PubMed]

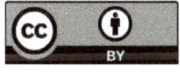

© 2020 by the authors. Licensee MDPI, Basel, Switzerland. This article is an open access article distributed under the terms and conditions of the Creative Commons Attribution (CC BY) license (http://creativecommons.org/licenses/by/4.0/).

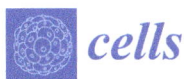

Article

VEGF-A-Cleavage by FSAP and Inhibition of Neo-Vascularization

Özgür Uslu [1], Joerg Herold [2] and Sandip M. Kanse [3],*

[1] Institute for Biochemistry, Justus-Liebig-University Giessen, 35392 Giessen, Germany; Oezguer1975@gmx.de
[2] Department of Angiology, Clinic for Vascular Medicine, Klinikum Darmstadt, 64283 Darmstadt, Germany; joerg_herold@hotmail.com
[3] Institute for Basic Medical Sciences, University of Oslo, Sognvannsveien 9, 0372 Oslo, Norway
* Correspondence: Sandip.kanse@medisin.uio.no

Received: 16 September 2019; Accepted: 4 November 2019; Published: 6 November 2019

Abstract: Alternative splicing leads to the secretion of multiple forms of vascular endothelial growth factor-A (VEGF-A) that differ in their activity profiles with respect to neovascularization. FSAP (factor VII activating protease) is the zymogen form of a plasma protease that is activated (FSAPa) upon tissue injury via the release of histones. The purpose of the study was to determine if FSAPa regulates VEGF-A activity in vitro and in vivo. FSAP bound to $VEGF_{165}$, but not $VEGF_{121}$, and $VEGF_{165}$ was cleaved in its neuropilin/proteoglycan binding domain. $VEGF_{165}$ cleavage did not alter its binding to VEGF receptors but diminished its binding to neuropilin. The stimulatory effects of $VEGF_{165}$ on endothelial cell proliferation, migration, and signal transduction were not altered by FSAP. Similarly, proliferation of VEGF receptor-expressing BAF3 cells, in response to $VEGF_{165}$, was not modulated by FSAP. In the mouse matrigel model of angiogenesis, FSAP decreased the ability of $VEGF_{165}$, basic fibroblast growth factor (bFGF), and their combination, to induce neovascularization. Lack of endogenous FSAP in mice did not influence neovascularization. Thus, FSAP inhibited $VEGF_{165}$-mediated angiogenesis in the matrigel model in vivo, where VEGF's interaction with the matrix and its diffusion are important.

Keywords: factor VII activating protease; HABP2; VEGF; matrigel; neo-vascularization; hind limb ischemia

---

1. Introduction

FSAP (factor VII activating protease) is a serine protease that circulates in plasma as an inactive zymogen. It belongs to the family of proteases that also includes the urokinase-plasminogen activator (uPA), tissue-PA (tPA), as well as hepatocyte growth factor activator (HGFA). Although a number of charged molecules can activate FSAP into the active protease (FSAPa), histones are the only endogenous molecules identified so far that can activate the zymogen form into FSAPa in plasma and in vivo [1]. In situations such as tissue injury [2], apoptosis, or necrosis [3], as well as when neutrophils undergo NETosis [4], the DNase activity in blood [5] is likely to release histones. FSAPa in turn can cleave and degrade histones and decrease their toxicity towards cells [3,4]. A single nucleotide polymorphism (SNP) in the FSAP gene, Marburg I (MI, G534E) is associated with a weak proteolytic activity [6] and an increased risk of carotid stenosis [7], stroke [8], venous thrombosis [9,10], liver fibrosis [11], and thyroid cancer [12]. The relationship to venous thrombosis [13] and thyroid cancer [14] was not replicated in a number of subsequent studies.

This relationship between the loss of FSAP activity and diseases is also replicated in FSAP-deficient ($Habp2^{-/-}$) mice. $Habp2^{-/-}$ mice show no explicit characteristics when maintained under standard pathogen-free laboratory conditions and do not exhibit any developmental abnormalities. These mice have been studied in two different models of vascular remodeling. In the wire-induced injury model of neointima formation, *Habp2*$^{-/-}$ mice formed a bigger neointima than wildtype (WT mice) [15]. In the model of hind limb ischemia, arteriogenesis in the adductor muscle was enhanced in *Habp2*$^{-/-}$ mice, whereas neovascularization was unchanged in the gastrocnemius muscle [16]. Thus, the lack of *Habp2* gene in mice promotes a more exacerbated repair response that is related to enhanced inflammation and increased activity of the pericellular proteolysis system [15,16].

The effects of FSAP in relation to human diseases and mouse models is likely to be related to proteolysis of different substrates. Although a number of substrates for FSAP have been identified [17] we will focus here only on pathways that are linked to vascular remodeling. Growth factors are cleaved by FSAP, which in some cases leads to a loss of activity, such as platelet derived growth factor-BB (PDGF-BB) [18]. PDGF-BB cleavage leads to an inhibition of vascular smooth muscle cells (VSMC) migration and proliferation, as well as neointima formation. FSAP inhibits basic fibroblast growth factor (bFGF)-mediated endothelial cell proliferation by binding to and/or slowly degrading the growth factor [19] and can also activate bFGF by releasing it from the matrix [20]. Activation of bone morphogenetic protein (BMP)-2 and the conversion of pro-BMP-2 into the active form of cytokine is also a function of FSAP that leads to differentiation of cells [21]. FSAP also cleaves protease activated receptors (PARs)-1 and -3 and influences vascular permeability in combination with hyaluronic fragments of different molecular weights [22]. PAR-1 was identified as a receptor on astrocytes and neurons that mediate the anti-apoptotic effects of FSAP in the context of stroke [23]. Stimulation of VSMC and endothelial cells by FSAP leads to an increased expression of proinflammatory genes in both cells types. Whereas the effect of FSAP could be clearly ascribed to PAR-1 on VSMC, this was clearly not the case for endothelial cells.

Vascular endothelial growth factor (VEGF) is a key factor for determining endothelial lineage, endothelial cell proliferation and migration, as well as recruitment of pericytes and vessel assembly [24]. It belongs to the cysteine knot family of growth factors that include the four genes of the PDGF family as well as placental growth factor (PLGF). Of the four genes encoding for VEGF, denoted A, B, C, and D, VEGF-A is considered to be the most important for hypoxia-driven angiogenesis and is secreted in multiple forms, such as $VEGF_{121}$, $VEGF_{165}$, and $VEGF_{189}$, by alternative splicing [25]. These isoforms have a common N-terminal region for receptor binding, whereas the C-terminal part that mediates binding to co-receptors such as neuropilin and cell- and matrix-associated proteoglycans (ECM) [26] is progressively longer. This C-terminal region has a cluster of negatively charged amino acids and has cleavage sites for uPA, plasmin, and matrix metalloproteinases [27], which regulate VEGF's association with the matrix and co-receptors and results in a different pattern of neovascularization.

With the knowledge that FSAP can cleave proteins at clusters of basic amino acids [17] and that it cleaves PDGF-BB [18], we hypothesized that the homologous protein VEGF-A is also cleaved, and its activity regulated by FSAP. We performed binding and cleavage studies with purified proteins to show that FSAP can indeed cleave long forms of VEGF in their heparin/neuropilin-binding domain and that, as expected, this disturbs their binding properties. However, no modulation of $VEGF_{165}$ activity in vitro on cellular functions was observed. An inhibiting effect of FSAP in the in vivo matrigel model of neovascularization model was observed, which supports the notion that this effect of FSAP may operate in vivo where matrix association, sequestration, and release of VEGF are decisive.

2. Material and Methods

FSAP preparations: The isolation of wild type-FSAP as well as the MI-SNP (G534E isoform) from human plasma, along with the preparation of enzymatically inactivated Phe-Pro-Arg-chloromethylketone (PPACK)-FSAP has been described before [18,28]. The buffer for storage of FSAP was 0.2 M arginine, 0.2 M lysine, 5 mM citrate, pH 4.5, and was also used at the appropriate dilution to exclude any influence of the vehicle. Because of the rapid auto-activation of the zymogen form of FSAP into FSAPa, under the experimental conditions used in this study, the term FSAP is synonymous for FSAPa.

Specific cleavage of VEGF isoforms: VEGF$_{165}$ or VEGF$_{121}$ (R & D Systems, Wiesbaden, Germany) (2 µg/mL) was incubated with FSAP (12 µg/mL) in Tris pH 7.4, 100 mM NaCl, 2 mM CaCl$_2$ for 1 h at 37 °C in the absence or presence of heparin (10 µg/mL) or aprotinin (15 µg/mL), and the reaction was stopped with SDS sample buffer. Western blots were performed under non-reducing and reducing conditions (β-mercaptoethanol; 10%, vol/vol) and VEGF was detected with a polyclonal goat antibody from R & D Systems. Cleaved VEGF was subjected to amino terminal sequencing using the automated Edman degradation procedure with an online phenylthiohydantoin derivative analyzer (Applied Biosystems, Darmstadt, Germany).

Binding interactions between FSAP, VEGFR2, VEGF, and neuropilin: VEGF$_{121}$ or VEGF$_{165}$ was immobilized in a Maxisorp microtiter 96-well plate (Nunc, Roskilde, Denmark) at a concentration of 1 µg/mL (50 mL) overnight at 4 °C in 50 mM NaHCO$_3$ buffer, pH 9.6. The plate was blocked with 3% (wt/vol) BSA in Tris pH 7.4, 100 mM NaCl. FSAP (0–2 µg/mL) was added to the wells with 0.3% (wt/vol) BSA for 2 h at 22 °C. After extensive washing, bound FSAP was detected with an antibody followed by peroxidase-linked secondary antibody. The binding of ligands to BSA-coated wells was used as a blank in all the experiments and was subtracted to obtain specific binding. Similarly, either neuropilin-1-Fc or VEGFR2-Fc (R & D Systems) were immobilized to study the binding of FSAP or VEGF.

Cellular assays: Human umbilical vein endothelial cells (HUVEC) were cultivated in ECBM medium (modified MCDB-151) containing 5% (vol/vol) FCS (Promocell, Heidelberg, Germany) on fibronectin-coated dishes. For regular growth of these cells, the medium was supplemented with amphotericin B (50 ng/mL), gentamicin (50 ng/mL), epidermal growth factor (0.1 ng/mL), and bFGF (1.0 ng/mL), as described by the manufacturer. Growth factors were preincubated with FSAP for 60 min at 37 °C before stimulation of serum starved cells, as described previously [18]. DNA synthesis was determined using the BrdU incorporation kit from Roche Diagnostics (Mannheim, Germany). Migration was tested in a Boyden chamber on a collagen type I coated membrane with 8 µm pores. Growth factors were preincubated with FSAP for 60 min at 37 °C before cell stimulation. Cells were incubated in medium containing 0.1% (vol/vol) FCS in the upper chamber, whereas the lower chamber received the same medium with different additives, as indicated. After an incubation period of 5 h at 37 °C, the upper side of the membrane was scraped to remove all cells. Thereafter, the membrane was fixed, stained, and the optical density of each well was measured to quantify cell migration. Cells were lysed in SDS-sample buffer and applied onto SDS-PAGE followed by western blotting and detection of phosphorylated ERK with a phospho-specific antibody with total ERK as a loading control (both from Cell Signaling Technology, Leiden, The Netherlands).

BAF3-VEGFR2 cells were obtained from Steven Stacker and Marc Achen (Ludwig Cancer Research Institute, Melbourne Branch, Australia) and BAF3-VEGFR1 cells were provided by Kari Alitalo (Ludwig Cancer Research Institute, Helsinki, Finland) and were cultured in RPMI-1640 medium containing murine interleukin (IL)-3 (Strathman Biotech, Hannover, Germany). Cell number was determined by the WST-1 assay (Roche Diagnostics).

Western blotting analysis: HUVEC were starved for 4 h in serum-free medium and then stimulated for 15 min with the appropriate agonist. Cells were pre-incubated with inhibitors for 30 min before induction with agonist. The experiments were stopped by adding SDS sample buffer containing 10 mM NaF, 1 mM orthovanadate, and 1 mM pyrophosphate, and the samples were processed for western blotting. SDS-PAGE was performed and proteins were transferred to Hybond nitrocellulose membranes (GE Healthcare, Freiberg, Germany). For analysis of western blotting, ECL prime chemiluminescence (GE Healthcare) was used. Tissue pieces were homogenized in a glass homogenizer in TBS (50 mM Tris, pH 7.4, containing 100 mM NaCl) with 1% (w/v) SDS. After centrifugation, the extracts were frozen at −80 °C until further analysis. Densitometric analysis was performed to calculate relative expression using ImageJ (NIH, Bethesda, Maryland, USA).

Matrigel model of in vivo angiogenesis: The matrigel model was performed essentially as described previously [29] and there were 7–8 mice per group. Growth factor-reduced matrigel (BD Biosciences) was supplemented with heparin (200 µg/mL), VEGF$_{165}$, and bFGF (200 ng/mL each), FSAP, MI-FSAP, or PPACK-FSAP (12 µg/mL), as well as the appropriate volume of buffer control. Without the presence of heparin, the neovascularization response is very weak in this model system. The concentration of each growth factor was halved when used in combination. Matrigel was applied subcutaneously into the right and left underside flank of 8–12 week old female C57/BL6 mice. The mice were sacrificed after 7 days and the matrigel plugs were removed, fixed with formalinaldehyde, and embedded in paraffin. Then, 7 µm serial sections were cut and mounted on slides, deparaffinized in xylene, and rehydrated through graded ethanol washes. After antigen retrieval with Tris-EDTA buffer (pH 9.0), the sections were stained with endothelial-specific lectin called bandeirea simplificifolia-1 (BS-1, FITC labelled) [30] and Cy3 labelled anti-α-SMA (α smooth muscle specific-actin) (Sigma) and DAPI. The number of red/green positive vessels counted per section from three different levels of the matrigel plugs and vascular density was expressed as number of vessels per mm^2. Percentage area of anti-α SMA, BS-1, and DAPI staining was also quantified using ImageJ. All three parameters essentially gave qualitatively very similar results, and only bona-fide vessel density results are presented here. We also localized von Willebrand factor (vWF), an alternative marker for endothelial cells (rabbit polyclonal, DAKO, Glostrup, Denmark), in some staining experiments. Both methods of endothelial cell quantification gave similar results.

Hind limb ischemia model and western blotting of VEGF-A: The model of hind limb ischemia and the resulting changes in arteriogenesis and angiogenesis have been described in detail in our earlier manuscript [16]. Western blotting with anti-VEGF-A and anti-COX IV was performed to adjust for differences in protein concentrations. Band density was measured using the image analysis system Quantity One system (Biorad, Munich, Germany). Experiments were performed in four mice per group.

Statistics and reproducibility: All biochemical and cellular experiments were performed in 3-5 independent experiments. Statistical significance was tested by using analysis of variance (ANOVA) with Bonferroni post-hoc test using the programme Graphpad Prism Biostatistics Software (Graphpad, San Diego, CA). A *p*-value < 0.05 was considered to be significant.

Study approval: All procedures involving experimental animals were approved by the local government animal care committee (GI 20/10-No. 66/2012) and complied with the Directive 2010/63/EU of the European Parliament.

3. Results

Binding and cleavage of VEGF-A by FSAP: In solid phase binding assays, FSAP bound to immobilized $VEGF_{165}$, but not to $VEGF_{121}$, in the presence of heparin (Figure 1A,B). Under non-reducing conditions, there was no change in the intensity or size of the $VEGF_{165}$ upon incubation with FSAP (Figure 1C,D); however, under reducing conditions, there was a decrease in VEGF immunoreactivity (Figure 1C,D). Cleavage was enhanced by heparin, which often functions as a co-factor for FSAP activity. Inhibition of FSAP by aprotinin reduced this cleavage. The enzymatically inactive PPACK-FSAP had no effect (Figure 1C). Cleavage of $VEGF_{165}$ was time-dependent (Figure 1D), but $VEGF_{121}$ was not cleaved at all (Supplementary Figure S1). The cleavage site was identified by amino acid sequencing and was found to be in the neuropilin/heparin-binding domain at position 124/125, which was distinct from the plasmin cleavage site at 110/111 (Figure 2). The cleavage site for plasmin and FSAP in relation to the disulphide bridges [31] is shown in Figure 2. Thus, FSAP cleaves $VEGF_{165}$ in the heparin/neuropilin-binding region.

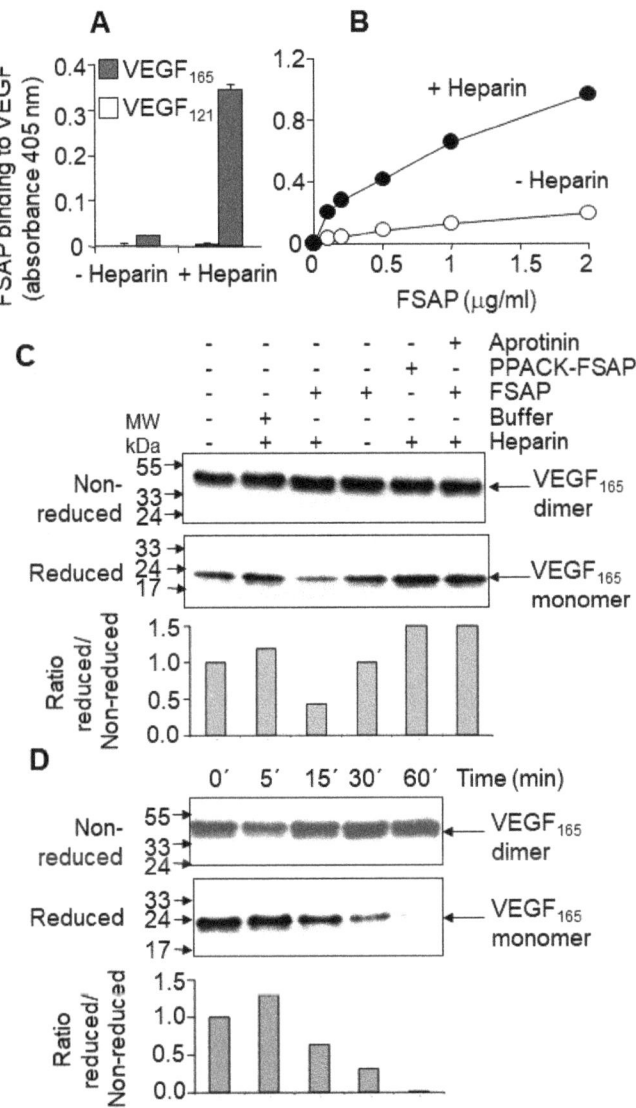

Figure 1. Binding of FSAP (factor VII activating protease) to VEGF (vascular endothelial growth factor) and its specific proteolytic cleavage: (**A**) $VEGF_{121}$ (open bars) or $VEGF_{165}$ (grey bars) was immobilized, and the binding of FSAP, in the absence or presence of heparin, was detected with an anti-FSAP antibody (mean ± SD of triplicate wells); (**B**) $VEGF_{165}$ was immobilized, and the binding of increasing concentrations of FSAP in the absence (open circles) or presence (filled circles) of heparin was determined. Error bars are smaller than the size of the symbols; (**C**) Mixtures of FSAP (or Phe-Pro-Arg-chloromethylketone (PPACK)-FSAP), buffer, heparin, $VEGF_{165}$, and aprotinin, as indicated, were incubated, and the reaction was analyzed by western blotting with an anti-VEGF antibody under reducing or non-reducing conditions; (**D**) FSAP, $VEGF_{165}$, and heparin were incubated for the indicated time intervals and the samples were analyzed for VEGF, as above. Densiometric analysis was performed to calculate the ratio of VEGF under reduced and non-reduced conditions.

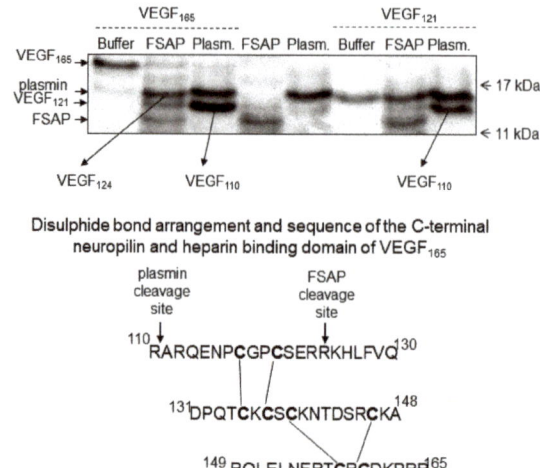

Figure 2. Sequencing of proteolytically cleaved VEGF: VEGF$_{165}$ or VEGF$_{121}$ (20 µg/mL) was incubated with FSAP (200 µg/mL) or plasmin (200 µg/mL) in the presence of heparin (10 µg/mL) for 2 h at 37 °C. The mixture was separated by SDS-PAGE under reducing conditions and processed for N-terminal sequencing. The FSAP and plasmin cleavage sites, as well as the disulphide bond assignments in the heparin/neuropilin-binding domain [31] sequence of VEGF$_{165}$ are indicated.

Interaction of FSAP with neuropilin and VEGFR-2: Neuropilins are co-receptors that bind to larger VEGF isoforms, such as VEGF$_{165}$, in a heparin-dependent manner, and regulate the activity of long forms of VEGF. Thus, the binding interactions between FSAP, VEGF$_{165}$, VEGFR, and neuropilin were investigated. FSAP bound strongly to neuropilin-1-Fc in a heparin-dependent manner, but there was no binding to VEGFR-2-Fc (Figure 3A). There was no difference in the binding of PPACK-FSAP, the MI-SNP of FSAP, or WT-FSAP (Figure 3A,B), indicating that the enzymatic activity of FSAP was not involved in the binding to neuropilin. VEGF$_{165}$ bound to both neuropilin and VEGFR2 in a heparin-dependent manner (Figure 3C). VEGF$_{165}$ binding to neuropilin-1-Fc was partially inhibited by FSAP in the absence or presence of heparin, but FSAP had no influence on binding of VEGF$_{165}$ to VEGFR-2-Fc (Figure 3C,D). Hence, FSAP binds to neuropilin, thereby cleaving VEGF$_{165}$ that, in turn, partially decreases its interactions with neuropilin but not VEGFR2.

Effect of FSAP on proliferation and migration of HUVEC or VEGFR-transfected BAF3 cells: Because FSAP can cleave VEGF$_{165}$ and inhibits its binding to neuropilin, the effect of FSAP-treated VEGF$_{165}$ on the activation of HUVEC was investigated in the absence or presence of heparin. FSAP did not influence bFGF- or VEGF$_{165}$-induced DNA synthesis or cell migration (Figure 4A,B). Phosphorylation of ERK in HUVEC with bFGF or VEGF pretreated with FSAP was not altered (Figure 5).

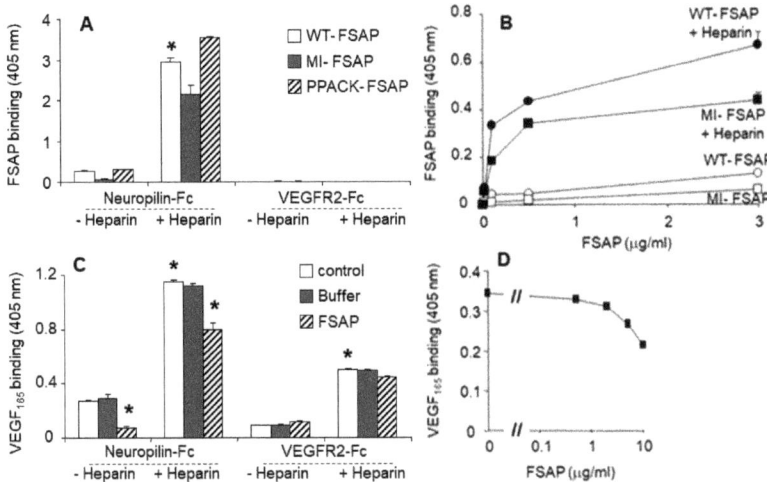

Figure 3. Interactions between FSAP, neuropilin, VEGFR2, and VEGF$_{165}$: (**A**) Neuropilin-1-Fc or VEGFR2-Fc was immobilized and the binding of wild type (WT)-FSAP (open bars), Marburg I (MI)-FSAP (G534E-SNP) (grey bars), or PPACK-FSAP (hatched bars) was determined in the absence or presence of heparin; (**B**) To immobilized neuropilin-1-Fc, increasing concentrations of WT-FSAP (circles) or MI-FSAP (squares) in the absence (open symbols) or presence (closed symbols) of heparin (filled circles) was added, and FSAP binding was determined; (**C**) Neuropilin-1-Fc or VEGFR2-Fc was immobilized, and the binding of VEGF$_{165}$ was determined in the absence or presence of heparin (open bars), buffer (grey bars), or FSAP (hatched bars); (**D**) Neuropilin-1-Fc was immobilized and the binding of VEGF$_{165}$ was determined in the presence of heparin and increasing concentrations of FSAP, as indicated. Results are shown as absorbance (mean + SD of triplicate wells). Error bars in 2B and 2D are smaller than the size of the symbols. * $p < 0.05$.

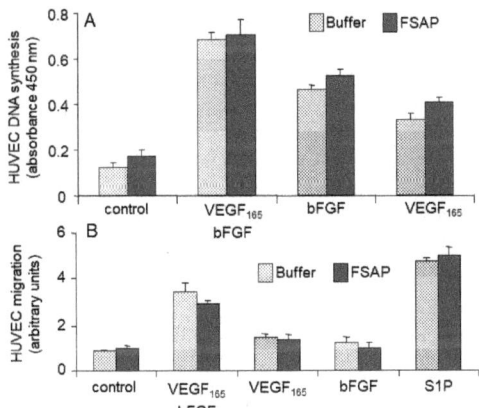

Figure 4. Effect of FSAP on proliferation and migration of human umbilical vein endothelial cells (HUVEC): basic fibroblast growth factor (bFGF) (40 ng/mL) and/or VEGF$_{165}$ (20 ng/mL) in the presence of FSAP (12 µg/mL) (dark bars) or buffer control (dotted bars), as well as heparin (10 µg/mL) was preincubated for 60 min at 37 °C, and the mixtures were used to stimulate serum-starved HUVEC. (**A**) DNA synthesis was determined using the BrdU incorporation kit; (**B**) Migration was tested in a Boyden chamber. Sphingosine-1-phosphate (S1P) was used a positive control and its concentration was 200 nM. Data are mean + SD of triplicate wells.

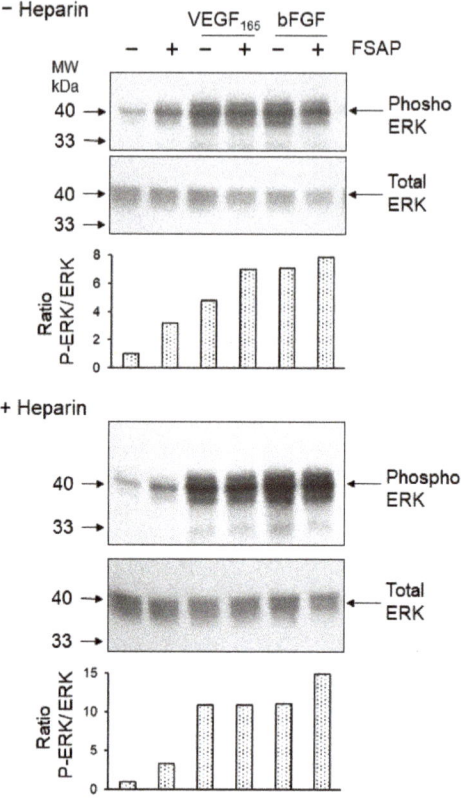

Figure 5. Effect of FSAP on ERK phosphorylation in HUVEC: Mixtures of FSAP (12 µg/mL), buffer, heparin (10 µg/mL), VEGF$_{165}$ (20 ng/mL), and/or (bFGF 50 ng/mL) were preincubated for 1 h at 37 °C in serum-free medium and then added to cells for 15 min. Cells extracts were analyzed by Western blotting for phosphorylated ERK. Analysis of total ERK was performed to confirm equal loading of gel with lysates. Relative phospho ERK levels were determined by densiometric analysis.

In order to further characterize this result, we also tested the activation of VEGFR-transfected BAF3 cells that are very sensitive to the effects of VEGF. Even in this very sensitive cellular system, FSAP did not inhibit VEGF$_{165}$- or VEGF$_{121}$-induced proliferation of BAF-3 cells transfected with VEGFR1 or VEGFR2 (Figure 6A,B). FSAP did not inhibit the effect of bFGF on HUVEC, which is in accordance with our previous results on VSMC [18], but is in contrast to earlier studies on HUVEC [19,20,32]. Expression of neuropilin-1 was observed on both cell types by flow cytometry (data not shown). Thus, in different cellular test systems, FSAP-mediated cleavage of VEGF$_{165}$ did not alter its ability to activate cellular functions.

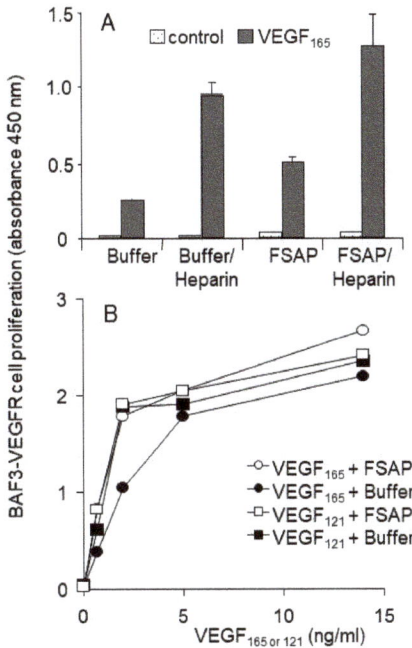

Figure 6. Effect of FSAP on VEGF-mediated proliferation of VEGFR expressing BAF3 cells: (**A**) VEGFR2-BAF3 cells were stimulated for 4 days with (dark bars) or without VEGF$_{165}$ (10 ng/mL) (dotted bars) in the absence or presence of FSAP (12 µg/mL), as well as heparin (10 µg/mL); (**B**) VEGFR1-BAF3 cells were stimulated with VEGF$_{165}$ (circles) or with VEGF$_{121}$ (squares) in the absence (filled) or presence (open) of FSAP (12 µg/mL), as well as heparin (10 µg/mL). Cell number was determined by the WST-1 assay. Mean + SD of triplicate wells is shown.

Effect of FSAP on growth factor-mediated neo-vascularization in matrigel plugs in vivo: We then tested the effect of FSAP in a model system where VEGF$_{165}$ interaction with the matrix is important. This model was based on measuring neovascularization in vivo into matrigel plugs that is essentially an extract of tumor extracellular matrix. VEGF$_{165}$ or bFGF, alone or in combination in the presence of heparin, stimulated the development of new vessels in matrigel, as determined by immunostaining for endothelial and smooth muscle cell markers (Figure 7A; endothelial-specific BS-1 (green) and α-SMA (α smooth muscle specific-actin) (red)). Quantification of the staining showed that the concomitant presence of FSAP reduced neovascularization induced by growth factors (Figure 7B). Enzymatically inactivated PPACK-FSAP did not inhibit growth factor-mediated neo-vascularization (Figure 7A,B), indicating the importance of the FSAP proteolytic activity for this effect. Similarly, the enzymatically inactive MI-isoform of FSAP did not inhibit VEGF$_{165}$/bFGF-mediated neo-vascularization (Supplementary Figure S2). The effect of VEGF$_{121}$-mediated neo-vascularization was not inhibited by FSAP (Supplementary Figure S2). Thus, exogenously applied FSAP could inhibit the effects of VEGF$_{165}$, bFGF, and their combination on neovascularization in matrigel plugs in vivo. Preliminary experiments showed that the neovascularization into matrigel in response to growth factors, in the absence of endogenous FSAP (*Habp2*$^{-/-}$ mice), was similar as in WT mice (data not shown).

Figure 7. *Cont.*

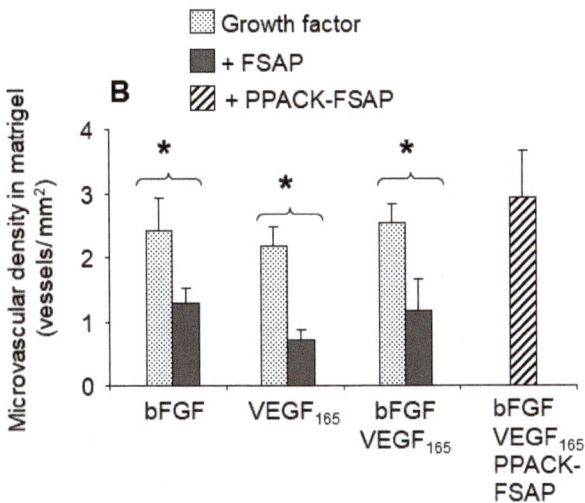

Figure 7. Effect of FSAP on microvascular density in matrigel plugs in vivo: (**A**) Photomicrographs of matrigel plugs after 7 days and stained for BS-1 (FITC, green), α-SMA (α smooth muscle specific-actin) (Cy3, red), and nuclei (DAPI, blue); (**B**) Microvascular density of plugs was determined, bars are means ± SEM (n = 7–8), * p < 0.05. Matrigel was supplemented with heparin and with either buffer (dotted bars), FSAP (black bars), or PPACK-FSAP (striped bars), as well as $VEGF_{165}$ or bFGF, as indicated.

VEGF expression in the Habp2$^{-/-}$ mice subjected to hind limb ischemia: We then examined whether the levels of the long forms of VEGF were higher in mice in the absence of endogenous FSAP (*Habp2$^{-/-}$* mice). For this, we used the hind limb ischemia model where angiogenesis is induced in the gastrocnemius muscle after femoral artery ligation [16]. Although, collateral growth in the adductor muscle was enhanced in *Habp2$^{-/-}$* mice, capillary density in the gastrocnemius muscle was not altered at 21 days. Western blotting showed that, at an earlier time point of day 3 after ligation, VEGF-A protein was significantly upregulated in the gastrocnemius muscle of *Habp2$^{-/-}$* mice compared to WT mice, whereas no increase was observed in the adductor muscle (Figure 8). At day 7, after ligation, this effect on VEGF-A protein was no longer evident. The VEGF-A isoform detected was largely the $VEGF_{121}$ dimer (30 kDa), and longer forms seemed not to be produced in this tissue. It was also possible that longer forms were produced and then cleaved to smaller forms. No change in VEGF-A mRNA was detected at the day 3 time point (Supplementary Figure S3). Thus, it was not possible to establish a causal link between the absence of endogenous FSAP and the increased presence of longer forms of VEGF in this experimental system.

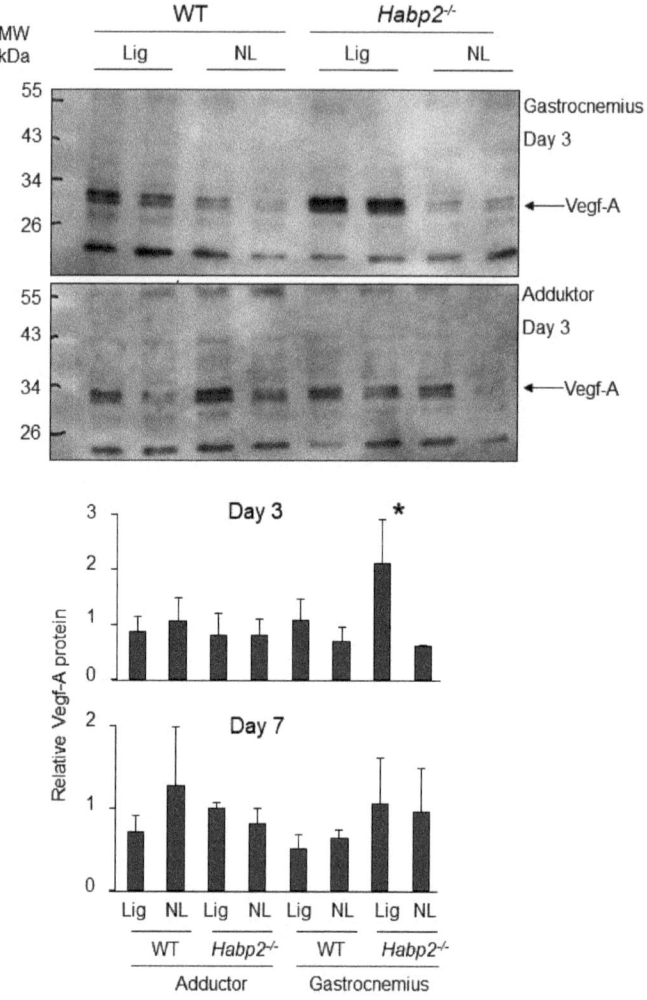

Figure 8. Changes in VEGF protein levels in the *Habp2*[-/-] mice after hind limb ischemia: In the hind limb muscles of WT- and *Habp2*[-/-] mice, VEGF-A protein was detected by western blotting at day 3 in the gastrocnemius muscle (top panel) and adductor muscles (bottom panel). VEGF-A was normalized to the expression of cytochrome C oxidase, as measured by western blotting on stripped blots. Relative VEGF-A levels were quantified by densitometry (means + SEM, $n = 4$, * $p < 0.05$).

4. Discussion

$VEGF_{165}$ was cleaved at position 124/125 in the heparin/neuropilin-binding region that resembles a classic, multi-basic, FSAP cleavage site. Because the disulphide bonds in this region were still intact, there was no difference in mobility of the protein under non-reducing conditions, only under reducing conditions. Only the larger forms of VEGF, 165 but not 121, bound to FSAP, thus conferring specificity to the process. FSAP also bound to neuropilin but not to VEGF-R2, and partially inhibited $VEGF_{165}$ binding to neuropilin. The binding and cleavage by FSAP was more pronounced in the presence of heparin, which is cofactor for FSAP. As previously reported, plasmin cleaved VEGF after position 110, thereby completely separating the receptor-binding domain from the heparin/neuropilin-binding domain [33,34]. Cleavage in the C-terminal region of VEGF$_{165}$ occurs naturally in vivo, and such cleaved forms have been observed in tumor ascites [35] as well as wound fluids [34]. Such cleavage is likely to reduce the association of VEGF long forms with the matrix and increase their mobility, thus raising the possibility of activating VEGF receptor as well as modulating their binding to co-receptors [27].

In proliferation, migration, and signal transduction assays on HUVEC, no consequence of the VEGF$_{165}$ cleavage was observed. This cleavage did not affect the induction of proliferation of VEGFR-transfected BAF3 cells either. This can be explained by the fact that the position of the cleavage in VEGF$_{165}$, in relation to the disulphide bond, was such that the molecule was still held together and preserved some of its characteristics. Other proteases such as urokinase, matrix metalloprotease (MMP), elastase, and tissue kallikrein also cleave the long forms of VEGF in this region and modulate its activity in different ways depending on the site of cleavage.

Matrigel-embedded growth factors provide a model to study neovascularization in vivo [29]. Growth factor-reduced matrigel is the matrix of mouse sarcoma, which contains 1851 unique proteins including classical matrix proteins such as laminin, collagen IV, entactin/nidogen, fibronectin, and heparan sulphate proteoglycans [36]. Heparin increases angiogenesis in this model by multiple mechanisms that probably include modifying growth factor's presentation to the cellular receptors [37]. In this model, FSAP inhibited the activity of VEGF$_{165}$, bFGF, and a combination of both, and microvascular density was decreased. We used BS1 and vWF as markers for endothelial cells and α-SMC actin as a marker for pericytes/VSMC. Individually, the staining of each marker was reduced by FSAP, indicating that FSAP directly inhibited both cell types. FSAP may also influence paracrine interactions between them, potentially, leading to the same end result. In this model, bFGF and VEGF$_{165}$ were known to upregulate PDGF-BB, and this in turn may have been responsible for the recruitment of the smooth muscle cells [38]. Smooth muscle cells and pericytes can indirectly contribute to the regulation of neo-vascularization through various paracrine/juxtacrine mechanisms [39], and we have previously shown that FSAP can inhibit PDGF-BB [18]. The inhibitory effect of FSAP on bFGF may be related to a complex interaction between FSAP and bFGF, as described before [19]. This result also illustrates the fact that the inhibitory effect of FSAP in this model was not limited to VEGF$_{165}$, and a completely different mechanism of action, independent of the growth factor, cannot be excluded.

In view of the lack of the effect of FSAP on VEGF-mediated proliferation and migration of endothelial cells in vitro, the strong reduction of angiogenesis in the matrigel model was remarkable. Because FSAP cleavage of VEGF$_{165}$ led to a VEGF$_{121}$-like molecule, the difference in the in vitro and in vivo results must be related to the difference between the two isoforms. It was possible that in the matrigel model, the VEGF was presented to the cells in a form that was bound to the matrix, and that the haptotaxis-effect was altered by FSAP. Evidence for proteolysis-mediated modulation of haptotaxis of matrix-anchored VEGF has been demonstrated before [40]. The cleavage of VEGF by FSAP may also alter the sequestration of the growth factor by the matrix or its spatial complexity, both of which are known to be important for VEGF activity [41]. VEGF can also activate leukocytes and other VEGFR-bearing cells, which may indirectly mediate the inhibition of angiogenesis by FSAP. An effect of VEGF in the matrigel model through changes in vascular permeability was also a possibility. The time course of the in vitro experiments, ranging from minutes to 24 h, were different from the in vivo matrigel experiments that lasted a few days, and this could also account for the differences in the results.

The induction of ischemia led to angiogenesis in the gastrocnemius muscle in the hind limb ischemia model. Mice without endogenous FSAP showed no changes in their angiogenesis response in this model, indicating that endogenous FSAP was not involved in this process [16]. However, collateral vessel growth was increased in the adductor muscle. Application of exogenous FSAP, directly into the adductor muscle, decreased collateral growth there, but increased angiogenesis in the gastrocnemius muscle. This was most likely a response to the decreased collateral growth in the vessels feeding the gastrocnemius muscle [16]. In the neointimal growth model, exogenous FSAP decreased neointima formation [15] and a lack of endogenous FSAP increased it [18]. Thus, in two independent models of vascular growth and repair, FSAP seemed to be involved in regulating vascular remodeling but not angiogenesis. This also fits with the lack of difference in neovascularization in $Habp2^{-/-}$ mice in the matrigel model (see Table 1 for an overview).

Table 1. Summary of the effects of FSAP on vascular growth and repair processes.

	$Habp2^{-/-}$ Mice: Lack of Endogenous FSAP	Local Application of Exogenous Purified FSAP
Neointima formation in response to intraluminal injury in the femoral artery	Increased [15]	Decreased [18]
Femoral artery ligation and stimulation of collateral development in the adductor muscle	Increased [16]	Decreased [16]
Femoral artery ligation and stimulation of angiogenesis in the gastrocnemius muscle	No change [16]	Increased, probably as a consequence of decreased collateral growth [16]
Matrigel/growth factor model of angiogenesis	No change (this study)	Decreased (this study)

We chose to study the hind limb ischemia model to investigate processing of long forms of VEGF because we have performed studies using this model in FSAP-deficient mice [16]. However, we did not detect any $VEGF_{165}$ in this tissue and it was not possible to find any direct evidence for changes in cleavage of this VEGF isoform. However, we did observe an increase in $VEGF_{121}$ in $Habp2^{-/-}$ in the absence of any increase in mRNA. Further experiments would be required to study VEGF isoform-specific mRNA and protein to provide compelling evidence for this hypothesis. In this model system there was an upregulation of uPA and MMP-9 at the mRNA and protein level in the gastrocnemius muscle, which could also account for the fact that only the short form of VEGF was detected [16]. Such experiments would be more conclusive in performed in relation to angiogenesis in the eye or the brain because they display the sharpest concentration gradients of $VEGF_{165}$ [27].

Although endogenous FSAP did not regulate angiogenesis and neovascularization, it did influence remodeling of vessels in general. $VEGF_{165}$ cleavage, binding properties towards neuropilin, and angiogenesis in matrigel were inhibited by exogenous FSAP. Thus, FSAP has the potential to modulate $VEGF_{165}$-mediated angiogenesis that may be relevant in some pathophysiological conditions.

Supplementary Materials: The following are available online at http://www.mdpi.com/2073-4409/8/11/1396/s1, Figure S1: Cleavage of $VEGF_{165}$ and $VEGF_{121}$ by FSAP, Figure S2: Microvascular density in matrigel plugs, Figure S3: *Vegf-A* mRNA in the hind limb ischemia model.

Author Contributions: Ö.U. and J.H. performed experiments, analyzed the data, and edited the manuscript. S.M.K. designed the research, obtained the funding, analyzed data, and drafted the manuscript.

Funding: Funding was from the Deutscheforschungsgemeinschaft, Germany.

Acknowledgments: We would like to thank Lars Muhl, Susanne Tannert-Otto, Thomas Schmidt Wöll, and Baerbel Fuehler for their excellent technical assistance. The gift of VEGFR cells from Steven Stacker and Marc Achen (Ludwig Cancer Research Institute, Melbourne Branch, Australia) and Kari Alitalo (Helsinki Branch, Finland) is greatly appreciated. This study was done as part of the MD/PhD thesis of Özgür Uslu at the Justus Liebig University, Giessen, Germany.

Conflicts of Interest: The authors have no financial or other conflicts of interest.

References

1. Yamamichi, S.; Fujiwara, Y.; Kikuchi, T.; Nishitani, M.; Matsushita, Y.; Hasumi, K. Extracellular histone induces plasma hyaluronan-binding protein (factor VII activating protease) activation in vivo. *Biochem. Biophys. Res. Commun.* **2011**, *409*, 483–488. [CrossRef] [PubMed]

2. Kanse, S.M.; Gallenmueller, A.; Zeerleder, S.; Stephan, F.; Rannou, O.; Denk, S.; Etscheid, M.; Lochnit, G.; Krueger, M.; Huber-Lang, M. Factor VII-activating protease is activated in multiple trauma patients and generates anaphylatoxin C5a. *J. Immunol.* **2012**, *188*, 2858–2865. [CrossRef] [PubMed]
3. Marsman, G.; von Richthofen, H.; Bulder, I.; Lupu, F.; Hazelzet, J.; Luken, B.M.; Zeerleder, S. DNA and factor VII-activating protease protect against the cytotoxicity of histones. *Blood Adv.* **2017**, *1*, 2491–2502. [CrossRef] [PubMed]
4. Grasso, S.; Neumann, A.; Lang, I.M.; Etscheid, M.; von Kockritz-Blickwede, M.; Kanse, S.M. Interaction of factor VII activating protease (FSAP) with neutrophil extracellular traps (NETs). *Thromb. Res.* **2018**, *161*, 36–42. [CrossRef] [PubMed]
5. Serpas, L.; Chan, R.W.Y.; Jiang, P.; Ni, M.; Sun, K.; Rashidfarrokhi, A.; Soni, C.; Sisirak, V.; Lee, W.S.; Cheng, S.H.; et al. Dnase1l3 deletion causes aberrations in length and end-motif frequencies in plasma DNA. *Proc. Natl. Acad. Sci. USA* **2019**, *116*, 641–649. [CrossRef]
6. Etscheid, M.; Muhl, L.; Pons, D.; Jukema, J.W.; Koenig, H.; Kanse, S.M. The Marburg I polymorphism of factor VII activating protease is associated with low proteolytic and low pro-coagulant activity. *Thromb. Res.* **2012**, *130*, 935–941. [CrossRef]
7. Willeit, J.; Kiechl, S.; Weimer, T.; Mair, A.; Santer, P.; Wiedermann, C.J.; Roemisch, J. Marburg I polymorphism of factor VII—Activating protease: A prominent risk predictor of carotid stenosis. *Circulation* **2003**, *107*, 667–670. [CrossRef]
8. Trompet, S.; Pons, D.; Kanse, S.M.; de Craen, A.J.; Ikram, M.A.; Verschuren, J.J.; Zwinderman, A.H.; Doevendans, P.A.; Tio, R.A.; de Winter, R.J.; et al. Factor VII Activating Protease Polymorphism (G534E) Is Associated with Increased Risk for Stroke and Mortality. *Stroke Res. Treat.* **2011**, *2011*, 424759. [CrossRef]
9. Ahmad-Nejad, P.; Dempfle, C.E.; Weiss, C.; Bugert, P.; Borggrefe, M.; Neumaier, M. The G534E-polymorphism of the gene encoding the factor VII-activating protease is a risk factor for venous thrombosis and recurrent events. *Thromb. Res.* **2012**, *130*, 441–444. [CrossRef]
10. Hoppe, B.; Tolou, F.; Dorner, T.; Kiesewetter, H.; Salama, A. Gene polymorphisms implicated in influencing susceptibility to venous and arterial thromboembolism: Frequency distribution in a healthy German population. *Thromb. Haemost.* **2006**, *96*, 465–470.
11. Wasmuth, H.E.; Tag, C.G.; Van de Leur, E.; Hellerbrand, C.; Mueller, T.; Berg, T.; Puhl, G.; Neuhaus, P.; Samuel, D.; Trautwein, C.; et al. The Marburg I variant (G534E) of the factor VII-activating protease determines liver fibrosis in hepatitis C infection by reduced proteolysis of platelet-derived growth factor BB. *Hepatology* **2009**, *49*, 775–780. [CrossRef] [PubMed]
12. Gara, S.K.; Jia, L.; Merino, M.J.; Agarwal, S.K.; Zhang, L.; Cam, M.; Patel, D.; Kebebew, E. Germline HABP2 Mutation Causing Familial Nonmedullary Thyroid Cancer. *N. Engl. J. Med.* **2015**, *373*, 448–455. [CrossRef] [PubMed]
13. Reiner, A.P.; Lange, L.A.; Smith, N.L.; Zakai, N.A.; Cushman, M.; Folsom, A.R. Common hemostasis and inflammation gene variants and venous thrombosis in older adults from the Cardiovascular Health Study. *J. Thromb. Haemost. JTH* **2009**, *7*, 1499–1505. [CrossRef] [PubMed]
14. Ngeow, J.; Eng, C. HABP2 in Familial Non-medullary Thyroid Cancer: Will the Real Mutation Please Stand Up? *J. Natl. Cancer Inst.* **2016**, *108*. [CrossRef] [PubMed]
15. Daniel, J.M.; Reichel, C.A.; Schmidt-Woell, T.; Dutzmann, J.; Zuchtriegel, G.; Krombach, F.; Herold, J.; Bauersachs, J.; Sedding, D.G.; Kanse, S.M. Factor VII-activating protease deficiency promotes neointima formation by enhancing leukocyte accumulation. *J. Thromb. Haemost. JTH* **2016**, *14*, 2058–2067. [CrossRef] [PubMed]
16. Herold, J.; Nowak, S.; Kostin, S.; Daniel, J.M.; Francke, A.; Subramaniam, S.; Braun-Dullaeus, R.C.; Kanse, S.M. Factor VII activating protease (FSAP) influences vascular remodeling in the mouse hind limb ischemia model. *Am. J. Transl. Res.* **2017**, *9*, 3084–3095.
17. Kara, E.; Manna, D.; Loset, G.A.; Schneider, E.L.; Craik, C.S.; Kanse, S. Analysis of the substrate specificity of Factor VII activating protease (FSAP) and design of specific and sensitive peptide substrates. *Thromb. Haemost.* **2017**, *117*, 1750–1760. [CrossRef]
18. Sedding, D.; Daniel, J.M.; Muhl, L.; Hersemeyer, K.; Brunsch, H.; Kemkes-Matthes, B.; Braun-Dullaeus, R.C.; Tillmanns, H.; Weimer, T.; Preissner, K.T.; et al. The G534E polymorphism of the gene encoding the factor VII-activating protease is associated with cardiovascular risk due to increased neointima formation. *J. Exp. Med.* **2006**, *203*, 2801–2807. [CrossRef]

19. Etscheid, M.; Beer, N.; Kress, J.A.; Seitz, R.; Dodt, J. Inhibition of bFGF/EGF-dependent endothelial cell proliferation by the hyaluronan-binding protease from human plasma. *Eur. J. Cell. Biol.* **2004**, *82*, 597–604. [CrossRef]
20. Kress, J.A.; Seitz, R.; Dodt, J.; Etscheid, M. Induction of intracellular signalling in human endothelial cells by the hyaluronan-binding protease involves two distinct pathways. *Biol. Chem.* **2006**, *387*, 1275–1283. [CrossRef]
21. Roedel, E.K.; Schwarz, E.; Kanse, S.M. The Factor VII-activating protease (FSAP) enhances the activity of bone morphogenetic protein-2 (BMP-2). *J. Biol. Chem.* **2013**, *288*, 7193–7202. [CrossRef] [PubMed]
22. Mambetsariev, N.; Mirzapoiazova, T.; Mambetsariev, B.; Sammani, S.; Lennon, F.E.; Garcia, J.G.; Singleton, P.A. Hyaluronic Acid binding protein 2 is a novel regulator of vascular integrity. *Arterioscler. Thromb. Vasc. Biol.* **2010**, *30*, 483–490. [CrossRef] [PubMed]
23. Joshi, A.U.; Orset, C.; Engelhardt, B.; Baumgart-Vogt, E.; Gerriets, T.; Vivien, D.; Kanse, S.M. Deficiency of Factor VII activating protease alters the outcome of ischemic stroke in mice. *Eur. J. Neurosci.* **2015**, *41*, 965–975. [CrossRef] [PubMed]
24. Apte, R.S.; Chen, D.S.; Ferrara, N. VEGF in Signaling and Disease: Beyond Discovery and Development. *Cell* **2019**, *176*, 1248–1264. [CrossRef]
25. Holmes, D.I.; Zachary, I. The vascular endothelial growth factor (VEGF) family: Angiogenic factors in health and disease. *Genome Biol.* **2005**, *6*, 209. [CrossRef]
26. Peng, K.; Bai, Y.; Zhu, Q.; Hu, B.; Xu, Y. Targeting VEGF-neuropilin interactions: A promising antitumor strategy. *Drug Discov. Today* **2019**, *24*, 656–664. [CrossRef]
27. Vempati, P.; Popel, A.S.; Mac Gabhann, F. Extracellular regulation of VEGF: Isoforms, proteolysis, and vascular patterning. *Cytokine Growth Factor Rev.* **2014**, *25*, 1–19. [CrossRef]
28. Kannemeier, C.; Al-Fakhri, N.; Preissner, K.T.; Kanse, S.M. Factor VII activating protease (FSAP) inhibits growth factor-mediated cell proliferation and migration of vascular smooth muscle cells. *FASEB J.* **2004**, *18*, 728–730. [CrossRef]
29. Pauly, R.R.; Passaniti, A.; Crow, M.; Kinsella, J.L.; Papadopoulos, N.; Monticone, R.; Lakatta, E.G.; Martin, G.R. Experimental models that mimic the differentiation and dedifferentiation of vascular cells. *Circulation* **1992**, *86*, III68-73.
30. Magee, J.C.; Stone, A.E.; Oldham, K.T.; Guice, K.S. Isolation, culture, and characterization of rat lung microvascular endothelial cells. *Am. J. Physiol.* **1994**, *267*, L433–L441. [CrossRef]
31. Keck, R.G.; Berleau, L.; Harris, R.; Keyt, B.A. Disulfide structure of the heparin binding domain in vascular endothelial growth factor: Characterization of posttranslational modifications in VEGF. *Arch. Biochem. Biophys.* **1997**, *344*, 103–113. [CrossRef] [PubMed]
32. Jeon, J.W.; Song, H.S.; Moon, E.J.; Park, S.Y.; Son, M.J.; Jung, S.Y.; Kim, J.T.; Nam, D.H.; Choi-Miura, N.H.; Kim, K.W.; et al. Anti-angiogenic action of plasma hyaluronan binding protein in human umbilical vein endothelial cells. *Int. J. Oncol.* **2006**, *29*, 209–215. [CrossRef] [PubMed]
33. Keyt, B.A.; Berleau, L.T.; Nguyen, H.V.; Chen, H.; Heinsohn, H.; Vandlen, R.; Ferrara, N. The carboxyl-terminal domain (111–165) of vascular endothelial growth factor is critical for its mitogenic potency. *J. Biol. Chem.* **1996**, *271*, 7788–7795. [CrossRef]
34. Roth, D.; Piekarek, M.; Paulsson, M.; Christ, H.; Krieg, T.; Bloch, W.; Davidson, J.M.; Eming, S.A. Plasmin modulates vascular endothelial growth factor-A-mediated angiogenesis during wound repair. *Am. J. Pathol.* **2006**, *168*, 670–684. [CrossRef] [PubMed]
35. Lee, S.; Jilani, S.M.; Nikolova, G.V.; Carpizo, D.; Iruela-Arispe, M.L. Processing of VEGF-A by matrix metalloproteinases regulates bioavailability and vascular patterning in tumors. *J. Cell. Biol.* **2005**, *169*, 681–691. [CrossRef] [PubMed]
36. Hughes, C.S.; Postovit, L.M.; Lajoie, G.A. Matrigel: A complex protein mixture required for optimal growth of cell culture. *Proteomics* **2010**, *10*, 1886–1890. [CrossRef]
37. Wake, H.; Mori, S.; Liu, K.; Takahashi, H.K.; Nishibori, M. Histidine-rich glycoprotein inhibited high mobility group box 1 in complex with heparin-induced angiogenesis in matrigel plug assay. *Eur. J. Pharmacol.* **2009**, *623*, 89–95. [CrossRef]
38. Kano, M.R.; Morishita, Y.; Iwata, C.; Iwasaka, S.; Watabe, T.; Ouchi, Y.; Miyazono, K.; Miyazawa, K. VEGF-A and FGF-2 synergistically promote neoangiogenesis through enhancement of endogenous PDGF-B-PDGFRβ signaling. *J. Cell. Sci.* **2005**, *118*, 3759–3768. [CrossRef]

39. Armulik, A.; Abramsson, A.; Betsholtz, C. Endothelial/pericyte interactions. *Circ. Res.* **2005**, *97*, 512–523. [CrossRef]
40. Chen, T.T.; Luque, A.; Lee, S.; Anderson, S.M.; Segura, T.; Iruela-Arispe, M.L. Anchorage of VEGF to the extracellular matrix conveys differential signaling responses to endothelial cells. *J. Cell. Biol.* **2010**, *188*, 595–609. [CrossRef]
41. Ekker, S.C.; Bedell, V.M. The ins and outs of VEGF signaling. *Blood* **2009**, *113*, 2123–2124. [CrossRef] [PubMed]

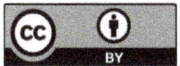

© 2019 by the authors. Licensee MDPI, Basel, Switzerland. This article is an open access article distributed under the terms and conditions of the Creative Commons Attribution (CC BY) license (http://creativecommons.org/licenses/by/4.0/).

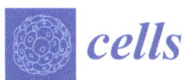

Article

Control of Angiogenesis via a VHL/miR-212/132 Axis

Zhiyong Lei [1,†], Timothy D. Klasson [2,†], Maarten M. Brandt [3], Glenn van de Hoek [4], Ive Logister [2], Caroline Cheng [2,3], Pieter A. Doevendans [1,5,6], Joost P. G. Sluijter [1,7,*] and Rachel H. Giles [2,*]

1. Department of Cardiology, Division Heart and Lungs, University Medical Center Utrecht, Heidelberglaan 100, 3584 CX Utrecht, The Netherlands
2. Department of Nephrology & Hypertension, Division Internal Medicine, University Medical Center Utrecht, Heidelberglaan 100, 3584 CX Utrecht, The Netherlands
3. Experimental Cardiology, Department of Cardiology, Thoraxcenter, Erasmus MC, University Medical Center Rotterdam, 3015 GD Rotterdam, The Netherlands
4. Department of Medical Genetics, University Medical Center Utrecht, Heidelberglaan 100, 3584 CX Utrecht, The Netherlands
5. Netherlands Heart Institute, Catharijnesingel 52, 3511 GC Utrecht, The Netherlands
6. Central Military Hospital Utrecht, Lundlaan 1, 3584 EZ Utrecht, The Netherlands
7. UMC Utrecht Regenerative Medicine Center, University Medical Center, 3584 CT Utrecht, The Netherlands
* Correspondence: j.sluijter@umcutrecht.nl (J.P.G.S.); r.giles@umcutrecht.nl (R.H.G.)
† These authors contributed equally to this work.

Received: 20 March 2020; Accepted: 15 April 2020; Published: 19 April 2020

Abstract: A common feature of tumorigenesis is the upregulation of angiogenesis pathways in order to supply nutrients via the blood for the growing tumor. Understanding how cells promote angiogenesis and how to control these processes pharmaceutically are of great clinical interest. Clear cell renal cell carcinoma (ccRCC) is the most common form of sporadic and inherited kidney cancer which is associated with excess neovascularization. ccRCC is highly associated with biallelic mutations in the von Hippel–Lindau (VHL) tumor suppressor gene. Although upregulation of the miR-212/132 family and disturbed VHL signaling have both been linked with angiogenesis, no evidence of a possible connection between the two has yet been made. We show that miRNA-212/132 levels are increased after loss of functional pVHL, the protein product of the VHL gene, in vivo and in vitro. Furthermore, we show that blocking miRNA-212/132 with anti-miRs can significantly alleviate the excessive vascular branching phenotype characteristic of $vhl^{-/-}$ mutant zebrafish. Moreover, using human umbilical vascular endothelial cells (HUVECs) and an endothelial cell/pericyte coculture system, we observed that VHL knockdown promotes endothelial cells neovascularization capacity in vitro, an effect which can be inhibited by anti-miR-212/132 treatment. Taken together, our results demonstrate an important role for miRNA-212/132 in angiogenesis induced by loss of VHL. Intriguingly, this also presents a possibility for the pharmaceutical manipulation of angiogenesis by modulating levels of MiR212/132.

Keywords: VHL loss of function; microRNA-212/132; angiogenesis

1. Introduction

Clear cell renal cell carcinoma (ccRCC), the most common form of sporadic and inherited kidney cancer, is highly associated with mutations in the von Hippel-Lindau (*VHL*) gene [1,2]. The protein product of the *VHL* gene (pVHL) is an E3 ubiquitin ligase involved in the degradation of hypoxia-inducible transcription factor subunits (HIF1α). Under normal oxygen tension, hydroxylated HIF1α can be recognized by the ubiquitin ligase complex containing pVHL and rapidly degraded. Upon hypoxia or loss of functional pVHL, HIF1α-subunits can no longer be hydroxylated and begin to accumulate. Stabilized HIF1α activates the expression of a large suite of downstream target genes (Erythropoietin (*EPO*), vascular endothelial growth factor (*VEGF*), etc), the actions of which are vital to promote angiogenesis. However, many of the changes initiated by the stabilization of HIF1α, such as increased angiogenesis, an upregulation of antiapoptotic signaling, and a shift to anaerobic glycolosis, can contribute to tumor growth and survival. People born with a mutation in one *VHL* allele may acquire somatic mutations in the second allele, resulting in consequent angiogenic symptoms and a variety of tumors, including ccRCC [3]. Another hallmark of ccRCC is the activated phosphatidylinositol-4,5-bisphosphate 3-kinase (PI3k)/AKT pathway signaling, higher levels of which is significantly correlated with a worse survival rate [2], although the mechanism by which this occurs is still not fully understood.

MicroRNAs (miRNAs) are small noncoding RNAs that posttranscriptionally regulate the expression of groups of target genes by inhibition of the translation of their targeting messenger RNAs (mRNAs) or marking these mRNAs for degradation. miRNAs are key regulators in many physiological and pathological processes [4], including the dynamic regulation of ccRCC during tumor progression [2]. By promoting the expression of vascular endothelial growth factor (*VEGF*), VHL/HIF1 signaling increases Cyclic adenosine monophosphate (cAMP) response element binding protein (CREB) levels, a transcription factor which upregulates the expression of pro-angiogenic miR-212/132 [5]. This implies that pVHL loss-of-function would stimulate miR-212/132 expression and therefore contribute to excessive angiogenesis. In this study, using a combination of cellular models, patient ccRCC material with biallelic loss of VHL and a previously described vhl$^{-/-}$ mutant zebrafish model, we show that miR-212/132 is upregulated after VHL knockdown or mutation and that this upregulation is at least partially responsible for pro-angiogenic effects. In order to grow, cancer tissues such as ccRCC have developed various strategies to provide sufficient blood supply by promoting angiogenesis [6]. Many of the common pharmaceutical treatments for ccRCC, such as sunitinib, use the strategy of reducing pathophysiological angiogenesis [7]. Conversely, many different strategies have been tested to improve perfusion of certain ischemic tissues or engineered tissue constructs by promoting neovascularization, which is essential for functional recovery of the organ after ischemic events or survival of transplanted engineered tissue constructs [8]. A scarcity of functional pVHL induces excessive vascular outgrowth, which further is enhanced by miR-212/132 expression, providing an exciting target for the modulation of angiogenesis.

2. Materials and Methods

2.1. MicroRNA In Situ Hybridization

microRNA in situ hybridization was performed with a modified microRNA in situ hybridization method as described [9]. Formalin-fixed paraffin-embedded tumor tissue from two ccRCCs and one healthy donor kidney dating from September 2006 were collected from the pathology archives of the University Medical Centre Utrecht (UMCU) after authorization of the UMCU institutional review board in accordance with Dutch medical ethical guidelines. Sequencing results of *VHL* identified no variants in the normal healthy kidney. However, in ccRCC #1, in addition to the already known germline deletion of *VHL* exons 1 and 2, an additional somatic mutation was found in the tumor (c.277delG/p.Gly93Ala_fs_x158). ccRCC #2 has a germline mutation c.266T> p.Leu89Pro and a somatic mutation of c.419-420delTC/p.Leu140Gln_fs_x142. Mutation analysis of these tumors has been previously published [10].

Paraffin samples were first deparaffinized with tissue clear (Cat# 1426, SAKURA) followed with 10 min of proteinase K treatment (5μg/ml, Cat# 03115828001, Roche). Hybridization was performed with 10 nM DIG-labeled miRCURY LNA miRNA detection probes in hybridization buffer (Urea (2 M), 2.5× SSC, 1× Denhardt's, 200 μg/ml yeast tRNA, 0.1% CHAPS, 0.1% Tween, and 50mg/ml heparin) for miR-132 (Cat# 38031-15, Exiqon). Sections were subsequently incubated with anti-DIG alkaline phosphatase antibody (1:1,500, Cat# 1093274, Roche). To block endogenous alkaline phosphatase activity, sections were incubated with levamisole solution (Cat. X3021, DAKO), followed by NBT/BCIP (Cat# K0598 DAKO) incubation for visualization. A light Eosin counter staining was performed to visualize histology of the tissue. Images were taken with an Olympus microscope (BX53) under bright field.

2.2. Cell Culture and Transfection

Human umbilical vascular endothelial cells (HUVECs) were cultured in EGM2 (Lonza, cat# cc-3156) according to manufacturer's instructions, and all experiments were performed before passage 7. HUVECS were either transfected with validated siVHL (ID: s14790), siPTEN (ID: s61222), silencer select negative control #1 (cat# 4390843), mirVana miRNA mimic negative control (cat# 4464085), hsa-miR-132-3p mimics (ID: MC10166), hsa-miR-212-3p mimics (ID: MC10340), mirVana miRNA inhibitor control1 (cat# 4464077), hsa-miR-132-3p inhibitor (ID: AM10166), or hsa-miR-212-3p inhibitor (ID: AM10340) (all from Life Technologies) using Lipofectamine 2000 (Life Technologies). The transfection was performed with a final concentration of 20 nM in opti-MEM reduced-serum medium (Cat# 31985062, Life Technologies) and replaced with fresh EGM2 after 6 hours. Cells were harvested 72 hours after transfection for protein or RNA analysis.

2.3. RNA Isolation and RT-PCR

Total RNA was isolated with Tripure Isolation Reagent following manufactory's instructions (Roche Applied Science) and treated with Dnase to remove potential genome DNA contaminations. cDNA was synthesized using the iScript^{TM} cDNA Synthesis Kit (Bio-Rad). Quantitative real-time polymerase chain reaction (qRT-PCR) was performed with iQ SYBR Green Supermix (Bio-Rad). The following primers were used for detection of human genes: *GAPDH* forward 5′-GGCATGGACTGTGGTCAT GA-3′ and reverse 5′-TTCACCACCATGGAGAAGGC-3′; *PTEN* forward 5′-TGGATTCGACTTAGACT TGACCT-3′ and reverse 5′-GGTGGGTTATGGTCTTCAAAAGG-3′; *VHL* forward 5′-CAGCTACCGA GGTCACCTTT-3′ and reverse 5′-CCGTCAACATTGAGAGATGG-3′; the following primers are used for *zebrafish*: *ptena* forward 5′-CCAGCCAGCGCAGGTATGTGTA-3′ and reverse 5′-GCGGCTGAGGAAAC TCGAAGATC-3′; *ptenb* forward 5′-GCTACCTTCTGAGGAATAAGCTGG-3′ and reverse 5′-CTTGATG TCCCCACACACAGGC-3′; *rpl13a* forward 5′-TCTGGAGGACTGTAAGAGGTATGC-3′ and reverse 5′-AGACGCACAATCTTGAGAGCAG-3′ (All primers from Integrated DNA Technologies, Coralville, IA, USA).

2.4. In Vitro Angiogenesis Assay

HUVECs (Lonza) and human brain vascular pericytes (Cat#1200, Sciencell) were cultured on gelatin-coated plates in EGM2 medium (Lonza cat# cc-3156) and DMEM (10% FCS; Lonza), respectively, in 5% CO_2 at 37 °C. Lentiviral transduced HUVECs expressing green fluorescent protein (GFP) and pericytes expressing red fluorescent protein (RFP) were used between passage 6–8. HUVECs were transfected either with siRNA or anti-miRs as described above. In order to monitor the effects of miR-132 and miR-212 in angiogenesis, transfected HUVEC-GFP and Pericytes-dsRed were suspended in a 2.5 mg/ml collagen type I (BD Biosciences) as described by Stratman [11]. Cocultures were imaged after 48 h and 120 h incubation in 5% CO_2 at 37 °C by fluorescence microscopy, followed by automated thresholding and skeletonization of the images using a commercial analysis system (Angiosys, Buckingham, UK). These images were used for automated tubule length measurement, junction measurement, and other analyses according to manufacturer's instructions.

2.5. Zebrafish

Experiments were conducted in accordance with Dutch guidelines for the care and use of laboratory animals, with the approval of the Animal Experimentation Committee (DEC) of the Royal Netherlands Academy of Arts and Sciences (KNAW). Mutant *zebrafish* possessed the previously described vhl^{hu2117} mutation [12]. For RNA collection, *zebrafish* embryos were collected at 5 dpf based on these phenotypes and RNA was collected using Trizol reagent (Ambion) as per manufacturer's instructions.

2.6. Injections and Visualizations

Wild-type and mutant *Zebrafish* embryos were injected at the 1–2-cell stage with 1 nL of 5 uM of the same miRNA mimics and antagonists used for the cell culture experiments described above. Mimics and antagonists were diluted in pure water with 0.1% phenol red for visualization and injected using a nanoject2000 microinjector (World Precision Instruments). *Zebrafish* were selected without bias at 5dpf and then imaged using an LSM700 microscope (Zeiss). DNA was then collected from theses embryos using lysis buffer, and then embryos were genotyped using a KASP™ genotyping system (LGC Genomics, Teddington, Middlesex, England) kit designed against the *vhl*^{hu2117} mutation or by sanger sequencing using the following primers: Fw: 5′-TAA GGG CTT AGC GCA TGT TC-3′ and Rv: 5′-CGA GTT AAA CGC GTA GAT AG-3′.

2.7. Statistical Analysis

Data was analyzed with Graphpad Prism 6 and comparisons were performed with student *t*-test or paired *t*-test between two groups and with ANOVA for more than two groups. Data are presented as mean ± SEM. *p*-values are indicated as follows: * $p < 0.05$; ** $p < 0.01$; *** $p < 0.001$; $p < 0.05$ is considered significant.

3. Results

miRNA-212/132 are transcribed as a single RNA transcript and subsequently processed into two different mature microRNA miR-132 and miR-212. Due to the different efficiency in pre-miR processing, miR-132 is the dominant family member, as shown in Figure 1F. In most of the tissues, the expression of miR-212 are hardly detectable with the only exception being the brain. For this reason, mir-132 was used as the primary target in this study. We first examined the expression of miR-132 in relation to VHL loss-of-function and (pseudo)-hypoxic signaling. We found that endothelial cells grown in hypoxic conditions display significantly elevated levels of miR-132 expression (Figure 1A). We observe similar effects in HUVECs transfected with siRNA targeting *VHL* mRNA relative to those treated with non-targeting siRNA (Figure 1B). miR-212/132 are well conserved in most species, including zebrafish (Supplementary Figure S1A). To confirm this effect in vivo, we used a previously established zebrafish model of *VHL* deficiency [12–14]. Like our cell models, *vhl*$^{-/-}$ zebrafish also show an increased level of expression of miR-132 (Figure 1C). In isogenic cell lines taken from human ccRCC *VHL*$^{-/-}$ tumors, the expression of miR-132 is reduced upon *VHL* reconstitution with ectopic *VHL* (Figure 1E). The reduction of miR-132 expression is present in all cell lines upon VHL introduction but less pronounced in the RCC10, which might be related to a cell-line-specific genetic alteration on top of the VHL disruption that affects the miR-132 pathway. To assess the functional consequences of miR-212/132 loss in these cells, we examined the expression of a known target mRNA of this miRNA family. PTEN, phosphatidylinositol-3,4,5-trisphosphate 3-phosphatase, antagonizes the activity of phosphatidylinositol-4,5-bisphosphate 3-kinase (PI3K), suppressing cellular proliferation, cell survival, and angiogenesis by inactivating the PI3K-driven AKT signaling pathway [15]. *PTEN* has been predicted to be a potential target of miR-212/132 in humans by targetscan (Supplemental Figure S1B), and the rat homologue of *PTEN* has been shown to be targeted by miR-212/132 in rat vascular smooth muscle cells [16]. Moreover, downregulation of PTEN has been significantly correlated with lower survival rate in ccRCC patients [2]. We reasoned that upregulated miR-212/132 upon mutation or silencing of *VHL* could result in the subsequent reduction of PTEN. We therefore examined PTEN expression in HUVEC cells transfected with miR-212/132 mimics and found that the expression of PTEN was significantly reduced in these cells (Figure 1D). In order to assess the relative effects of miR-212 versus miR-132, we examined the differential expression of these miRNA in different mouse tissues. miR-212 is found at extremely low levels in the tissues tested, except brain tissue (Figure 1F). Based on this information, we examined miR-132 expression in histology slides taken from ccRCC tumors using microRNA in situ hybridization. In agreement with our previous qPCR results, we observed widespread overexpression of miR-132 in tumor material from ccRCC samples with biallelic *VHL* mutations proven by sequencing (Figure 1E). These results demonstrate that miR-132 is increased in response to the pseudo-hypoxia induced by the lack of functional pVHL, which eventually leads to overexpression of miR-132.

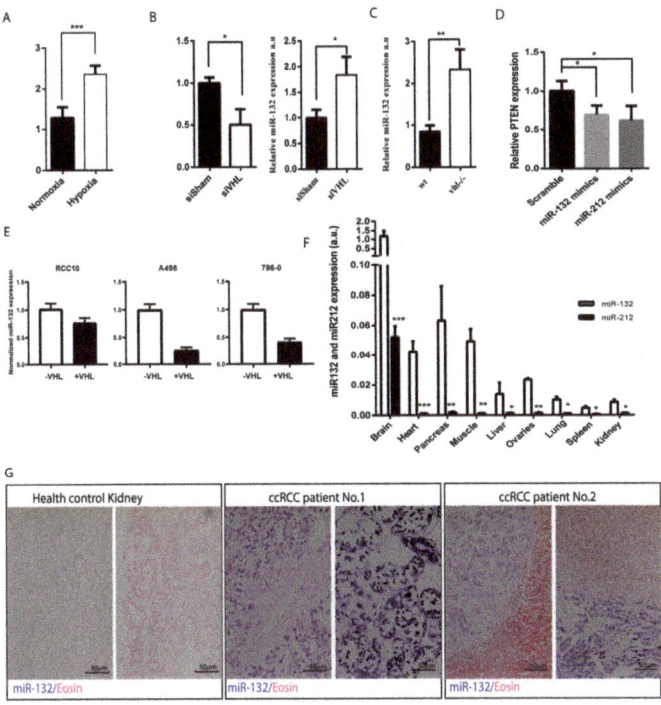

Figure 1. Characterization of miR-132 expression under hypoxic and pseudo-hypoxic conditions: (**A**) The expression of miR-132 in human umbilical vascular endothelial cells (HUVECs) under normoxia and hypoxia as compared by qPCR. (**B**) The expression of von Hippel–Lindau (VHL) in HUVECs after transfection with siRNA against VHL and the expression of miR-132 in siSham and siVHL transfected HUVECs as compared by qPCR. (**C**) The expression of miR-132 in wildtype (WT) and vhl$^{-/-}$ mutant zebrafish as compared by qPCR. (**D**) The expression of known miR 132 target PTEN (phosphatidylinositol-3,4,5-trisphosphate 3-phosphatase) in HUVECs treated with miR-132/212 mimics versus control as compared by qPCR. (**E**) The expression of miR-132 in established VHL$^{-/-}$ lines RCC10, A498, and 786-0 as well as the same lines reconstituted with ectopic VHL. The presented data is a mean of 3 in-depended PCR experiments with counting error. (**F**) Relative expression of miR-132 and 212 in different tissues in mouse. Note miR-132 expression is considerably higher than miR-212. $n = 3$. (**G**) The expression of miR-132 in healthy kidney tissue and ccRCC from two patients with known bilateral VHL mutations in their tumor as shown by miR-132 in situ hybridization. miR-132 in situ is in purple blue. Light eosin counterstaining appears pink. * $p < 0.05$; ** $p < 0.01$; *** $p < 0.001$

To assess the functional consequences of miR-212/132 expression in a *VHL*-null environment, we used an in vitro coculture assay designed to gauge angiogenesis. In agreement with the important role of VHL in HIF1 degradation, knockdown of VHL in HUVEC/pericyte coculture shows significantly more vascular junctions, tubule number, and total tubular length as compared to siSham control treatment (Figure 2A–C). To evaluate whether the pro-angiogenic effects of *VHL* silencing are mediated by a downstream increase in miR-212/132, GFP-labelled HUVECs were treated with anti-miRs against miR-212/132 in combination with siRNA targeting *VHL*. Inhibiting the action of miR-212/132 reduced the excessive angiogenetic response induced by the silencing of *VHL* significantly (Figure 2D), suggesting that VHL-regulated angiogenesis is at least partially mediated by the upregulation of miR-212/132.

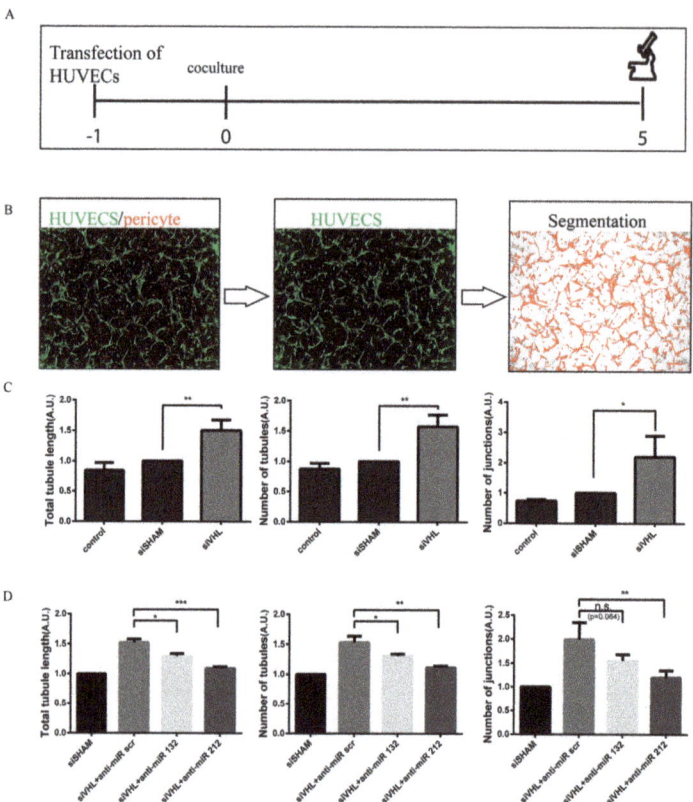

Figure 2. Reduced levels of VHL enhances endothelial cell neovascularization capacity and can be inhibited by blocking miR-132 or miR-212. (**A**) Schematic outline of the coculture experiment with HUVECs and pericytes. (**B**) Representative images showing the analysis process of tubular structures in the endothelial cells and pericytes coculture assay. (**C**) VHL siRNA knockdown in HUVECs enhances endothelial cell neovascularization capacity. (**D**) Blocking miR-132/212 inhibits neovascularization enhancement induced by VHL knockdown. Cell images are used to produce skeletonized 2D images which can be analyzed automatically. * $p < 0.05$; ** $p < 0.01$; *** $p < 0.001$

$vhl^{-/-}$ zebrafish embryos display a phenotype of post-vascularization branching/sprouting around the intersomitic vessels in the tails. Counting these sprouts is known as a quantitative measure of angiogenesis in zebrafish [13]. $vhl^{-/-}$ zebrafish were injected at a one-cell stage with anti-miRs directed against miR-132 or miR-212, and four days later, tails of the living fish were imaged with a confocal microscope (Figure 3A). The cloaca of the zebrafish is placed in the center of the image, and the branches sprouting from the inter-somitic vessels were counted for the four vessels anterior and the four vessels posterior to the cloaca (Figure 3B). Anti-miR injections against miR-212/132 significantly reduced the extent of intersomitic vessel sprouting in $vhl^{-/-}$ fish (Figure 3C,D). In addition, injecting wild-type zebrafish with miR-212/132 mimics partially recapitulated the *vhl* mutant vessel sprouting phenotype (Supplemental Figure S1C,D). In light of the fact that miR-212/132 expression is therefore linked to vessel sprouting in $vhl^{-/-}$ zebrafish, we proceeded to look at the expression of PTEN in our VHL-null models, as we had previously done in HUVECs. Zebrafish, as opposed to mammals, have two copies of the *pten* gene: *ptena* and *ptenb*. Zebrafish with loss of both *ptena* and *ptenb* [17] also display a vessel sprouting phenotype that phenocopies the one found in zebrafish injected with miR-212/132 mimics. *ptenb* is a predicted target of miR-212/132 in targetscan but not *ptena* (Supplemental Figure S1E). Accordingly, we found significantly reduced *ptenb* expression in $vhl^{-/-}$ zebrafish with no significant changes observed in *ptena* (Figure 4E).

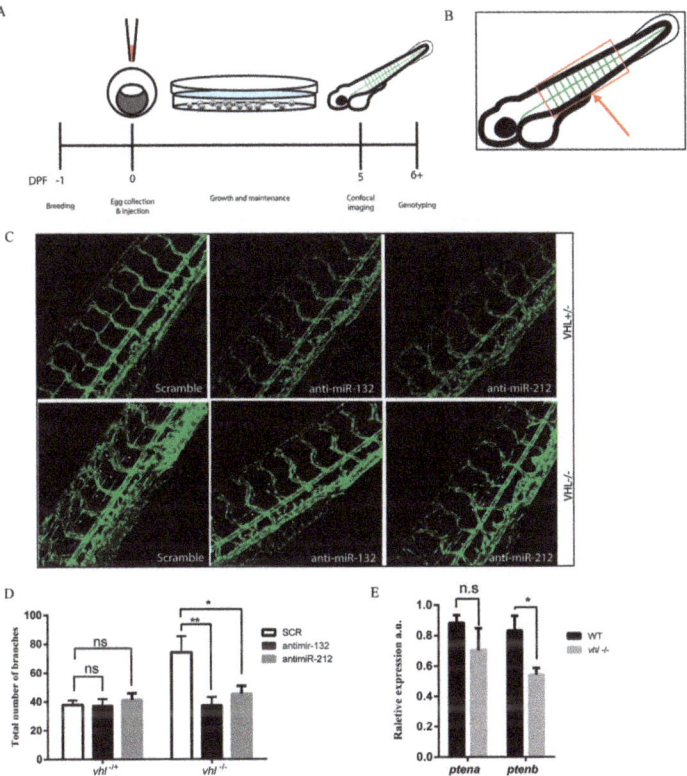

Figure 3. Inhibition of miR-132 or miR-212 suppresses VHL loss of function-induced vasculature outgrowth in zebrafish. (**A**) Schematic outline of the zebrafish embryo microinjection experiment. microRNA mimics and anti-miRs are injected into the yolk of the eggs on day 0 and imaged with a confocal microscope on day 5. (**B**) Schematic cartoon showing the area of the zebrafish embryo that is imaged after microinjection. The cloaca is marked with a red arrow. The imaging area is shown with a red box. The vessels of the tail are shown in green. (**C**) Representative images of zebrafish tail vascular structures in $vhl^{+/-}$ and $vhl^{-/-}$ zebrafish after injection with scrambled or miR-132 and miR-212 inhibitors. White arrows designate examples of structures which have been scored as branches. (**D**) Quantification of vascular branching in zebrafish tail structures after injection with scrambled control inhibitors, miR-132 inhibitors, or miR-212 inhibitors. (**E**) The expression levels of ptena and ptenb in WT and $vhl^{-/-}$ zebrafish determined by qPCR. * $p < 0.05$; ** $p < 0.01$.

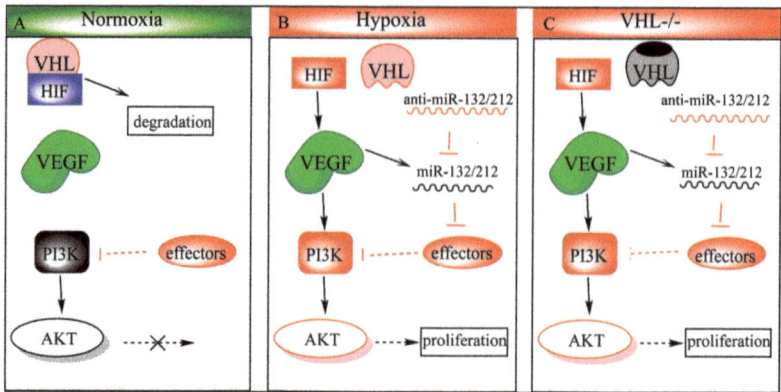

Figure 4. Proposed mechanism of miR-132/212 in modulation of the VHL/phosphatidylinositol-4, 5-bisphosphate 3-kinase (PI3K)/Protein kinase B(AKT)pathways. (**A**) During normoxia, hypoxia-inducible transcription factor 1 (HIF1) is ubiquitinated by the VHL-ubiquinition complex, targeting it for degradation. Some effectors, such as *PTEN*, antagonizes PI3k to prevent AKT from being activated. (**B**) Upon hypoxia, HIF1 can no longer be hydroxylated, which prohibits VHL-regulated degradation, and allows stabilized HIF1 to translocate to the nucleus, upregulating its downstream targets such as *vascular endothelial growth factor (VEGF)*. VEGF in turn activates the PI3k-AKT pathway and upregulates miR-132/212 expression as well. Upregulated miR-132/212 inhibits effector (e.g., *PTEN*) expression, which in turn prolongs AKT activity. (**C**) VHL loss-of-function phenocopies hypoxic conditions even in the presence of oxygen (pseudo-hypoxia).

4. Discussion

In this study, we used patient material, human cells, and zebrafish to examine the role of the miRNA-212/132 family in ccRCC tumor neovascularization caused by the loss-of-functional pVHL. We observed that miR-212/132 is upregulated in response to *VHL* mutation both in zebrafish model systems and in human patient ccRCC tumor material carrying biallelic inactivating *VHL* mutations. We demonstrated that the excessive angiogenesis attributable to *VHL* mutation is strongly affected by miR-212/132. Indeed, targeting these miRNAs with anti-miRs can significantly reduce angiogenesis in both in vitro and in vivo models of *VHL* deficiency. We identified the tumor suppressor PTEN as one of the targets affected by miRNA-212/132 in *VHL*-null models. Taken together, our results implicate miRNA-212/132 as an important intermediate in angiogenesis after loss-of-functional pVHL or tissue hypoxia.

The miR-212/132 family is clustered in the genome and is highly conserved in vertebrates. miR-212/132 is initially expressed as one primary miRNA and then processed into two mature miRNA with the same target-defining "seed" sequence [18]. This miRNA family plays a number of roles in the promotion of angiogenesis. Mice without functional miR-212/132 show impaired arteriogenesis response after hindlimb ischemia [19]. The pro-angiogenic potential of miR-132 has been used to increase angiogenesis in endothelial cell grafts and after ischemic injury [20]. miR-212/132 frequently act as a promoter of cell proliferation, and increases in their expression levels have also been suggested as contributors to tumorigenesis in addition to their angiogenic role. miR-132 has previously been shown to induce neovascularization in the endothelium by targeting p120 Ras GTPase-activating protein [5]. In addition, anti-miR-132 has also been shown to reduce tumor burden in a mouse xenograft model of human breast carcinoma [5].

This study supports the previously reported role of miR-212/132 in angiogenesis and expands upon its role in the context of VHL-regulated hypoxia signaling. When VHL is mutated or downregulated, miR-212/132 is consequently upregulated. miR-212/132 targeting of mRNA such as *PTEN* ensures that downstream effectors are upregulated. For example, in the case of *PTEN*, PI3K may activate AKT, leading to an increase in proliferation. Indeed, cysts taken from VHL patients display hyperactivation of PI3K signaling [21]. Due to technical reasons, we were not able to detect this increased AKT signaling directly in our zebrafish model. In addition, $Pten^{-/-} Vhl^{-/-}$ double mutant mice develop benign squamous metaplasia and cystadenoma [21] and display kidney cysts that are very similar to those taken from the kidneys of human VHL patients, while mouse models with Vhl mutations only do not develop renal tumors [22]. Uncontrolled proliferation and angiogenesis are hallmarks of cancer, and many tumors contain mutations leading to hyperactivation of signaling networks which act to promote these processes [23–25]. Differential expression of miRNA has been previously reported in tumors including ccRCC [26] and is widely believed to be an important player in tumorigenesis [27–29]. A group of miRs, termed hypoxamiRs, has been shown to be upregulated in hypoxia and play a role in the modulation of cellular responses to a lack of oxygen. The hypoxamiRs include miR-21; 23; 24; 26; 103/107; 373; and, most well studied, miR-210. Hypoxia is also considered a hallmark of the microenvironment of solid tumors, and a number of hypoxamiRs have been implicated in tumorigenesis [30,31]. Thus, the action of miRNA may play an important role in tumorigenesis and therefore presents an interesting potential target for the treatment of cancer.

One of the hallmarks of ccRCC is resistance to cytotoxic treatment. Antiapoptotic signaling is upregulated after HIF1α hyper-stabilization in ccRCC tumors. Many experimental treatments focus on inhibiting the action of downstream antiapoptosis proteins such as mammalian target of rapamycin (mTOR), an important pro-survival protein induced by activated AKT signaling [32]. Our results and the results of other studies suggest that miR-212/132 may act as a promoter of tumorigenesis by targeting inhibitors of proliferation, survival, and angiogenesis, presenting an interesting opportunity for pharmaceutical intervention. Currently, medications which target miRNA are largely unexplored as an avenue by which to target cancer. Here, we have shown that antagonizing the activity of this miRNA family can reduce angiogenesis in relevant models of VHL deficiency. $PTEN$, which we have confirmed to be a target of the miR-212/132 family in these models, is frequently mutated in cancer. Another miRNA, miRNA-21, has previously been shown to target PTEN in multiple cancer types and has been implicated in tumorigenesis [33]. Loss of PTEN leads to upregulation of mTOR signaling, and mTOR inhibitors have been used to treat multiple cancer types. Therefore, we envision that treatments designed to antagonize the effect of miRNA-212/132 or other miRNA might be able to reduce the angiogenic burden of tumors in patients, to reduce tumor resistance to other chemotherapeutic agents, or to slow or halt tumor growth.

Conversely, treatments with miR-212/132 might also be a useful method to promote angiogenesis and to increase neovascularization in the cases where neovascularization would be helpful, such as certain ischemic tissues or newly transplanted engineered tissue constructs. In fact, ex vivo transfection of mir-132 into endothelial cells has been shown to be beneficial for transplantation and vascularization of transplanted endothelial cells [34]. Based on our results and the results of other studies, further work is warranted in this area.

Supplementary Materials: The following are available online at http://www.mdpi.com/2073-4409/9/4/1017/s1, Figure S1: Upreguation of miR-132/212 improve neovascularization in WT Zebrafish.

Author Contributions: Z.L., T.D.K., J.P.G.S., and R.H.G. conceived and designed the experiments. T.D.K., Z.L., M.M.B., G.v.d.H. and I.L. performed the experiments. C.C., P.A.D., J.P.G.S. and R.H.G supervise the study. T.D.K., Z.L., and M.M.B. analysed the data. T.D.K., Z.L., P.A.D., C.C., J.P.G.S., and R.H.G. wrote the paper. All authors have read and agreed to the published version of the manuscript.

Funding: This research forms part of the Project P1.05 LUST of the research program of the BioMedical Materials institute, cofunded by the Dutch Ministry of Economic Affairs. We furthermore acknowledge the financial support of the European Community's Seventh Framework Programme FP7 under grant agreement numbers 305608 (EURONOMICS) and 241955 (SYSCILIA); the Dutch Kidney Foundation Consortium CP11.18 "KOUNCIL"; and the Netherlands CardioVascular Research Initiative (CVON): the Dutch Heart Foundation, Dutch Federation of University Medical Centers, the Netherlands Organization for Health Research and Development, and the Royal Netherlands Academy of Sciences, CUREPLaN foundation Leducq (P.D.). This project was supported by the project EVICARE (No.725229) of the European Research Council (ERC) to J.P.G.S; by NOW-CAS grant (116006102) to P.D. and J.S.

Conflicts of Interest: The authors declare no conflict of interest.

References

1. Baldewijns, M.M.; van Vlodrop, I.J.; Vermeulen, P.B.; Soetekouw, P.M.; van Engeland, M.; de Bruine, A.P. VHL and HIF signalling in renal cell carcinogenesis. *J. Pathol.* **2010**, *221*, 125–138. [CrossRef]
2. Cancer Genome Atlas Network. Comprehensive molecular characterization of human colon and rectal cancer. *Nature* **2012**, *487*, 330–337. [CrossRef]
3. Frantzen, C.; Kruizinga, R.C.; van Asselt, S.J.; Zonnenberg, B.A.; Lenders, J.W.; de Herder, W.W.; Walenkamp, A.M.; Giles, R.H.; Hes, F.J.; Sluiter, W.J.; et al. Pregnancy-related hemangioblastoma progression and complications in von Hippel-Lindau disease. *Neurology* **2012**, *79*, 793–796. [CrossRef] [PubMed]
4. Shen, J.; Hung, M.C. Signaling-mediated regulation of MicroRNA processing. *Cancer Res.* **2015**. [CrossRef] [PubMed]
5. Anand, S.; Majeti, B.K.; Acevedo, L.M.; Murphy, E.A.; Mukthavaram, R.; Scheppke, L.; Huang, M.; Shields, D.J.; Lindquist, J.N.; Lapinski, P.E.; et al. MicroRNA-132-mediated loss of p120RasGAP activates the endothelium to facilitate pathological angiogenesis. *Nat. Med.* **2010**, *16*, 909–914. [CrossRef] [PubMed]
6. Qian, C.N. Hijacking the vasculature in ccRCC—Co-option, remodelling and angiogenesis. *Nat. Rev. Urol.* **2013**, *10*, 300–304. [CrossRef] [PubMed]
7. Schmid, T.A.; Gore, M.E. Sunitinib in the treatment of metastatic renal cell carcinoma. *Adv. Urol.* **2016**, *8*, 348–371. [CrossRef] [PubMed]
8. Rouwkema, J.; Rivron, N.C.; van Blitterswijk, C.A. Vascularization in tissue engineering. *Trends Biotechnol.* **2008**, *26*, 434–441. [CrossRef]
9. Lei, Z.; van Mil, A.; Xiao, J.; Metz, C.H.G.; van Eeuwijk, E.C.M.; Doevendans, P.A.; Sluijter, J.P.G. MMISH: Multicolor microRNA in situ hybridization for paraffin embedded samples. *Biotechnol. Rep. (Amst)* **2018**, *18*, e00255. [CrossRef]
10. Nordstrom-O'Brien, M.; van der Luijt, R.B.; van Rooijen, E.; van den Ouweland, A.M.; Majoor-Krakauer, D.F.; Lolkema, M.P.; van Brussel, A.; Voest, E.E.; Giles, R.H. Genetic analysis of von Hippel-Lindau disease. *Hum. Mutat.* **2010**, *31*, 521–537. [CrossRef]
11. Stratman, A.N.; Malotte, K.M.; Mahan, R.D.; Davis, M.J.; Davis, G.E. Pericyte recruitment during vasculogenic tube assembly stimulates endothelial basement membrane matrix formation. *Blood* **2009**, *114*, 5091–5101. [CrossRef] [PubMed]
12. Van Rooijen, E.; Voest, E.E.; Logister, I.; Korving, J.; Schwerte, T.; Schulte-Merker, S.; Giles, R.H.; van Eeden, F.J. Zebrafish mutants in the von Hippel-Lindau tumor suppressor display a hypoxic response and recapitulate key aspects of Chuvash polycythemia. *Blood* **2009**, *113*, 6449–6460. [CrossRef] [PubMed]
13. Van Rooijen, E.; Voest, E.E.; Logister, I.; Bussmann, J.; Korving, J.; van Eeden, F.J.; Giles, R.H.; Schulte-Merker, S. von Hippel-Lindau tumor suppressor mutants faithfully model pathological hypoxia-driven angiogenesis and vascular retinopathies in zebrafish. *Dis. Models Mech.* **2010**, *3*, 343–353. [CrossRef]
14. Van Rooijen, E.; Santhakumar, K.; Logister, I.; Voest, E.; Schulte-Merker, S.; Giles, R.; van Eeden, F. A zebrafish model for VHL and hypoxia signaling. *Methods Cell Biol.* **2011**, *105*, 163–190. [CrossRef] [PubMed]
15. Jiang, B.H.; Liu, L.Z. PI3K/PTEN signaling in angiogenesis and tumorigenesis. *Adv. Cancer Res.* **2009**, *102*, 19–65. [CrossRef]
16. Jin, W.; Reddy, M.A.; Chen, Z.; Putta, S.; Lanting, L.; Kato, M.; Park, J.T.; Chandra, M.; Wang, C.; Tangirala, R.K.; et al. Small RNA sequencing reveals microRNAs that modulate angiotensin II effects in vascular smooth muscle cells. *J. Biol. Chem.* **2012**, *287*, 15672–15683. [CrossRef]
17. Choorapoikayil, S.; Weijts, B.; Kers, R.; de Bruin, A.; den Hertog, J. Loss of Pten promotes angiogenesis and enhanced vegfaa expression in zebrafish. *Dis. Models Mech.* **2013**, *6*, 1159–1166. [CrossRef]
18. Remenyi, J.; Hunter, C.J.; Cole, C.; Ando, H.; Impey, S.; Monk, C.E.; Martin, K.J.; Barton, G.J.; Hutvagner, G.; Arthur, J.S. Regulation of the miR-212/132 locus by MSK1 and CREB in response to neurotrophins. *Biochem. J.* **2010**, *428*, 281–291. [CrossRef]
19. Lei, Z.; van Mil, A.; Brandt, M.M.; Grundmann, S.; Hoefer, I.; Smits, M.; El Azzouzi, H.; Fukao, T.; Cheng, C.; Doevendans, P.A.; et al. MicroRNA-132/212 family enhances arteriogenesis after hindlimb ischaemia through modulation of the Ras-MAPK pathway. *J. Cell. Mol. Med.* **2015**. [CrossRef]

20. Gomes, R.S.; das Neves, R.P.; Cochlin, L.; Lima, A.; Carvalho, R.; Korpisalo, P.; Dragneva, G.; Turunen, M.; Liimatainen, T.; Clarke, K.; et al. Efficient pro-survival/angiogenic miRNA delivery by an MRI-detectable nanomaterial. *ACS Nano* **2013**, *7*, 3362–3372. [CrossRef]
21. Frew, I.J.; Minola, A.; Georgiev, S.; Hitz, M.; Moch, H.; Richard, S.; Vortmeyer, A.O.; Krek, W. Combined VHLH and PTEN mutation causes genital tract cystadenoma and squamous metaplasia. *Mol. Cell. Biol.* **2008**, *28*, 4536–4548. [CrossRef] [PubMed]
22. Ma, W.; Tessarollo, L.; Hong, S.-B.; Baba, M.; Southon, E.; Back, T.C.; Spence, S.; Lobe, C.G.; Sharma, N.; Maher, G.W. Hepatic vascular tumors, angiectasis in multiple organs, and impaired spermatogenesis in mice with conditional inactivation of the VHL gene. *Cancer Res.* **2003**, *63*, 5320–5328. [PubMed]
23. Kumar, A.; Rajendran, V.; Sethumadhavan, R.; Purohit, R. AKT kinase pathway: A leading target in cancer research. *Sci. World J.* **2013**, *2013*, 756134. [CrossRef] [PubMed]
24. Hubbard, P.A.; Moody, C.L.; Murali, R. Allosteric modulation of Ras and the PI3K/AKT/mTOR pathway: Emerging therapeutic opportunities. *Front. Physiol.* **2014**, *5*, 478. [CrossRef] [PubMed]
25. Samatar, A.A.; Poulikakos, P.I. Targeting RAS-ERK signalling in cancer: Promises and challenges. *Nat. Rev. Drug Discov.* **2014**, *13*, 928–942. [CrossRef]
26. Ge, Y.Z.; Wu, R.; Xin, H.; Zhu, M.; Lu, T.Z.; Liu, H.; Xu, Z.; Yu, P.; Zhao, Y.C.; Li, M.H.; et al. A tumor-specific microRNA signature predicts survival in clear cell renal cell carcinoma. *J. Cancer Res. Clin. Oncol.* **2015**. [CrossRef]
27. Acunzo, M.; Romano, G.; Wernicke, D.; Croce, C.M. MicroRNA and cancer—A brief overview. *Adv. Biol. Regul.* **2015**, *57*, 1–9. [CrossRef]
28. Braicu, C.; Cojocneanu-Petric, R.; Chira, S.; Truta, A.; Floares, A.; Petrut, B.; Achimas-Cadariu, P.; Berindan-Neagoe, I. Clinical and pathological implications of miRNA in bladder cancer. *Int. J. Nanomed.* **2015**, *10*, 791–800. [CrossRef]
29. Qin, X.; Xu, H.; Gong, W.; Deng, W. The Tumor Cytosol miRNAs, Fluid miRNAs, and Exosome miRNAs in lung cancer. *Front. Oncol.* **2014**, *4*, 357. [CrossRef]
30. Greco, S.; Martelli, F. MicroRNAs in hypoxia response. *Antioxid. Redox Signal.* **2014**, *21*, 1164–1166. [CrossRef]
31. Gee, H.E.; Ivan, C.; Calin, G.A.; Ivan, M. HypoxamiRs and cancer: From biology to targeted therapy. *Antioxid. Redox Signal.* **2014**, *21*, 1220–1238. [CrossRef] [PubMed]
32. Lin, Y.C.; Lu, L.T.; Chen, H.Y.; Duan, X.; Lin, X.; Feng, X.H.; Tang, M.J.; Chen, R.H. SCP phosphatases suppress renal cell carcinoma by stabilizing PML and inhibiting mTOR/HIF signaling. *Cancer Res.* **2014**, *74*, 6935–6946. [CrossRef]
33. Leslie, N.R.; Foti, M. Non-genomic loss of PTEN function in cancer: Not in my genes. *Trends Pharm. Sci.* **2011**, *32*, 131–140. [CrossRef] [PubMed]
34. Devalliere, J.; Chang, W.G.; Andrejecsk, J.W.; Abrahimi, P.; Cheng, C.J.; Jane-wit, D.; Saltzman, W.M.; Pober, J.S. Sustained delivery of proangiogenic microRNA-132 by nanoparticle transfection improves endothelial cell transplantation. *FASEB J.* **2014**, *28*, 908–922. [CrossRef] [PubMed]

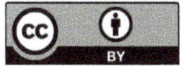

© 2020 by the authors. Licensee MDPI, Basel, Switzerland. This article is an open access article distributed under the terms and conditions of the Creative Commons Attribution (CC BY) license (http://creativecommons.org/licenses/by/4.0/).

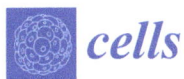

Review

An Emerging Role for isomiRs and the microRNA Epitranscriptome in Neovascularization

Reginald V.C.T. van der Kwast [1], Paul H.A. Quax [1] and A. Yaël Nossent [1,2,*]

1. Department of Surgery and Einthoven Laboratory for Experimental Vascular Medicine, Leiden University Medical Center, 2333 ZA Leiden, The Netherlands; rvdkwast@lumc.nl (R.V.C.T.v.d.K.); P.H.A.Quax@lumc.nl (P.H.A.Q.)
2. Department of Laboratory Medicine and Department of Internal Medicine II, Medical University of Vienna, 1090 Vienna, Austria
* Correspondence: a.y.nossent@lumc.nl

Received: 29 November 2019; Accepted: 21 December 2019; Published: 25 December 2019

Abstract: Therapeutic neovascularization can facilitate blood flow recovery in patients with ischemic cardiovascular disease, the leading cause of death worldwide. Neovascularization encompasses both angiogenesis, the sprouting of new capillaries from existing vessels, and arteriogenesis, the maturation of preexisting collateral arterioles into fully functional arteries. Both angiogenesis and arteriogenesis are highly multifactorial processes that require a multifactorial regulator to be stimulated simultaneously. MicroRNAs can regulate both angiogenesis and arteriogenesis due to their ability to modulate expression of many genes simultaneously. Recent studies have revealed that many microRNAs have variants with altered terminal sequences, known as isomiRs. Additionally, endogenous microRNAs have been identified that carry biochemically modified nucleotides, revealing a dynamic microRNA epitranscriptome. Both types of microRNA alterations were shown to be dynamically regulated in response to ischemia and are able to influence neovascularization by affecting the microRNA's biogenesis, or even its silencing activity. Therefore, these novel regulatory layers influence microRNA functioning and could provide new opportunities to stimulate neovascularization. In this review we will highlight the formation and function of isomiRs and various forms of microRNA modifications, and discuss recent findings that demonstrate that both isomiRs and microRNA modifications directly affect neovascularization and vascular remodeling.

Keywords: microRNA; isomiRs; epitranscriptome; neovascularization; angiogenesis; arteriogenesis; A-to-I editing; m6A; RNA modifications; RNA methylation

---

1. Introduction

Ischemic cardiovascular disease (CVD) is the leading cause of death in worldwide and was responsible for approximately 17.8 million deaths in 2017 [1,2]. Additionally, it is estimated that current standard therapies are unsuitable or insufficient for 30% of patients [3,4]. Therefore, there is a critical need for new therapeutic treatments for ischemic CVD.

A potential strategy to treat patients with ischemia is to stimulate neovascularization, which is the body's natural repair mechanism to restore blood flow to ischemic tissues. Postnatal neovascularization is comprised of angiogenesis, the sprouting of new capillaries from existing vessels, and arteriogenesis, the maturation of preexisting collateral arterioles into fully functional arteries. Both angiogenesis and arteriogenesis are highly multifactorial processes that involve multiple types of vascular and immune cells. In order to improve neovascularization as a whole, therapeutic strategies which simultaneously target both angiogenesis and arteriogenesis are needed [5,6].

During the last decade, microRNAs have emerged as multifactorial regulators of neovascularization [7–9]. MicroRNAs are short non-coding RNAs of approximately 22 nucleotides that inhibit translation of messenger RNAs (mRNAs). A single microRNA can have hundreds of mRNAs in its 'targetome', often regulating an entire network or pathway simultaneously [10]. MicroRNAs are typically defined as one specific sequence of RNA nucleotides, however, recent studies have shown that this 'canonical' microRNA sequence is often altered. These microRNA alterations can be grouped into two types: (i) isomiRs, which are microRNAs with altered terminal sequences and (ii) biochemical modifications of specific nucleotides within microRNAs, which collectively are referred to as the microRNA epitranscriptome. Both types of microRNA variations appear actively regulated in response to ischemia and can directly influence neovascularization associated processes, as we will discuss below. The microRNA epitranscriptome unveils a whole new regulatory layer that could provide novel therapeutic options for ischemic CVD. In this review we will first briefly introduce the processes involved in angiogenesis and arteriogenesis, after which we will highlight various ways in which a microRNA can be altered, and discuss recent findings which demonstrate that these microRNA alterations can affect neovascularization associated processes.

2. Neovascularization—Angiogenesis and Arteriogenesis

After the occlusion of a large artery, blood flow to the downstream tissues is hampered, causing ischemia. Blood flow towards the ischemic tissue can be restored by a process called arteriogenesis. Arteriogenesis is the growth and maturation of collateral arteries from a pre-existing arteriole network, which connects all major arteries in the body [5]. Arteriogenesis is triggered by an increase in shear stress in the arterioles, which occurs after an arterial occlusion causes redirection of blood flow through the arterioles. The increased shear stress causes endothelial cells (ECs) in the arteriole wall to express adhesion molecules and secrete cytokines, leading to the attraction of circulating monocytes and other immune cells [11–15]. These inflammatory cells produce and secrete proteases, growth factors, and cytokines which enable remodeling of the vessel wall and stimulate migration and proliferation of vascular ECs and smooth muscle cells (SMCs) [16–18]. This results in an increase in vessel diameter, until fluid sheer stress decreases which halts the arteriogenic process. Finally, the vascular SMCs and fibroblasts secrete matrix components to reconstitute the vessel wall [19,20].

The process of angiogenesis, on the other hand, is the sprouting of a new capillary from the existing vasculature in order to redistribute local blood flow towards ischemic areas. Unlike arteriogenesis, angiogenesis is driven by the hypoxia caused by ischemia, and revolves around resolving local ischemia rather than restoring arterial blood flow after the occlusion of a vessel. Angiogenesis is initiated when an angiogenic stimulus, produced by hypoxic cells, activates the vascular endothelial layer. Activated ECs will start to proliferate and migrate towards the stimulus, such as vascular endothelial growth factor (VEGF), resulting in a new capillary [21]. Next to ECs, other cell types are important regulators of angiogenesis. Vascular SMCs, pericytes, fibroblasts and immune cells play key roles by supporting and modulating EC function and secreting the proangiogenic stimuli to start the process [22–24].

Since both angiogenesis and arteriogenesis are highly multifactorial processes, the simultaneous stimulation of both processes requires a multifactorial regulator, like microRNAs [7,8].

3. MicroRNAs

MicroRNAs are endogenous, small non-coding RNA molecules that inhibit translation of mRNAs. The microRNA's target selection is predominantly determined by the microRNA's 'seed sequence', nucleotides 2–8 at the 5'-end of a microRNA [25,26], which bind their target mRNAs via Watson–Crick base-pairing. Due to this relatively small targeting sequence, a single microRNA's 'targetome' can consist of hundreds of mRNAs, enabling microRNAs to regulate multifactorial processes [10].

The biogenesis of microRNAs starts with the transcription of the microRNA containing gene, yielding a primary microRNA (pri-miR) which then undergoes several steps of maturation to form the mature and functional microRNA (Figure 1) [27]. First, the pri-miR is cleaved in the nucleus by Drosha to generate a hairpin-shaped precursor microRNA (pre-miR) [28]. The pre-miR is then translocated to the cytoplasm where a final cleavage is performed by Dicer, yielding a microRNA duplex [29]. Either side of the duplex can associate with Argonaute proteins and become a functional mature microRNA after incorporation into the RNA-induced silencing complex (RISC) [30]. Mature microRNAs are named after their side, 5′ or 3′, in the pri-miR hairpin (e.g., miR-#-5p or -3p).

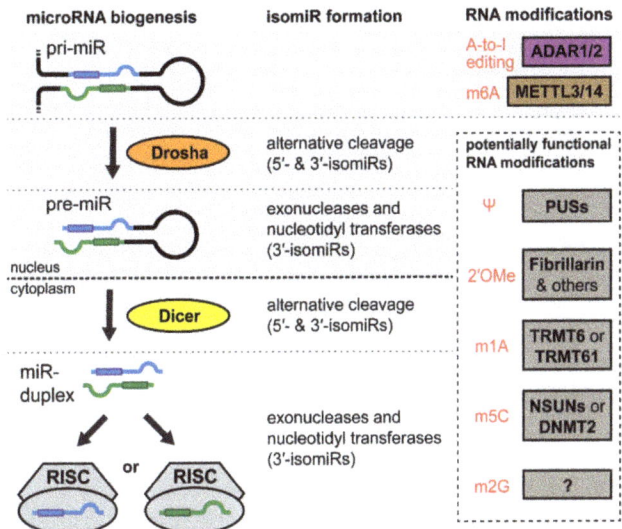

Figure 1. MicroRNA biogenesis and alterations that induce isomiR formation or microRNA nucleotide modifications. Transcription of the microRNA containing gene forms the primary microRNA (pri-miR). Drosha cleaves the pri-miR to generate the precursor microRNA (pre-miR). The pre-miR cleaved by Dicer in the cytoplasm yielding the microRNA duplex. Either side of the duplex can be incorporated into the RNA-induced silencing complex (RISC) to become a functional mature microRNA. IsomiRs can be formed during microRNA biogenesis when Drosha or Dicer cleave in alternative locations, or when exonucleases or nucleotidyl transferases remove or add nucleotides to the 3′-end of the pre-miR or the mature microRNA. RNA nucleotide modifications with known or potential functional implications on microRNA biogenesis or functioning are shown in red with their 'writers' next to them.

MicroRNA biogenesis is strictly regulated, even at a microRNA-specific level, by numerous factors, including DNA methylation, activity modulation of key maturation proteins and many RNA-binding proteins [29,31–33]. As a result, microRNA expression is often highly tissue specific and is dynamically regulated during key physiological processes, including the response to ischemia [29,34].

In 2007, the importance of microRNAs in neovascularization was demonstrated for the first time when several studies showed that Dicer-dependent microRNAs were required for angiogenesis [35–37]. Since then, microRNAs have been shown to play a functional role in all processes involved in neovascularization, including production and secretion of angiogenic stimuli, as well as EC, SMC, fibroblast and immune cell proliferation, migration and activation, which have recently been reviewed in references [8,38–40]. Several of these vasoactive microRNAs have also been well described to play an important role in vascular remodeling during ischemic cardiovascular diseases [8,41].

For example, Bonauer et al. showed that miR-92a is highly expressed in human ECs and functions as negative regulator of angiogenesis [42]. Inhibition of miR-92a increased angiogenesis in vivo and improved blood flow recovery after hindlimb ischemia [42]. Furthermore, administration of miR-92a inhibitors in porcine models for myocardial infarction demonstrated that miR-92 inhibition prevents adverse infarct remodeling and ischemia/reperfusion injury [43,44]. Phase 1 trials aimed to improve wound healing with a future potential clinical application towards heart failure treatment have recently been completed for miR-92a inhibitor MRG 110 (NCT03603431) [45].

Both miR-126-3p and -5p are also highly expressed in ECs where they promote angiogenesis by stimulating EC proliferation and VEGF signaling and regulating leukocyte adhesion [46–49]. Inhibition of miR-126-3p was shown to decrease recovery after myocardial infarction and hindlimb ischemia in mice [47,50,51]. Furthermore, miR-126 levels are decreased in patients with ischemic coronary artery disease [52]. Similarly, miR-10a also stimulates angiogenesis by promoting VEGF signaling in ECs and regulating their inflammatory phenotype [53–57].

MiR-21-5p regulates proliferation and apoptosis of vascular wall smooth muscle cells [58,59] and promotes fibrosis by stimulating fibroblast survival and growth factor secretion [60]. Preclinical studies have shown that inhibition of miR-21-5p can prevent maladaptive vascular remodeling and heart failure [59,60]. These findings suggest that the miR-21-5p inhibitor RG-012, which is currently being tested in a phase 2 clinical trial to prevent kidney fibrosis in patients with Alport syndrome (NCT02855268), could potentially be used for the treatment of CVD.

Additionally, it is noteworthy that several groups of genomically clustered microRNAs have been identified that are able to broadly regulate neovascularization in response to ischemia: Knockout of the miR-17/92 gene cluster (located on chromosome 14 in mice and on human chromosome 13) increased both angiogenesis and arteriogenesis [61,62], while the inhibition of individual microRNAs from the 14q32 microRNA cluster (located on chromosome 12F1 in mice and on human chromosome 14) was shown to independently stimulate both angiogenesis and arteriogenesis [9].

4. IsomiRs and the microRNA Epitranscriptome

Typically, microRNAs have been defined as a single sequence of RNA nucleotides, and are listed as such in the principle public microRNA database, miRbase [63]. However, recent studies have shown that this 'canonical' microRNA sequence can be altered. These microRNA alterations can be separated into two types: isomiRs and RNA nucleotide modifications.

IsomiRs are microRNA sequence variants that have one or more nucleotides added or deleted at their 5'- and/or 3'-ends compared to the canonical microRNA sequence.

RNA nucleotide modifications are biochemical modifications of the standard RNA nucleotides, which are performed by enzymes present in all living organisms. Recent studies have demonstrated that these RNA nucleotide modifications have a functional regulatory role and form what has been named the 'epitranscriptome' [64]. While many different RNA nucleotide modifications exist, only a few have been studied in the context of microRNAs: Adenosine-to-inosine editing (A-to-I editing) and N6-adenosine methylation (m6A) and 2'-O-methylation (2'OMe).

Below, we will discuss those studies that demonstrate that isomiRs and microRNA A-to-I editing and m6A can be actively regulated and play a directing role in neovascularization, as well as other modifications (including 2'OMe) that are likely to have a similar role.

5. IsomiRs

5.1. IsomiRs

IsomiRs were discovered when microRNA sequencing studies observed that many microRNAs had sequence variants with one or more nucleotides added or deleted from the 5'- and/or 3'-ends compared to the 'canonical' microRNA sequence [65,66]. While initially dismissed as errors or artifacts, isomiRs have since been shown to be functional microRNAs which actively associate with the RISC complex and inhibit mRNA translation of their targets [67–70]. Furthermore, sequencing studies have shown that isomiRs are widespread and represent approximately 50% of the microRNA transcripts present in cells and tissue [71,72].

IsomiRs are primarily generated by cleavage variations of either DROSHA or DICER during microRNA biogenesis (Figure 1) [68,73]. IsomiRs with altered 3'-end sequences, 3'-isomiRs, can also be created by exonucleases which remove 3' nucleotides, or by nucleotidyl transferases, which catalyze the addition of 3′ nucleotides. The number and type of isomiRs that arise from a single locus varies per microRNA, but approximately 75% of microRNA loci give rise to at least one isomiR [74].

In general, 3′-isomiRs are more abundant than 5′-isomiRs, however, a number of microRNAs do have prevalent 5′-isomiRs [75–78]. Since a microRNA's 5′-end determines its seed sequence, 5′-isomiRs have an altered targetome compared to the canonical microRNA sequence and are thus functionally different (Figure 2) [67,79–81]. While 3′-isomiRs do not have an altered seed sequence, their 3′-end variability has been associated with altered microRNA stability and turnover [82–86]. Furthermore, recent findings have shown that changes in microRNA length due to 3′-end variation can affect microRNA targeting strength and activity in specific cases [87,88]. Combined, these findings highlight the importance to take isomiRs into account during microRNA research.

		Mechanisms of formation	Potential effects
pri-miR-21 sequence	CGGGUAGCUUAUCAGACUGAUGUUGACUGU		
canonical miR-21-5p	5′ UAGCUUAUCAGACUGAUGUUGA 3′	• canonical biogenesis	• canonical function
5′-isomiRs	AGCUUAUCAGACUGAUGUUGA GUAGCUUAUCAGACUGAUGUUGA	• alternative cleavage by Dicer or Drosha	• altered targetome • length-dependent effects
3′-isomiRs	UAGCUUAUCAGACUGAUGUUGAC UAGCUUAUCAGACUGAUG UAGCUUAUCAGACUGAUGUUGAA	• alternative cleavage by Dicer or Drosha • exonuclease or nucleotidyl transferase activity	• altered stability and/or turnover • length-dependent effects
5′- & 3′-isomiRs	AGCUUAUCAGACUGAUGUUGAC UAGCUUAUCAGACUGAUGUUGACA AGCUUAUCAGACUGAUGUUGACA	• alternative cleavage by Dicer and/or Drosha • exonuclease or nucleotidyl transferase activity	• altered targetome • altered stability and/or turnover • length-dependent effects

Figure 2. Different types of isomiRs, their mechanism of formation and their potential functional effects. The sequence of miR-21 and some of its isomiRs are shown to exemplify the different isomiR types. In each case, the seed sequence is underlined (red if altered) and red nucleotides are due to nucleotidyl transferase activity. Relative to the canonical microRNA, 5′-isomiRs generally have an altered targetome due to shift in seed sequence whereas 3′-isomiRs can affect the microRNAs stability or turnover. Both types of isomiRs affect the length of the microRNA and can thus incur length-dependent effects.

5.2. IsomiRs in Neovascularization Associated Cells and Processes

Due to the prevalence of isomiRs, most microRNAs that are known regulators of neovascularization have isomiRs. In fact, the microRNA loci with the most known isomiRs are miR-21-5p (Figure 2) and miR-10a-5p, two microRNAs with well-established roles in vascular biology and neovascularization [53–57], which have at least 40 isomiRs each [74]. MiR-21-5p isomiRs were found to be highly expressed in endothelial cells, as well as, miR-126-5p and -3p and their isomiRs, which are also well-established vasoactive microRNAs [8,89–91]. Combined, the miR-21-5p and miR-126 transcripts accounted for almost 40% of the total endothelial microRNA transcripts detected, including at least two 5′-isomiRs with physiologically relevant abundance [89,91]. One of these studies reported that approximately 55% of the total microRNA transcripts detected in human umbilical vein endothelial cells (HUVECs) were in fact isomiRs originating from 230 distinct microRNA loci [89]. For 33 of these microRNA loci, the isomiR variant was the most abundant form, rather than the canonical sequence. Since isomiRs often have altered stability and turnover [83–86], these abundant isomiRs could help regulate vasoactive microRNA expression. Furthermore, abundant 5′-isomiRs are likely to be functionally important due to their altered seed sequence and thus targetome.

IsomiR expression profiles can vary based on cell type and in response to biological stimuli, including stimuli associated with neovascularization [75,76,78,92]. For example, Voellenke et al. examined isomiR expression of normoxic and hypoxic human umbilical vein endothelial cells (HUVECs) using deep sequencing [89]. While the study lacked the power to identify any statistically significant patterns, the authors did observe that hypoxic conditions altered isomiR expression. Furthermore, Nejad et al. demonstrated that treating fibroblasts with interferon-beta, a regulatory factor in both angiogenesis and arteriogenesis [93–95], specifically decreased expression of the longer 3′-isomiRs from 13 microRNA loci, while the shorter isomiRs were generally upregulated [96]. Among the regulated microRNAs was miR-222-3p, which has been shown to regulate angiogenesis and inflammation-mediated vascular remodeling [97,98]. Interestingly, the longer 3'-isomiRs of miR-222-3p (>22 nt) were previously found to increase apoptotic activity, whereas the shorter isomiRs did not, suggesting the altered 3'-isomiR profiles could also be functionally important [88]. However, the exact factors that mediate the isomiR-specific regulation remain to be uncovered. It is likely that, similar to canonical microRNA biogenesis, isomiR biogenesis is regulated by a multitude of factors, including factors which specifically regulate individual isomiRs [29,31,68].

We have recently performed a focused study on the 5'-isomiR of miR-411-5p from the vasoactive 14q32 microRNA cluster in order to collect direct evidence that isomiRs are actively regulated during ischemia-induced neovascularization [99]. We found that miR-411's isomiR expression profile was tissue-specific and that canonical miR-411-5p was less abundant than its 5'-isomiR in human vascular ECs, fibroblasts and in whole human venous tissue. We discovered that the expression of the 5'-isomiR is decreased relative to canonical miR-411-5p expression in response to acute ischemia, both in cells and in a murine model for effective neovascularization after ischemia [99]. Strikingly, the relative 5'-isomiR expression was upregulated instead in ischemic veins from patients with critical limb ischemia due to peripheral artery disease (PAD). We demonstrated that the 5'-isomiR has a different targetome than the canonical miR-411-5p and inhibits translation of, among others, the pro-angiogenic Angiopoietin-1. Finally, we showed that the 5'-isomiR decreases vascular cell migration while the canonical miR-411-5p does not [99]. Combined these data show that isomiR formation is indeed a functional pathway, which is actively regulated during ischemia, with direct implications for neovascularization.

Table 1 presents a summary of the key studies that demonstrate the prevalence and importance of isomiRs.

Table 1. Key studies demonstrating the prevalence and importance of isomiRs.

Topic	Key Findings	References
Prevalence of isomiRs	• Generally, isomiRs represent ~50% of microRNA transcripts in cells and tissues (~55% in HUVECs)	[71,72,89,91]
	• ~75% of microRNA loci can produce at least 1 isomiR	[74]
Potential functional effect of isomiRs	• 5'-isomiRs have altered targetome due to a shifted seed sequence compared to the cannonical microRNA	[67,79–81,99]
	• 3'-isomiRs can have altered microRNA stability and turnover	[82–86]
	• isomiRs with different length can have altered targeting strength and activity	[87,88]
Abundant vasoactive microRNAs with isomiRs	• miR-21-5p (at least 43 potential isomiRs, also in HUVECs)	[74,89,91]
	• miR-10a-5p (at least 41 isomiRs)	[74]
	• miR-126 (highly abundant in HUVECs together with miR-21-5p and its isomiRs)	[89,91]
	• miR-222-3p (has functionally different 3'-isomiRs)	[88,96]
	• miR-411-5p (5'-isomiR has altered functionality and anti-angiogenic properties)	[99]
Regulation of isomiRs	• IsomiR expression profiles can vary based on cell type and in response to biological stimuli	[75,76,78,92]
	• Hypoxic HUVECs display altered isomiR expression	[89]
	• Independent regulation of miR-411-5p and its 5'-isomiR in response to ischemia	[99]

HUVECs: human umbilical vein endothelial cells.

6. Adenosine-to-Inosine Editing

6.1. Adenosine-to-Inosine Editing

A-to-I editing is the biochemical modification of adenosines into inosines by deamination. Unlike adenosine, inosine preferentially binds to cytidine and is therefore generally interpreted as guanosine by the cellular machinery [100]. This form of RNA editing can have a number of consequences on RNA functioning, ranging from destabilizing the RNA molecules' secondary structure to altering a protein amino acid sequence due to editing of the mRNA's coding sequence [101–103]. In mammals, A-to-I editing accounts for more than 90% of all RNA editing events and is catalyzed by either ADAR1 or ADAR2 (adenosine deaminase acting on RNA 1 or 2), which are expressed throughout the body [104–106]. The removal of the editing activity of either ADAR1 or ADAR2 in mice leads to premature lethality, demonstrating that A-to-I editing is of vital importance [107–109]. However, the precise regulatory mechanisms governing this critical cellular process have yet to be fully elucidated [110]. Changes to ADAR levels or its activity were shown to affect global editing, but these observations do not always correlate well with frequencies of individual editing events [111,112]. Therefore, it is evident that additional regulatory mechanisms exist that modulate A-to-I editing in a site-specific manner.

ADARs specifically target double stranded RNA structures, including those found in pri-miRs (Figure 1). The editing of a pri-miR can profoundly influence microRNA maturation, resulting in changes in mature microRNA expression [113–115]. However, when editing alters the microRNA's seed sequence, this can completely change the mature microRNA's target selection, resulting in the regulation of a different targetome [116].

6.2. MicroRNA A-to-I Editing in Neovascularization

MicroRNA editing is a widespread phenomenon which also affects many vasoactive microRNAs, as demonstrated recently in a study by Li et al. The authors mapped microRNA A-to-I editing at an unprecedented scale and found 2711 potential pri-miR editing sites within approximately 80% of all human pri-miRs [117]. MicroRNA editing profiles were also found to be tissue-specific, which is in agreement with previous findings [113,115,118]. Furthermore, 367 potential editing sites were found within human mature microRNAs, often located in the seed sequence [117].

In the field of cancer research, several microRNA editing events were shown to have a functional effect on cell migration and/or proliferation [119–121], which are also crucial processes in both angiogenesis and arteriogenesis [20,21]. For example, seed sequence editing of miR-455-5p was shown to alter its targetome, causing edited miR-455-5p to decrease tumor cell proliferation and migration, while the unedited version had the opposite effect [122]. Furthermore, editing of the seed sequence of miR-200b enhanced tumor cell proliferation and migration, in contrast to the unedited version [120]. Interestingly, higher miR-200b editing levels were associated with a poorer prognosis in cancer patients, highlighting the possibility that microRNA editing can be clinically relevant as a biomarker or therapeutic target.

We have recently demonstrated that microRNA-editing can also directly regulate neovascularization. We showed that A-to-I-editing of miR-487b-3p, another microRNA from the vasoactive 14q32 microRNA cluster, is increased in ischemic muscle tissues undergoing neovascularization after induction of hindlimb ischemia [123]. MiR-487b-3p editing was also found in all human vascular ECs, SMCs, and fibroblasts. The edited mature miR-487b-3p has a unique targetome and promotes angiogenesis, in contrast to the canonical miR-487b-3p [123]. In a follow-up study, we demonstrate that vasoactive microRNA editing is a widespread phenomenon that enhances neovascularization in response to ischemia (manuscript submitted).

7. N6-Adenosine Methylation

7.1. N6-Adenosine Methylation

The modification of adenosine to N^6-methyladenosine (m6A) is perhaps the most prevalent RNA nucleotide modification in eukaryotic cells and is present in more than 25% of human transcripts [124,125]. m6A is installed by the methyltransferase complex containing 'writer' METTL3 (Methyltransferase Like 3) and RNA-binding platform METTL14 [126], supported by cofactors WTAP (Wilms' tumor 1-associating protein) and KIAA1429 [127,128]. Strikingly, m6A levels are dynamically regulated throughout all stages of life, with the help of m6A demethylases, or 'erasers', FTO (fat mass and obesity-associated protein), and ALKBH5 (alkB homolog 5) [129,130]. m6A methylation has been shown to affect almost every aspect of RNA metabolism, from expression and processing in the nucleus to translation and degradation in the cytoplasm [131–133]. The importance of its functions is illustrated by studies that demonstrate that individual knockout of either METTL3, METTL14 or WTAP causes prenatal lethality in mice [134–136]. While m6A can alter RNA folding and structure [137,138], most of m6A's biological functions are mediated through a group of 'reader' proteins that specifically recognize the methylated adenosine on RNA, including the YTHD (YT521-B homology domain) and the IGF2BP (insulin-like growth factor-2 mRNA-binding protein) families [127,139–141].

While most m6A research has focused predominantly on mRNAs, several studies have demonstrated that m6A is important for microRNA biogenesis. Alarcon et al. demonstrated that pri-miRs are marked by the METTL3-dependent m6A (Figure 1). Pri-miR m6A marks are read by m6A-binding protein hnRNPA2B1 that, in turn, stimulates initiation of DICER-mediated processing through recruitment of DICER's cofactor DGCR8 [142,143]. Intriguingly, a study by Berulava et al. demonstrated that well over 200 mature microRNAs contain m6A in a human embryonic kidney cell line (HEK293). While m6A does not affect canonical base pairing, several studies have suggested that it may block the noncanonical A:G base pairing, which could affect mRNA-microRNA interaction strength [138,144]. This is supported by a recent study that found that an m6A modified miR-200c-3p resulted in significantly less suppression of its target genes than unmethylated miR-200c-3p [145]. Furthermore, recent studies also suggest that m6A of mRNAs can influence their 'targetability' by microRNAs by promoting or preventing the binding of certain RNA-binding proteins that block microRNA-mediated transcript destabilization [141,146].

7.2. Importance of m6A in the Cardio-Vasculature and in Vasoactive MicroRNAs

Two recent studies have demonstrated the importance of m6A in cardiovascular homeostasis. Dorn et al. demonstrates that METTL3-dependant m6A helps modulate cardiac homeostasis and hypertrophic stress responses in mice [147]. The overexpression of METTL3 was shown to cause spontaneous hypertrophy, whereas METTL3 knockdown leads to maladaptive remodeling and signs of heart failure. Mathiyalagan et al. demonstrated that m6A is increased in failing mammalian hearts and in hypoxic cardiomyocytes [148]. Furthermore, increasing the expression of m6A eraser FTO in ischemic mouse hearts attenuates the ischemia-induced increase in m6A and decrease in cardiac contractile function. These findings highlight a key role for m6A in ischemic cardiovascular disease.

Pri-miR m6A marks were shown to be required for the appropriate processing of most pri-miRs to mature miRNAs, including vasoactive microRNAs [142,143]. Furthermore, m6A of the above mentioned vasoactive miR-126 and miR-222 was shown to affect cell migration and/or proliferation in cancer cells. A study by Ma et al., demonstrated that the pri-miR of miR-126 undergoes METTL14-dependent m6A, which facilitates its processing to mature miR-126 [149]. Decreased METTL14-dependent m6A of pri-miR-126 led to the reduced expression of miR-126, which in turn increased cancer cell migration and invasion [149]. Han et al. showed that METTL3-dependant m6A of pri-miR-222 increases its maturation to mature miR-222, resulting in the reduction of PTEN, and ultimately leading to the proliferation of bladder cancer [150]. Furthermore, METTL3 was increased in bladder cancer and correlated with poor patient prognosis [150].

Combined, the abundance of m6A, its importance in microRNA biogenesis and functioning, and the dysregulation of m6A during ischemia and cardiovascular disease, suggest that m6A of microRNAs could play an important role in ischemic cardiovascular disease and neovascularization.

8. Other Modifications in the microRNA Epitranscriptome

As mentioned above, numerous other RNA nucleotide modifications exist, however, their presence and function in small RNAs (16–28 nucleotides long), which consist mostly of microRNAs [151], remains understudied [152]. An important reason for this is that conventional methods to detect RNA modifications are often unsuitable for small RNAs [152,153]. Recently, Lan et al. optimized a screening based on mass spectrometry which allowed them to provide the first overview of RNA nucleotide modifications in mammalian small RNAs using human HEK293T cells [154]. Besides inosine and m6A, 22 additional distinct nucleotide modifications were found, 13 of which consisted of different types or combinations of RNA methylations [154]. While little is known about the effect of these RNA nucleotide modifications on the functioning of small RNA, and thus microRNA, several have been studied in other RNA types.

Below, we will report the key findings of these studied RNA modifications and highlight which properties could potentially affect microRNA function. Furthermore, the discussed nucleotide modifications and their potential effects on microRNAs are summarized in Table 2.

Table 2. Known or postulated effects of nucleotide modification within microRNAs.

Nucleotide Modification	Abbreviation	Writers	Erasers	Potential Effects on microRNAs
Adenosine-to-inosine editing	A-to-I editing	ADAR1 or ADAR2	-	• pri-miR editing can profoundly influence maturation • seed sequence editing can alter targetome
N6-methyl-adenosine	m6A	METTL3/14	ALKBH5 FTO	• regulates pri-miR processing • hampered nonstandard A:G base pairing may affect silencing activity
Pseudouridine	Ψ	PUSs	-	• stronger base pairing with adenosine might affect silencing activity *
2'-O-methyl-nucleosides	2'OMe	Methyl-transferases	-	• may protect from A-to-I editing * • may affect stability and turnover * • enhanced RNA-RNA duplex stability might affect silencing activity *
N1-methyl-adenosine	m1A	TRMT6 & 61	ALKBH3	• positive charge can dramatically alter interactions with proteins * • disrupts RNA base pairing which can affect silencing activity *
N3-methyl-cytosine	m5C	NSUNs DNMT2	-	• may enhance stability *
N2-methyl-guanosine	m2G	unclear	-	• allows noncanonical base pairing which may affect silencing activity *

* effects are postulated effects based on observations in other RNA types.

8.1. Pseudouridine (Ψ)

Pseudouridine (Ψ) is one of the most abundant RNA modifications [155,156]. Ψ is highly conserved and is generated from isomerization of uridine, catalyzed by pseudouridine synthases (PUSs) [155,156]. Recent advances in high-resolution detection methods have demonstrated that Ψ-nucleotides are found in many, if not all, species of RNA [156,157]. Pseudouridylation was shown to be important for ribosomal RNA biogenesis, pre-mRNA splicing, and translation fidelity [155,156]. Compared to a uracil, Ψ forms a stronger base pairing interaction with adenosine, which allows it to alter RNA secondary structures, suggesting that microRNA pseudouridylation could affect mRNA silencing [158,159]. Furthermore, transcriptome wide pseudouridylation was shown to increase under stress conditions, including serum deprivation, a key component of ischemia [160].

8.2. 2′-O-Methylnucleosides

It is known that 2′-O-methylation (2′OMe) can reside on all four ribonucleosides and is widely conserved [161,162]. Furthermore, 2′OMe is performed by methyltransferases like Fibrillarin and many, if not all, 2′OMe-events are directed by small nucleolar RNAs [64,163,164]. 2′OMe appears essential in processing ribosomal RNAs, small nuclear RNAs, and transfer RNAs, but it has also been found in mRNAs and even in microRNAs, by our group among others [123,161,165]. While the precise location and function of 2′OMe sites in many RNA types are currently unclear, 2′OMe in general has a stabilizing effect and can influence interactions with proteins or other RNAs [161,162]. 2′OMe may in fact protect adenosine residues from A-to-I editing [165–167]. Interestingly, we found that both 2′OMe and A-to-I editing of the same adenosine residue in pri-miR-487b are increased simultaneously under ischemia [123]. However, further studies are required to examine whether both RNA modifications can be found on a single copy of miR-487b-3p. Finally, 2′OMe also greatly enhances the stability of RNA-RNA duplexes, a quality that is often utilized to enhance the stability and specificity of synthetic antisense RNA-oligonucleotides, with similar implications for 2′OMe of microRNAs [168–171].

8.3. N1-Methyladenosine (m1A)

Recent methodological advances have demonstrated that m1A is a transcriptome-wide modification [172,173]. Several members of the TRMT family (tRNA methyltransferase family) have already been shown to be m1A writers and additional writers are thought to exist [172–174]. Similar to m6A, m1A is reversible and can be demethylated by erasers ALKBH1 and 3 (alkB homolog 1 and 3) [173,175]. Furthermore, m1A levels are dynamically regulated by various types of cellular stress and correlate with upregulation of translation in general [172,173]. This modification carries a positive charge and can therefore alter both protein–RNA interactions and RNA secondary structures dramatically [131], which can potentially lead to disruption of microRNA biogenesis [29]. Furthermore, m1A appears to disrupts RNA base-pairing and induces local RNA duplex melting, suggesting that m1A may also affect microRNA-target interactions [132,176].

8.4. N5-Methylcytosine (m5C)

While best known as a DNA modification in the epigenome, m5C can be installed on RNAs too by members from the NSUN family (nucleolar protein/sun RNA methyltransferase family) and by DNMT2 (DNA methyltransferase-2) and is therefore also part of the epitranscriptome [177–181]. m5C has been found in both noncoding and coding RNAs in mammals and a few studies have shown that m5C has functional implications [177,182,183]. For example, m5C of tRNAs was shown to protect tRNAs against stress-induced cleavage [180,184,185]. Furthermore, the depletion of m5C methyltransferase Nsun7 in mice resulted in a concomitant decrease of expression of specific non-coding RNAs, suggesting m5C marks can enhance RNA stability [186].

8.5. N2-Methylguanosine (m2G)

In tRNAs and rRNAs, m2G is a relatively common RNA modification, however, which m2G writers are responsible in humans remains unclear [187,188]. Interestingly, the study by Lan et al. demonstrated that m2G is also relatively common in small RNAs [154]. Our knowledge about this RNA modification is still very limited due to a lack of high-throughput detection methods [188,189]. However, studies have shown that m2G can form both canonical and non-canonical Watson–Crick base pairing interactions, allowing m2G to regulate the stability of tRNA tertiary structures and potentially influence microRNA silencing activity [188,190].

9. Dynamic Regulation of the Epitranscriptome

The epitranscriptome is dynamically regulated. This is abundantly clear for m6A modifications due to the discovery of both m6A writers and erasers [147,148]. Not all modifications may be reversible like m6A, but most, if not all, other modifications do appear to be regulated. Several studies have shown that RNA alterations are modulated under stress and pathological conditions [64,191,192]. For example, the deposition and distribution of m6A were increased in response to heat shock and DNA damage [193–195]. Total transcriptomic pseudourydilation increased in response to heat shock, nutrient deprivation, and serum deprivation [157,160]. Further, m1A levels in mammalian cells also increased in response to heat shock, but decreased after nutrient starvation [172]. Furthermore, cellular m5C levels are decreased in response external stress and cytotoxic stress which affects protein translation rates [196,197]. Additionally, the expression of methyltransferase Fibrillarin is increased in many cancers to facilitate additional 2'OMe of ribosomal RNAs [162,198,199], while mRNA A-to-I editing is induced by both hypoxia and inflammation [200]. Importantly, we have shown that both A-to-I editing and 2'OMe also increase in microRNAs during ischemia [123,201]. These findings suggest that the microRNA epitranscriptome is likely to also be dynamically regulated and functional in pathological conditions, and could provide novel targets for therapeutic intervention.

Several studies have also indicated that certain RNA nucleotide modifications regulate each other. As mentioned previously, 2'OMe was found to protect adenosine residues from A-to-I editing [165–167]. A different study demonstrated that replacing an adenosine which can be A-to-I edited by m6A also prevents editing almost completely in an in vitro assay [202]. Furthermore, it was recently demonstrated that transcript m6A levels are negatively correlated with the A-to-I editing levels of the transcript, even when they are not competing for the same nucleotide [203]. The depletion of m6A resulted in upregulated A-to-I editing on the m6A-depleted transcripts, confirming a transcriptome wide interplay between m6A and A-to-I editing [203]. These findings highlight the complexity of the epitranscriptome and the importance of studying multiple RNA modifications simultaneously in order to examine known interactions and to identify novel interactions.

10. Concluding Remarks

During the past decade, both isomiRs and the epitranscriptome have emerged as novel and dynamic layers of regulation of gene expression. Both types of microRNA alterations have been shown to modulate key physiological responses, including neovascularization by affecting the microRNA's biogenesis, stability and function. MicroRNAs have already been established as multifactorial regulators of both angiogenesis and arteriogenesis [7–9], and therefore this additional regulatory layer may provide new options for therapeutic neovascularization. The therapeutic potential of both isomiRs and the microRNA epitranscriptome is highlighted by the findings that 5'-isomiR formation of miR-411-5p and A-to-I editing of miR-487b-3p are actively regulated in response to ischemia in vivo, resulting in novel microRNAs with anti- or pro-angiogenic properties, respectively [99,123]. Therefore, altered microRNAs could provide novel targets for therapeutic inhibition or overexpression to stimulate neovascularization after ischemic CVD.

The first therapeutic small RNA (Patisiran) was granted FDA approval in 2018 and the first phase 2 clinical trials with microRNA-oriented RNA therapeutics are currently ongoing, highlighting that microRNA therapeutics are on their way to clinical practice [45]. Over the last decade, important advances have been made in development of microRNA therapeutics, however, several key issues remain, which have been expertly reviewed in the studies by Lucas et al. and Rupaimoole et al. [41,204]. These issues include maximizing the effect of the therapeutics' effect on the diseased tissue, while minimizing the off-target binding and toxicity. Now that the prevalence and functionality of microRNA alterations are becoming clear, further research is warranted to understand which altered microRNAs could pose off-target risks during design and development of microRNA-based therapeutics. However, uncovering the intricate mechanisms which govern regulation of microRNA alterations could also reveal novel therapeutic targets to modulate microRNA functioning.

Alternatively, tissue- and pathology-specific regulation of the microRNA alterations could potentially be used as a biomarker for cardiovascular disease, considering that isomiR expression profiles were found sufficient to distinguish between cancer subtypes [205].

Finally, while the abundance and function of many nucleotide modifications have not been studied in microRNAs yet, it is likely that most, if not all, will prove clinically relevant. The unique properties of certain nucleotide modifications, like for example m6A, could be exploited to enhance the specificity of microRNA-therapeutics when targeting microRNAs carrying such modifications. It is important to note that further advances in technology and methodology are required to expand our knowledge of the microRNA epitranscriptome [154,206]. However, given the surge of interest in this field, we expect many more clinically relevant microRNA alteration events to be discovered in the near future.

Author Contributions: Conceptualization—R.V.C.T.v.d.K., P.H.A.Q. and A.Y.N.; Writing—Original Draft—R.V.C.T.v.d.K.; Writing—Review & Editing—R.V.C.T.v.d.K., P.H.A.Q. and A.Y.N.; Funding Acquisition—A.Y.N. All authors have read and agreed to the published version of the manuscript.

Funding: R.V.C.T.v.d.K. was supported by a grant from the Dutch Heart Foundation (E. Dekker Senior Postdoc Grant, A.Y.N., 2014T102). A.Y.N. was supported by the LUMC Johanna Zaaijer Fund (2017) and the Austrian Science Fund FWF (Lise Meitner Grant, A.Y.N., M2578-B30).

Conflicts of Interest: The authors declare no conflict of interest

References

1. Timmis, A.; Townsend, N.; Gale, C.; Grobbee, R.; Maniadakis, N.; Flather, M.; Wilkins, E.; Wright, L.; Vos, R.; Bax, J.; et al. European Society of Cardiology: Cardiovascular Disease Statistics 2017. *Eur Heart J.* **2018**, *39*, 508–579. [CrossRef] [PubMed]
2. Kaptoge, S.; Pennells, L.; De Bacquer, D.; Cooney, M.T.; Kavousi, M.; Stevens, G.; Riley, L.M.; Savin, S.; Khan, T.; Altay, S.; et al. World Health Organization cardiovascular disease risk charts: Revised models to estimate risk in 21 global regions. *Lancet Glob. Health* **2019**, *7*, e1332–e1345. [CrossRef]
3. Dormandy, J.; Heeck, L.; Vig, S. Acute limb ischemia. *Semin. Vasc. Surg.* **1999**, *12*, 148–153. [PubMed]
4. Powell, R.J.; Comerota, A.J.; Berceli, S.A.; Guzman, R.; Henry, T.D.; Tzeng, E.; Velazquez, O.; Marston, W.A.; Bartel, R.L.; Longcore, A.; et al. Interim analysis results from the RESTORE-CLI, a randomized, double-blind multicenter phase II trial comparing expanded autologous bone marrow-derived tissue repair cells and placebo in patients with critical limb ischemia. *J. Vasc. Surg.* **2011**, *54*, 1032–1041. [CrossRef] [PubMed]
5. Van Oostrom, M.C.; van Oostrom, O.; Quax, P.H.; Verhaar, M.C.; Hoefer, I.E. Insights into mechanisms behind arteriogenesis: What does the future hold? *J. Leukoc. Biol.* **2008**, *84*, 1379–1391. [CrossRef] [PubMed]
6. Raval, Z.; Losordo, D.W. Cell Therapy of Peripheral Arterial Disease: From Experimental Findings to Clinical Trials. *Circ. Res.* **2013**, *112*, 1288–1302. [CrossRef]
7. Weber, C. MicroRNAs: From basic mechanisms to clinical application in cardiovascular medicine. *Arterioscler. Thromb. Vasc. Biol.* **2013**, *33*, 168–169. [CrossRef]
8. Welten, S.M.; Goossens, E.A.; Quax, P.H.; Nossent, A.Y. The multifactorial nature of microRNAs in vascular remodelling. *Cardiovasc. Res.* **2016**, *110*, 6–22. [CrossRef]
9. Welten, S.M.; Bastiaansen, A.J.; de Jong, R.C.; de Vries, M.R.; Peters, E.H.; Boonstra, M.; Sheikh, S.P.; La, M.N.; Kandimalla, E.R.; Quax, P.H.; et al. Inhibition of 14q32 MicroRNAs miR-329, miR-487b, miR-494 and miR-495 Increases Neovascularization and Blood Flow Recovery after Ischemia. *Circ. Res.* **2014**, *115*, 696–708. [CrossRef]
10. Friedman, R.C.; Farh, K.K.; Burge, C.B.; Bartel, D.P. Most mammalian mRNAs are conserved targets of microRNAs. *Genome Res.* **2009**, *19*, 92–105. [CrossRef]
11. Heil, M.; Schaper, W. Pathophysiology of collateral development. *Coron. Artery Dis.* **2004**, *15*, 373–378. [CrossRef] [PubMed]
12. Hoefer, I.E.; van Royen, N.; Rectenwald, J.E.; Deindl, E.; Hua, J.; Jost, M.; Grundmann, S.; Voskuil, M.; Ozaki, C.K.; Piek, J.J.; et al. Arteriogenesis proceeds via ICAM-1/Mac-1- mediated mechanisms. *Circ. Res.* **2004**, *94*, 1179–1185. [CrossRef] [PubMed]
13. Scholz, D.; Ito, W.; Fleming, I.; Deindl, E.; Sauer, A.; Wiesnet, M.; Busse, R.; Schaper, J.; Schaper, W. Ultrastructure and molecular histology of rabbit hind-limb collateral artery growth (arteriogenesis). *Virchows Arch.* **2000**, *436*, 257–270. [CrossRef] [PubMed]

14. Hoefer, I.E.; van Royen, N.; Rectenwald, J.E.; Bray, E.J.; Abouhamze, Z.; Moldawer, L.L.; Voskuil, M.; Piek, J.J.; Buschmann, I.R.; Ozaki, C.K. Direct evidence for tumor necrosis factor-alpha signaling in arteriogenesis. *Circulation* **2002**, *105*, 1639–1641. [CrossRef] [PubMed]
15. Kosaki, K.; Ando, J.; Korenaga, R.; Kurokawa, T.; Kamiya, A. Fluid shear stress increases the production of granulocyte-macrophage colony-stimulating factor by endothelial cells via mRNA stabilization. *Circ. Res.* **1998**, *82*, 794–802. [CrossRef] [PubMed]
16. Bergmann, C.E.; Hoefer, I.E.; Meder, B.; Roth, H.; van Royen, N.; Breit, S.M.; Jost, M.M.; Aharinejad, S.; Hartmann, S.; Buschmann, I.R. Arteriogenesis depends on circulating monocytes and macrophage accumulation and is severely depressed in op/op mice. *J. Leukoc. Biol.* **2006**, *80*, 59–65. [CrossRef] [PubMed]
17. Stabile, E.; Burnett, M.S.; Watkins, C.; Kinnaird, T.; Bachis, A.; la Sala, A.; Miller, J.M.; Shou, M.; Epstein, S.E.; Fuchs, S. Impaired arteriogenic response to acute hindlimb ischemia in CD4-knockout mice. *Circulation* **2003**, *108*, 205–210. [CrossRef]
18. Van Weel, V.; Toes, R.E.; Seghers, L.; Deckers, M.M.; de Vries, M.R.; Eilers, P.H.; Sipkens, J.; Schepers, A.; Eefting, D.; van Hinsbergh, V.W.; et al. Natural killer cells and CD4+ T-cells modulate collateral artery development. *Arterioscler. Thromb. Vasc. Biol.* **2007**, *27*, 2310–2318. [CrossRef]
19. Wolf, C.; Cai, W.J.; Vosschulte, R.; Koltai, S.; Mousavipour, D.; Scholz, D.; Afsah-Hedjri, A.; Schaper, W.; Schaper, J. Vascular remodeling and altered protein expression during growth of coronary collateral arteries. *J. Mol. Cell. Cardiol.* **1998**, *30*, 2291–2305. [CrossRef]
20. Buschmann, I.; Schaper, W. Arteriogenesis Versus Angiogenesis: Two Mechanisms of Vessel Growth. *News Physiol Sci.* **1999**, *14*, 121–125. [CrossRef]
21. Carmeliet, P. Mechanisms of angiogenesis and arteriogenesis. *Nat. Med.* **2000**, *6*, 389–395. [CrossRef] [PubMed]
22. Schwartz, C.J.; Mitchell, J.R. Cellular infiltration of the human arterial adventitia associated with atheromatous plaques. *Circulation* **1962**, *26*, 73–78. [CrossRef] [PubMed]
23. Newman, A.C.; Nakatsu, M.N.; Chou, W.; Gershon, P.D.; Hughes, C.C.W. The requirement for fibroblasts in angiogenesis: Fibroblast-derived matrix proteins are essential for endothelial cell lumen formation. *Mol. Biol. Cell* **2011**, *22*, 3791–3800. [CrossRef] [PubMed]
24. Noonan, D.M.; De Lerma Barbaro, A.; Vannini, N.; Mortara, L.; Albini, A. Inflammation, inflammatory cells and angiogenesis: Decisions and indecisions. *Cancer Metastasis Rev.* **2008**, *27*, 31–40. [CrossRef] [PubMed]
25. Brennecke, J.; Stark, A.; Russell, R.B.; Cohen, S.M. Principles of microRNA-target recognition. *PLoS Biol.* **2005**, *3*, e85. [CrossRef]
26. Lewis, B.P.; Shih, I.H.; Jones-Rhoades, M.W.; Bartel, D.P.; Burge, C.B. Prediction of mammalian microRNA targets. *Cell* **2003**, *115*, 787–798. [CrossRef]
27. Lee, Y.; Jeon, K.; Lee, J.T.; Kim, S.; Kim, V.N. MicroRNA maturation: Stepwise processing and subcellular localization. *EMBO J.* **2002**, *21*, 4663–4670. [CrossRef]
28. Lee, Y.; Ahn, C.; Han, J.; Choi, H.; Kim, J.; Yim, J.; Lee, J.; Provost, P.; Radmark, O.; Kim, S.; et al. The nuclear RNase III Drosha initiates microRNA processing. *Nature* **2003**, *425*, 415–419. [CrossRef]
29. Ha, M.; Kim, V.N. Regulation of microRNA biogenesis. *Nat. Rev. Mol. Cell Biol.* **2014**, *15*, 509–524. [CrossRef]
30. Kobayashi, H.; Tomari, Y. RISC assembly: Coordination between small RNAs and Argonaute proteins. *Biochim. Biophys. Acta* **2016**, *1859*, 71–81. [CrossRef]
31. Treiber, T.; Treiber, N.; Plessmann, U.; Harlander, S.; Daiss, J.L.; Eichner, N.; Lehmann, G.; Schall, K.; Urlaub, H.; Meister, G. A Compendium of RNA-Binding Proteins that Regulate MicroRNA Biogenesis. *Mol. Cell* **2017**, *66*, 270. [CrossRef] [PubMed]
32. Saito, Y.; Liang, G.; Egger, G.; Friedman, J.M.; Chuang, J.C.; Coetzee, G.A.; Jones, P.A. Specific activation of microRNA-127 with downregulation of the proto-oncogene BCL6 by chromatin-modifying drugs in human cancer cells. *Cancer Cell* **2006**, *9*, 435–443. [CrossRef] [PubMed]
33. Vrba, L.; Munoz-Rodriguez, J.L.; Stampfer, M.R.; Futscher, B.W. miRNA gene promoters are frequent targets of aberrant DNA methylation in human breast cancer. *PLoS ONE* **2013**, *8*, e54398. [CrossRef] [PubMed]
34. Downie Ruiz Velasco, A.; Welten, S.M.J.; Goossens, E.A.C.; Quax, P.H.A.; Rappsilber, J.; Michlewski, G.; Nossent, A.Y. Posttranscriptional Regulation of 14q32 MicroRNAs by the CIRBP and HADHB during Vascular Regeneration after Ischemia. *Mol. Ther. Nucleic Acids* **2019**, *14*, 329–338. [CrossRef] [PubMed]

35. Kuehbacher, A.; Urbich, C.; Zeiher, A.M.; Dimmeler, S. Role of Dicer and Drosha for endothelial microRNA expression and angiogenesis. *Circ. Res.* **2007**, *101*, 59–68. [CrossRef]
36. Suarez, Y.; Fernandez-Hernando, C.; Pober, J.S.; Sessa, W.C. Dicer dependent microRNAs regulate gene expression and functions in human endothelial cells. *Circ. Res.* **2007**, *100*, 1164–1173. [CrossRef]
37. Suarez, Y.; Fernandez-Hernando, C.; Yu, J.; Gerber, S.A.; Harrison, K.D.; Pober, J.S.; Iruela-Arispe, M.L.; Merkenschlager, M.; Sessa, W.C. Dicer-dependent endothelial microRNAs are necessary for postnatal angiogenesis. *Proc. Natl. Acad. Sci. USA* **2008**, *105*, 14082–14087. [CrossRef]
38. Kir, D.; Schnettler, E.; Modi, S.; Ramakrishnan, S. Regulation of angiogenesis by microRNAs in cardiovascular diseases. *Angiogenesis* **2018**, *21*, 699–710. [CrossRef]
39. Lin, X.; Zhan, J.K.; Wang, Y.J.; Tan, P.; Chen, Y.Y.; Deng, H.Q.; Liu, Y.S. Function, Role, and Clinical Application of MicroRNAs in Vascular Aging. *BioMed Res. Int.* **2016**, *2016*, 6021394. [CrossRef]
40. Sun, L.L.; Li, W.D.; Lei, F.R.; Li, X.Q. The regulatory role of microRNAs in angiogenesis-related diseases. *J. Cell Mol. Med.* **2018**, *22*, 4568–4587. [CrossRef]
41. Lucas, T.; Bonauer, A.; Dimmeler, S. RNA Therapeutics in Cardiovascular Disease. *Circ. Res.* **2018**, *123*, 205–220. [CrossRef] [PubMed]
42. Bonauer, A.; Carmona, G.; Iwasaki, M.; Mione, M.; Koyanagi, M.; Fischer, A.; Burchfield, J.; Fox, H.; Doebele, C.; Ohtani, K.; et al. MicroRNA-92a controls angiogenesis and functional recovery of ischemic tissues in mice. *Science* **2009**, *324*, 1710–1713. [CrossRef] [PubMed]
43. Hinkel, R.; Penzkofer, D.; Zuhlke, S.; Fischer, A.; Husada, W.; Xu, Q.F.; Baloch, E.; van Rooij, E.; Zeiher, A.M.; Kupatt, C.; et al. Inhibition of microRNA-92a protects against ischemia/reperfusion injury in a large-animal model. *Circulation* **2013**, *128*, 1066–1075. [CrossRef] [PubMed]
44. Bellera, N.; Barba, I.; Rodriguez-Sinovas, A.; Ferret, E.; Asin, M.A.; Gonzalez-Alujas, M.T.; Perez-Rodon, J.; Esteves, M.; Fonseca, C.; Toran, N.; et al. Single intracoronary injection of encapsulated antagomir-92a promotes angiogenesis and prevents adverse infarct remodeling. *J. Am. Heart Assoc.* **2014**, *3*, e000946. [CrossRef] [PubMed]
45. Hanna, J.; Hossain, G.S.; Kocerha, J. The Potential for microRNA Therapeutics and Clinical Research. *Front. Genet.* **2019**, *10*, 478. [CrossRef] [PubMed]
46. Fish, J.E.; Santoro, M.M.; Morton, S.U.; Yu, S.; Yeh, R.F.; Wythe, J.D.; Ivey, K.N.; Bruneau, B.G.; Stainier, D.Y.; Srivastava, D. miR-126 regulates angiogenic signaling and vascular integrity. *Dev. Cell* **2008**, *15*, 272–284. [CrossRef] [PubMed]
47. Wang, S.; Aurora, A.B.; Johnson, B.A.; Qi, X.; McAnally, J.; Hill, J.A.; Richardson, J.A.; Bassel-Duby, R.; Olson, E.N. The endothelial-specific microRNA miR-126 governs vascular integrity and angiogenesis. *Dev. Cell* **2008**, *15*, 261–271. [CrossRef]
48. Schober, A.; Nazari-Jahantigh, M.; Wei, Y.; Bidzhekov, K.; Gremse, F.; Grommes, J.; Megens, R.T.; Heyll, K.; Noels, H.; Hristov, M.; et al. MicroRNA-126-5p promotes endothelial proliferation and limits atherosclerosis by suppressing Dlk1. *Nat. Med.* **2014**, *20*, 368–376. [CrossRef]
49. Harris, T.A.; Yamakuchi, M.; Ferlito, M.; Mendell, J.T.; Lowenstein, C.J. MicroRNA-126 regulates endothelial expression of vascular cell adhesion molecule 1. *Proc. Natl. Acad. Sci. USA* **2008**, *105*, 1516–1521. [CrossRef]
50. Van Solingen, C.; Seghers, L.; Bijkerk, R.; Duijs, J.M.; Roeten, M.K.; van Oeveren-Rietdijk, A.M.; Baelde, H.J.; Monge, M.; Vos, J.B.; de Boer, H.C.; et al. Antagomir-mediated silencing of endothelial cell specific microRNA-126 impairs ischemia-induced angiogenesis. *J. Cell Mol. Med.* **2009**, *13*, 1577–1585. [CrossRef]
51. Katare, R.; Rawal, S.; Munasinghe, P.E.; Tsuchimochi, H.; Inagaki, T.; Fujii, Y.; Dixit, P.; Umetani, K.; Kangawa, K.; Shirai, M.; et al. Ghrelin Promotes Functional Angiogenesis in a Mouse Model of Critical Limb Ischemia Through Activation of Proangiogenic MicroRNAs. *Endocrinology* **2016**, *157*, 432–445. [CrossRef] [PubMed]
52. Fichtlscherer, S.; De Rosa, S.; Fox, H.; Schwietz, T.; Fischer, A.; Liebetrau, C.; Weber, M.; Hamm, C.W.; Roxe, T.; Muller-Ardogan, M.; et al. Circulating microRNAs in patients with coronary artery disease. *Circ. Res.* **2010**, *107*, 677–684. [CrossRef] [PubMed]
53. Wang, X.; Ling, C.C.; Li, L.; Qin, Y.; Qi, J.; Liu, X.; You, B.; Shi, Y.; Zhang, J.; Jiang, Q.; et al. MicroRNA-10a/10b represses a novel target gene mib1 to regulate angiogenesis. *Cardiovasc. Res.* **2016**, *110*, 140–150. [CrossRef] [PubMed]

54. Hergenreider, E.; Heydt, S.; Treguer, K.; Boettger, T.; Horrevoets, A.J.; Zeiher, A.M.; Scheffer, M.P.; Frangakis, A.S.; Yin, X.; Mayr, M.; et al. Atheroprotective communication between endothelial cells and smooth muscle cells through miRNAs. *Nat. Cell Biol.* **2012**, *14*, 249–256. [CrossRef] [PubMed]
55. Fang, Y.; Shi, C.; Manduchi, E.; Civelek, M.; Davies, P.F. MicroRNA-10a regulation of proinflammatory phenotype in athero-susceptible endothelium in vivo and in vitro. *Proc. Natl. Acad Sci. USA* **2010**, *107*, 13450–13455. [CrossRef]
56. Hassel, D.; Cheng, P.; White, M.P.; Ivey, K.N.; Kroll, J.; Augustin, H.G.; Katus, H.A.; Stainier, D.Y.; Srivastava, D. MicroRNA-10 regulates the angiogenic behavior of zebrafish and human endothelial cells by promoting vascular endothelial growth factor signaling. *Circ. Res.* **2012**, *111*, 1421–1433. [CrossRef]
57. Liu, L.Z.; Li, C.; Chen, Q.; Jing, Y.; Carpenter, R.; Jiang, Y.; Kung, H.F.; Lai, L.; Jiang, B.H. MiR-21 induced angiogenesis through AKT and ERK activation and HIF-1alpha expression. *PLoS ONE* **2011**, *6*, e19139. [CrossRef]
58. Maegdefessel, L.; Azuma, J.; Toh, R.; Deng, A.; Merk, D.R.; Raiesdana, A.; Leeper, N.J.; Raaz, U.; Schoelmerich, A.M.; McConnell, M.V.; et al. MicroRNA-21 blocks abdominal aortic aneurysm development and nicotine-augmented expansion. *Sci. Transl. Med.* **2012**, *4*, 122ra122. [CrossRef]
59. Ji, R.; Cheng, Y.; Yue, J.; Yang, J.; Liu, X.; Chen, H.; Dean, D.B.; Zhang, C. MicroRNA expression signature and antisense-mediated depletion reveal an essential role of MicroRNA in vascular neointimal lesion formation. *Circ. Res.* **2007**, *100*, 1579–1588. [CrossRef]
60. Thum, T.; Gross, C.; Fiedler, J.; Fischer, T.; Kissler, S.; Bussen, M.; Galuppo, P.; Just, S.; Rottbauer, W.; Frantz, S.; et al. MicroRNA-21 contributes to myocardial disease by stimulating MAP kinase signalling in fibroblasts. *Nature* **2008**, *456*, 980–984. [CrossRef]
61. Kaluza, D.; Kroll, J.; Gesierich, S.; Manavski, Y.; Boeckel, J.N.; Doebele, C.; Zelent, A.; Rossig, L.; Zeiher, A.M.; Augustin, H.G.; et al. Histone deacetylase 9 promotes angiogenesis by targeting the antiangiogenic microRNA-17-92 cluster in endothelial cells. *Arterioscler. Thromb. Vasc. Biol.* **2013**, *33*, 533–543. [CrossRef] [PubMed]
62. Landskroner-Eiger, S.; Qiu, C.; Perrotta, P.; Siragusa, M.; Lee, M.Y.; Ulrich, V.; Luciano, A.K.; Zhuang, Z.W.; Corti, F.; Simons, M.; et al. Endothelial miR-17 approximately 92 cluster negatively regulates arteriogenesis via miRNA-19 repression of WNT signaling. *Proc. Natl. Acad. Sci. USA* **2015**, *112*, 12812–12817. [CrossRef] [PubMed]
63. Kozomara, A.; Birgaoanu, M.; Griffiths-Jones, S. miRBase: From microRNA sequences to function. *Nucleic Acids Res.* **2019**, *47*, D155–D162. [CrossRef] [PubMed]
64. Hoernes, T.P.; Erlacher, M.D. Translating the epitranscriptome. *Wiley Interdiscip. Rev. RNA* **2017**, *8*. [CrossRef] [PubMed]
65. Landgraf, P.; Rusu, M.; Sheridan, R.; Sewer, A.; Iovino, N.; Aravin, A.; Pfeffer, S.; Rice, A.; Kamphorst, A.O.; Landthaler, M.; et al. A mammalian microRNA expression atlas based on small RNA library sequencing. *Cell* **2007**, *129*, 1401–1414. [CrossRef]
66. Blow, M.J.; Grocock, R.J.; van Dongen, S.; Enright, A.J.; Dicks, E.; Futreal, P.A.; Wooster, R.; Stratton, M.R. RNA editing of human microRNAs. *Genome Biol.* **2006**, *7*, R27. [CrossRef]
67. Cloonan, N.; Wani, S.; Xu, Q.; Gu, J.; Lea, K.; Heater, S.; Barbacioru, C.; Steptoe, A.L.; Martin, H.C.; Nourbakhsh, E.; et al. MicroRNAs and their isomiRs function cooperatively to target common biological pathways. *Genome Biol.* **2011**, *12*, R126. [CrossRef]
68. Neilsen, C.T.; Goodall, G.J.; Bracken, C.P. IsomiRs—The overlooked repertoire in the dynamic microRNAome. *Trends Genet.* **2012**, *28*, 544–549. [CrossRef]
69. Llorens, F.; Banez-Coronel, M.; Pantano, L.; del Rio, J.A.; Ferrer, I.; Estivill, X.; Marti, E. A highly expressed miR-101 isomiR is a functional silencing small RNA. *BMC Genom.* **2013**, *14*, 104. [CrossRef]
70. Loher, P.; Londin, E.R.; Rigoutsos, I. IsomiR expression profiles in human lymphoblastoid cell lines exhibit population and gender dependencies. *Oncotarget* **2014**, *5*, 8790–8802. [CrossRef]
71. McCall, M.N.; Kim, M.S.; Adil, M.; Patil, A.H.; Lu, Y.; Mitchell, C.J.; Leal-Rojas, P.; Xu, J.; Kumar, M.; Dawson, V.L.; et al. Toward the human cellular microRNAome. *Genome Res.* **2017**, *27*, 1769–1781. [CrossRef] [PubMed]
72. Tan, G.C.; Chan, E.; Molnar, A.; Sarkar, R.; Alexieva, D.; Isa, I.M.; Robinson, S.; Zhang, S.; Ellis, P.; Langford, C.F.; et al. 5′ isomiR variation is of functional and evolutionary importance. *Nucleic Acids Res.* **2014**, *42*, 9424–9435. [CrossRef] [PubMed]

73. Bofill-De Ros, X.; Yang, A.; Gu, S. IsomiRs: Expanding the miRNA repression toolbox beyond the seed. *Biochim. Biophys. Acta Gene Regul. Mech.* **2019**. [CrossRef] [PubMed]
74. Telonis, A.G.; Loher, P.; Jing, Y.; Londin, E.; Rigoutsos, I. Beyond the one-locus-one-miRNA paradigm: microRNA isoforms enable deeper insights into breast cancer heterogeneity. *Nucleic Acids Res.* **2015**, *43*, 9158–9175. [CrossRef] [PubMed]
75. Burroughs, A.M.; Ando, Y.; de Hoon, M.J.; Tomaru, Y.; Nishibu, T.; Ukekawa, R.; Funakoshi, T.; Kurokawa, T.; Suzuki, H.; Hayashizaki, Y.; et al. A comprehensive survey of 3′ animal miRNA modification events and a possible role for 3′ adenylation in modulating miRNA targeting effectiveness. *Genome Res.* **2010**, *20*, 1398–1410. [CrossRef] [PubMed]
76. Wyman, S.K.; Knouf, E.C.; Parkin, R.K.; Fritz, B.R.; Lin, D.W.; Dennis, L.M.; Krouse, M.A.; Webster, P.J.; Tewari, M. Post-transcriptional generation of miRNA variants by multiple nucleotidyl transferases contributes to miRNA transcriptome complexity. *Genome Res.* **2011**, *21*, 1450–1461. [CrossRef]
77. Lee, L.W.; Zhang, S.; Etheridge, A.; Ma, L.; Martin, D.; Galas, D.; Wang, K. Complexity of the microRNA repertoire revealed by next-generation sequencing. *RNA* **2010**, *16*, 2170–2180. [CrossRef]
78. Newman, M.A.; Mani, V.; Hammond, S.M. Deep sequencing of microRNA precursors reveals extensive 3′ end modification. *RNA* **2011**, *17*, 1795–1803. [CrossRef]
79. Mercey, O.; Popa, A.; Cavard, A.; Paquet, A.; Chevalier, B.; Pons, N.; Magnone, V.; Zangari, J.; Brest, P.; Zaragosi, L.E.; et al. Characterizing isomiR variants within the microRNA-34/449 family. *FEBS Lett.* **2017**, *591*, 693–705. [CrossRef]
80. Karali, M.; Persico, M.; Mutarelli, M.; Carissimo, A.; Pizzo, M.; Singh Marwah, V.; Ambrosio, C.; Pinelli, M.; Carrella, D.; Ferrari, S.; et al. High-resolution analysis of the human retina miRNome reveals isomiR variations and novel microRNAs. *Nucleic Acids Res.* **2016**, *44*, 1525–1540. [CrossRef]
81. Manzano, M.; Forte, E.; Raja, A.N.; Schipma, M.J.; Gottwein, E. Divergent target recognition by coexpressed 5′-isomiRs of miR-142-3p and selective viral mimicry. *RNA* **2015**, *21*, 1606–1620. [CrossRef] [PubMed]
82. Marzi, M.J.; Ghini, F.; Cerruti, B.; de Pretis, S.; Bonetti, P.; Giacomelli, C.; Gorski, M.M.; Kress, T.; Pelizzola, M.; Muller, H.; et al. Degradation dynamics of microRNAs revealed by a novel pulse-chase approach. *Genome Res.* **2016**, *26*, 554–565. [CrossRef] [PubMed]
83. Guo, Y.; Liu, J.; Elfenbein, S.J.; Ma, Y.; Zhong, M.; Qiu, C.; Ding, Y.; Lu, J. Characterization of the mammalian miRNA turnover landscape. *Nucleic Acids Res.* **2015**, *43*, 2326–2341. [CrossRef] [PubMed]
84. Gutierrez-Vazquez, C.; Enright, A.J.; Rodriguez-Galan, A.; Perez-Garcia, A.; Collier, P.; Jones, M.R.; Benes, V.; Mizgerd, J.P.; Mittelbrunn, M.; Ramiro, A.R.; et al. 3′ Uridylation controls mature microRNA turnover during CD4 T-cell activation. *RNA* **2017**, *23*, 882–891. [CrossRef] [PubMed]
85. Katoh, T.; Hojo, H.; Suzuki, T. Destabilization of microRNAs in human cells by 3′ deadenylation mediated by PARN and CUGBP1. *Nucleic Acids Res.* **2015**, *43*, 7521–7534. [CrossRef]
86. Katoh, T.; Sakaguchi, Y.; Miyauchi, K.; Suzuki, T.; Kashiwabara, S.; Baba, T.; Suzuki, T. Selective stabilization of mammalian microRNAs by 3′ adenylation mediated by the cytoplasmic poly(A) polymerase GLD-2. *Genes Dev.* **2009**, *23*, 433–438. [CrossRef]
87. Yamane, D.; Selitsky, S.R.; Shimakami, T.; Li, Y.; Zhou, M.; Honda, M.; Sethupathy, P.; Lemon, S.M. Differential hepatitis C virus RNA target site selection and host factor activities of naturally occurring miR-122 3 variants. *Nucleic Acids Res.* **2017**, *45*, 4743–4755. [CrossRef]
88. Yu, F.; Pillman, K.A.; Neilsen, C.T.; Toubia, J.; Lawrence, D.M.; Tsykin, A.; Gantier, M.P.; Callen, D.F.; Goodall, G.J.; Bracken, C.P. Naturally existing isoforms of miR-222 have distinct functions. *Nucleic Acids Res.* **2017**, *45*, 11371–11385. [CrossRef]
89. Voellenkle, C.; Rooij, J.; Guffanti, A.; Brini, E.; Fasanaro, P.; Isaia, E.; Croft, L.; David, M.; Capogrossi, M.C.; Moles, A.; et al. Deep-sequencing of endothelial cells exposed to hypoxia reveals the complexity of known and novel microRNAs. *RNA* **2012**, *18*, 472–484. [CrossRef]
90. Chistiakov, D.A.; Orekhov, A.N.; Bobryshev, Y.V. The role of miR-126 in embryonic angiogenesis, adult vascular homeostasis, and vascular repair and its alterations in atherosclerotic disease. *J. Mol. Cell. Cardiol.* **2016**, *97*, 47–55. [CrossRef]
91. Guduric-Fuchs, J.; O'Connor, A.; Cullen, A.; Harwood, L.; Medina, R.J.; O'Neill, C.L.; Stitt, A.W.; Curtis, T.M.; Simpson, D.A. Deep sequencing reveals predominant expression of miR-21 amongst the small non-coding RNAs in retinal microvascular endothelial cells. *J. Cell. Biochem.* **2012**, *113*, 2098–2111. [CrossRef] [PubMed]

92. Fernandez-Valverde, S.L.; Taft, R.J.; Mattick, J.S. Dynamic isomiR regulation in Drosophila development. *RNA* **2010**, *16*, 1881–1888. [CrossRef] [PubMed]
93. Schirmer, S.H.; Fledderus, J.O.; Bot, P.T.; Moerland, P.D.; Hoefer, I.E.; Baan, J., Jr.; Henriques, J.P.; van der Schaaf, R.J.; Vis, M.M.; Horrevoets, A.J.; et al. Interferon-beta signaling is enhanced in patients with insufficient coronary collateral artery development and inhibits arteriogenesis in mice. *Circ. Res.* **2008**, *102*, 1286–1294. [CrossRef] [PubMed]
94. Yildirim, C.; Nieuwenhuis, S.; Teunissen, P.F.; Horrevoets, A.J.; van Royen, N.; van der Pouw Kraan, T.C. Interferon-Beta, a Decisive Factor in Angiogenesis and Arteriogenesis. *J. Interferon Cytokine Res. Off. J. Int. Soc. Interferon Cytokine Res.* **2015**, *35*, 411–420. [CrossRef] [PubMed]
95. Schirmer, S.H.; Bot, P.T.; Fledderus, J.O.; van der Laan, A.M.; Volger, O.L.; Laufs, U.; Bohm, M.; de Vries, C.J.; Horrevoets, A.J.; Piek, J.J.; et al. Blocking interferon-beta stimulates vascular smooth muscle cell proliferation and arteriogenesis. *J. Biol. Chem.* **2010**, *285*, 34677–34685. [CrossRef] [PubMed]
96. Nejad, C.; Pillman, K.A.; Siddle, K.J.; Pepin, G.; Anko, M.L.; McCoy, C.E.; Beilharz, T.H.; Quintana-Murci, L.; Goodall, G.J.; Bracken, C.P.; et al. miR-222 isoforms are differentially regulated by type-I interferon. *RNA* **2018**, *24*, 332–341. [CrossRef] [PubMed]
97. Poliseno, L.; Tuccoli, A.; Mariani, L.; Evangelista, M.; Citti, L.; Woods, K.; Mercatanti, A.; Hammond, S.; Rainaldi, G. MicroRNAs modulate the angiogenic properties of HUVECs. *Blood* **2006**, *108*, 3068–3071. [CrossRef]
98. Dentelli, P.; Rosso, A.; Orso, F.; Olgasi, C.; Taverna, D.; Brizzi, M.F. microRNA-222 controls neovascularization by regulating signal transducer and activator of transcription 5A expression. *Arterioscler. Thromb. Vasc. Biol.* **2010**, *30*, 1562–1568. [CrossRef]
99. Van der Kwast, R.; Woudenberg, T.; Quax, P.H.A.; Nossent, A.Y. MicroRNA-411 and Its 5'-IsomiR Have Distinct Targets and Functions and Are Differentially Regulated in the Vasculature under Ischemia. *Mol. Ther. J. Am. Soc. Gene Ther.* **2019**. [CrossRef]
100. Wagner, R.W.; Smith, J.E.; Cooperman, B.S.; Nishikura, K. A double-stranded RNA unwinding activity introduces structural alterations by means of adenosine to inosine conversions in mammalian cells and Xenopus eggs. *Proc. Natl. Acad. Sci. USA* **1989**, *86*, 2647–2651. [CrossRef]
101. Gommans, W.M. A-to-I editing of microRNAs: Regulating the regulators? *Semin. Cell Dev. Biol.* **2012**, *23*, 251–257. [CrossRef] [PubMed]
102. Kume, H.; Hino, K.; Galipon, J.; Ui-Tei, K. A-to-I editing in the miRNA seed region regulates target mRNA selection and silencing efficiency. *Nucleic Acids Res.* **2014**, *42*, 10050–10060. [CrossRef] [PubMed]
103. Savva, Y.A.; Rieder, L.E.; Reenan, R.A. The ADAR protein family. *Genome Biol.* **2012**, *13*, 252. [CrossRef] [PubMed]
104. Nishikura, K. A-to-I editing of coding and non-coding RNAs by ADARs. *Nat. Rev. Mol. Cell Biol.* **2016**, *17*, 83–96. [CrossRef]
105. Mallela, A.; Nishikura, K. A-to-I editing of protein coding and noncoding RNAs. *Crit. Rev. Biochem. Mol. Biol.* **2012**, *47*, 493–501. [CrossRef]
106. Nigita, G.; Veneziano, D.; Ferro, A. A-to-I RNA Editing: Current Knowledge Sources and Computational Approaches with Special Emphasis on Non-Coding RNA Molecules. *Front. Bioeng. Biotechnol.* **2015**, *3*. [CrossRef]
107. Wang, Q.; Khillan, J.; Gadue, P.; Nishikura, K. Requirement of the RNA editing deaminase ADAR1 gene for embryonic erythropoiesis. *Science* **2000**, *290*, 1765–1768. [CrossRef]
108. Higuchi, M.; Maas, S.; Single, F.N.; Hartner, J.; Rozov, A.; Burnashev, N.; Feldmeyer, D.; Sprengel, R.; Seeburg, P.H. Point mutation in an AMPA receptor gene rescues lethality in mice deficient in the RNA-editing enzyme ADAR2. *Nature* **2000**, *406*, 78–81. [CrossRef]
109. Brusa, R.; Zimmermann, F.; Koh, D.S.; Feldmeyer, D.; Gass, P.; Seeburg, P.H.; Sprengel, R. Early-onset epilepsy and postnatal lethality associated with an editing-deficient GluR-B allele in mice. *Science* **1995**, *270*, 1677–1680. [CrossRef]
110. Hong, H.; Lin, J.; Chen, L. Regulatory factors governing adenosine-to-inosine (A-to-I) RNA editing. *Biosci Rep.* **2015**, *35*. [CrossRef]
111. Lai, F.; Chen, C.X.; Lee, V.M.; Nishikura, K. Dramatic increase of the RNA editing for glutamate receptor subunits during terminal differentiation of clonal human neurons. *J. Neurochem.* **1997**, *69*, 43–52. [CrossRef] [PubMed]

112. Liu, Y.; Emeson, R.B.; Samuel, C.E. Serotonin-2C receptor pre-mRNA editing in rat brain and in vitro by splice site variants of the interferon-inducible double-stranded RNA-specific adenosine deaminase ADAR1. *J. Biol. Chem.* **1999**, *274*, 18351–18358. [CrossRef] [PubMed]
113. Yang, W.; Chendrimada, T.P.; Wang, Q.; Higuchi, M.; Seeburg, P.H.; Shiekhattar, R.; Nishikura, K. Modulation of microRNA processing and expression through RNA editing by ADAR deaminases. *Nat. Struct. Mol. Biol.* **2006**, *13*, 13–21. [CrossRef] [PubMed]
114. Kawahara, Y.; Zinshteyn, B.; Chendrimada, T.P.; Shiekhattar, R.; Nishikura, K. RNA editing of the microRNA-151 precursor blocks cleavage by the Dicer-TRBP complex. *EMBO Rep.* **2007**, *8*, 763–769. [CrossRef]
115. Kawahara, Y.; Megraw, M.; Kreider, E.; Iizasa, H.; Valente, L.; Hatzigeorgiou, A.G.; Nishikura, K. Frequency and fate of microRNA editing in human brain. *Nucleic Acids Res.* **2008**, *36*, 5270–5280. [CrossRef]
116. Kawahara, Y.; Zinshteyn, B.; Sethupathy, P.; Iizasa, H.; Hatzigeorgiou, A.G.; Nishikura, K. Redirection of silencing targets by adenosine-to-inosine editing of miRNAs. *Science* **2007**, *315*, 1137–1140. [CrossRef]
117. Li, L.; Song, Y.; Shi, X.; Liu, J.; Xiong, S.; Chen, W.; Fu, Q.; Huang, Z.; Gu, N.; Zhang, R. The landscape of miRNA editing in animals and its impact on miRNA biogenesis and targeting. *Genome Res.* **2018**, *28*, 132–143. [CrossRef]
118. Vitsios, D.M.; Davis, M.P.; van Dongen, S.; Enright, A.J. Large-scale analysis of microRNA expression, epi-transcriptomic features and biogenesis. *Nucleic Acids Res.* **2016**. [CrossRef]
119. Wang, Y.; Liang, H. When MicroRNAs Meet RNA Editing in Cancer: A Nucleotide Change Can Make a Difference. *Bioessays News Rev. Mol. Cell. Dev. Biol.* **2018**, *40*. [CrossRef]
120. Wang, Y.; Xu, X.; Yu, S.; Jeong, K.J.; Zhou, Z.; Han, L.; Tsang, Y.H.; Li, J.; Chen, H.; Mangala, L.S.; et al. Systematic characterization of A-to-I RNA editing hotspots in microRNAs across human cancers. *Genome Res.* **2017**, *27*, 1112–1125. [CrossRef]
121. Cho, C.J.; Myung, S.J.; Chang, S. ADAR1 and MicroRNA.; A Hidden Crosstalk in Cancer. *Int. J. Mol. Sci.* **2017**, *18*, 799. [CrossRef] [PubMed]
122. Shoshan, E.; Mobley, A.K.; Braeuer, R.R.; Kamiya, T.; Huang, L.; Vasquez, M.E.; Salameh, A.; Lee, H.J.; Kim, S.J.; Ivan, C.; et al. Reduced adenosine-to-inosine miR-455-5p editing promotes melanoma growth and metastasis. *Nat. Cell Biol.* **2015**, *17*, 311–321. [CrossRef] [PubMed]
123. Van der Kwast, R.V.C.T.; van Ingen, E.; Parma, L.; Peters, H.A.B.; Quax, P.H.A.; Nossent, A.Y. Adenosine-to-Inosine Editing of MicroRNA-487b Alters Target Gene Selection After Ischemia and Promotes Neovascularization. *Circ. Res.* **2018**, *122*, 444–456. [CrossRef] [PubMed]
124. Dominissini, D.; Moshitch-Moshkovitz, S.; Schwartz, S.; Salmon-Divon, M.; Ungar, L.; Osenberg, S.; Cesarkas, K.; Jacob-Hirsch, J.; Amariglio, N.; Kupiec, M.; et al. Topology of the human and mouse m6A RNA methylomes revealed by m6A-seq. *Nature* **2012**, *485*, 201–206. [CrossRef]
125. Meyer, K.D.; Saletore, Y.; Zumbo, P.; Elemento, O.; Mason, C.E.; Jaffrey, S.R. Comprehensive analysis of mRNA methylation reveals enrichment in 3′ UTRs and near stop codons. *Cell* **2012**, *149*, 1635–1646. [CrossRef]
126. Wang, P.; Doxtader, K.A.; Nam, Y. Structural Basis for Cooperative Function of Mettl3 and Mettl14 Methyltransferases. *Mol. Cell* **2016**, *63*, 306–317. [CrossRef]
127. Yang, Y.; Hsu, P.J.; Chen, Y.S.; Yang, Y.G. Dynamic transcriptomic m(6)A decoration: Writers, erasers, readers and functions in RNA metabolism. *Cell Res.* **2018**, *28*, 616–624. [CrossRef]
128. Schwartz, S.; Mumbach, M.R.; Jovanovic, M.; Wang, T.; Maciag, K.; Bushkin, G.G.; Mertins, P.; Ter-Ovanesyan, D.; Habib, N.; Cacchiarelli, D.; et al. Perturbation of m6A writers reveals two distinct classes of mRNA methylation at internal and 5′ sites. *Cell Rep.* **2014**, *8*, 284–296. [CrossRef]
129. Zheng, G.; Dahl, J.A.; Niu, Y.; Fedorcsak, P.; Huang, C.M.; Li, C.J.; Vagbo, C.B.; Shi, Y.; Wang, W.L.; Song, S.H.; et al. ALKBH5 is a mammalian RNA demethylase that impacts RNA metabolism and mouse fertility. *Mol. Cell* **2013**, *49*, 18–29. [CrossRef]
130. Jia, G.; Fu, Y.; Zhao, X.; Dai, Q.; Zheng, G.; Yang, Y.; Yi, C.; Lindahl, T.; Pan, T.; Yang, Y.G.; et al. N6-methyladenosine in nuclear RNA is a major substrate of the obesity-associated FTO. *Nat. Chem. Biol.* **2011**, *7*, 885–887. [CrossRef]
131. Roundtree, I.A.; Evans, M.E.; Pan, T.; He, C. Dynamic RNA Modifications in Gene Expression Regulation. *Cell* **2017**, *169*, 1187–1200. [CrossRef] [PubMed]
132. Zhao, B.S.; Roundtree, I.A.; He, C. Post-transcriptional gene regulation by mRNA modifications. *Nat. Rev. Mol. Cell Biol.* **2017**, *18*, 31–42. [CrossRef] [PubMed]

133. Nachtergaele, S.; He, C. The emerging biology of RNA post-transcriptional modifications. *RNA Biol.* **2017**, *14*, 156–163. [CrossRef] [PubMed]
134. Yoon, K.J.; Ringeling, F.R.; Vissers, C.; Jacob, F.; Pokrass, M.; Jimenez-Cyrus, D.; Su, Y.; Kim, N.S.; Zhu, Y.; Zheng, L.; et al. Temporal Control of Mammalian Cortical Neurogenesis by m(6)A Methylation. *Cell* **2017**, *171*, 877–889. [CrossRef] [PubMed]
135. Wang, Y.; Li, Y.; Toth, J.I.; Petroski, M.D.; Zhang, Z.; Zhao, J.C. N6-methyladenosine modification destabilizes developmental regulators in embryonic stem cells. *Nat. Cell Biol.* **2014**, *16*, 191–198. [CrossRef] [PubMed]
136. Horiuchi, K.; Umetani, M.; Minami, T.; Okayama, H.; Takada, S.; Yamamoto, M.; Aburatani, H.; Reid, P.C.; Housman, D.E.; Hamakubo, T.; et al. Wilms' tumor 1-associating protein regulates G2/M transition through stabilization of cyclin A2 mRNA. *Proc. Natl. Acad. Sci. USA* **2006**, *103*, 17278–17283. [CrossRef]
137. Liu, N.; Zhou, K.I.; Parisien, M.; Dai, Q.; Diatchenko, L.; Pan, T. N6-methyladenosine alters RNA structure to regulate binding of a low-complexity protein. *Nucleic Acids Res.* **2017**, *45*, 6051–6063. [CrossRef]
138. Liu, N.; Dai, Q.; Zheng, G.; He, C.; Parisien, M.; Pan, T. N(6)-methyladenosine-dependent RNA structural switches regulate RNA-protein interactions. *Nature* **2015**, *518*, 560–564. [CrossRef]
139. Huang, H.; Weng, H.; Sun, W.; Qin, X.; Shi, H.; Wu, H.; Zhao, B.S.; Mesquita, A.; Liu, C.; Yuan, C.L.; et al. Recognition of RNA N(6)-methyladenosine by IGF2BP proteins enhances mRNA stability and translation. *Nat. Cell Biol.* **2018**, *20*, 285–295. [CrossRef]
140. Wang, X.; Zhao, B.S.; Roundtree, I.A.; Lu, Z.; Han, D.; Ma, H.; Weng, X.; Chen, K.; Shi, H.; He, C. N(6)-methyladenosine Modulates Messenger RNA Translation Efficiency. *Cell* **2015**, *161*, 1388–1399. [CrossRef]
141. Wang, X.; Lu, Z.; Gomez, A.; Hon, G.C.; Yue, Y.; Han, D.; Fu, Y.; Parisien, M.; Dai, Q.; Jia, G.; et al. N6-methyladenosine-dependent regulation of messenger RNA stability. *Nature* **2014**, *505*, 117–120. [CrossRef] [PubMed]
142. Alarcon, C.R.; Goodarzi, H.; Lee, H.; Liu, X.; Tavazoie, S.; Tavazoie, S.F. HNRNPA2B1 Is a Mediator of m(6)A-Dependent Nuclear RNA Processing Events. *Cell* **2015**, *162*, 1299–1308. [CrossRef] [PubMed]
143. Alarcon, C.R.; Lee, H.; Goodarzi, H.; Halberg, N.; Tavazoie, S.F. N6-methyladenosine marks primary microRNAs for processing. *Nature* **2015**, *519*, 482–485. [CrossRef] [PubMed]
144. Dai, Q.; Fong, R.; Saikia, M.; Stephenson, D.; Yu, Y.T.; Pan, T.; Piccirilli, J.A. Identification of recognition residues for ligation-based detection and quantitation of pseudouridine and N6-methyladenosine. *Nucleic Acids Res.* **2007**, *35*, 6322–6329. [CrossRef]
145. Konno, M.; Koseki, J.; Asai, A.; Yamagata, A.; Shimamura, T.; Motooka, D.; Okuzaki, D.; Kawamoto, K.; Mizushima, T.; Eguchi, H.; et al. Distinct methylation levels of mature microRNAs in gastrointestinal cancers. *Nat. Commun.* **2019**, *10*, 3888. [CrossRef]
146. Muller, S.; Glass, M.; Singh, A.K.; Haase, J.; Bley, N.; Fuchs, T.; Lederer, M.; Dahl, A.; Huang, H.; Chen, J.; et al. IGF2BP1 promotes SRF-dependent transcription in cancer in a m6A- and miRNA-dependent manner. *Nucleic Acids Res.* **2019**, *47*, 375–390. [CrossRef]
147. Dorn, L.E.; Lasman, L.; Chen, J.; Xu, X.; Hund, T.J.; Medvedovic, M.; Hanna, J.H.; van Berlo, J.H.; Accornero, F. The N(6)-Methyladenosine mRNA Methylase METTL3 Controls Cardiac Homeostasis and Hypertrophy. *Circulation* **2019**, *139*, 533–545. [CrossRef]
148. Mathiyalagan, P.; Adamiak, M.; Mayourian, J.; Sassi, Y.; Liang, Y.; Agarwal, N.; Jha, D.; Zhang, S.; Kohlbrenner, E.; Chepurko, E.; et al. FTO-Dependent N(6)-Methyladenosine Regulates Cardiac Function During Remodeling and Repair. *Circulation* **2019**, *139*, 518–532. [CrossRef]
149. Ma, J.Z.; Yang, F.; Zhou, C.C.; Liu, F.; Yuan, J.H.; Wang, F.; Wang, T.T.; Xu, Q.G.; Zhou, W.P.; Sun, S.H. METTL14 suppresses the metastatic potential of hepatocellular carcinoma by modulating N(6)-methyladenosine-dependent primary MicroRNA processing. *Hepatology* **2017**, *65*, 529–543. [CrossRef]
150. Han, J.; Wang, J.Z.; Yang, X.; Yu, H.; Zhou, R.; Lu, H.C.; Yuan, W.B.; Lu, J.C.; Zhou, Z.J.; Lu, Q.; et al. METTL3 promote tumor proliferation of bladder cancer by accelerating pri-miR221/222 maturation in m6A-dependent manner. *Mol. Cancer* **2019**, *18*, 110. [CrossRef]
151. Cech, T.R.; Steitz, J.A. The noncoding RNA revolution-trashing old rules to forge new ones. *Cell* **2014**, *157*, 77–94. [CrossRef] [PubMed]
152. Kim, Y.K.; Heo, I.; Kim, V.N. Modifications of small RNAs and their associated proteins. *Cell* **2010**, *143*, 703–709. [CrossRef] [PubMed]

153. Zhang, X.; Cozen, A.E.; Liu, Y.; Chen, Q.; Lowe, T.M. Small RNA Modifications: Integral to Function and Disease. *Trends Mol. Med.* **2016**, *22*, 1025–1034. [CrossRef] [PubMed]
154. Lan, M.D.; Xiong, J.; You, X.J.; Weng, X.C.; Zhou, X.; Yuan, B.F.; Feng, Y.Q. Existence of Diverse Modifications in Small-RNA Species Composed of 16-28 Nucleotides. *Chem. Eur. J.* **2018**, *24*, 9949–9956. [CrossRef] [PubMed]
155. Charette, M.; Gray, M.W. Pseudouridine in RNA: What, where, how, and why. *Iubmb Life* **2000**, *49*, 341–351. [CrossRef] [PubMed]
156. Karijolich, J.; Yi, C.; Yu, Y.T. Transcriptome-wide dynamics of RNA pseudouridylation. *Nat. Rev. Mol. Cell Biol.* **2015**, *16*, 581–585. [CrossRef]
157. Schwartz, S.; Bernstein, D.A.; Mumbach, M.R.; Jovanovic, M.; Herbst, R.H.; Leon-Ricardo, B.X.; Engreitz, J.M.; Guttman, M.; Satija, R.; Lander, E.S.; et al. Transcriptome-wide mapping reveals widespread dynamic-regulated pseudouridylation of ncRNA and mRNA. *Cell* **2014**, *159*, 148–162. [CrossRef]
158. Arnez, J.G.; Steitz, T.A. Crystal structure of unmodified tRNA(Gln) complexed with glutaminyl-tRNA synthetase and ATP suggests a possible role for pseudo-uridines in stabilization of RNA structure. *Biochemistry* **1994**, *33*, 7560–7567. [CrossRef]
159. Cohn, W.E. Pseudouridine, a carbon-carbon linked ribonucleoside in ribonucleic acids: Isolation, structure, and chemical characteristics. *J. Biol. Chem.* **1960**, *235*, 1488–1498.
160. Carlile, T.M.; Rojas-Duran, M.F.; Zinshteyn, B.; Shin, H.; Bartoli, K.M.; Gilbert, W.V. Pseudouridine profiling reveals regulated mRNA pseudouridylation in yeast and human cells. *Nature* **2014**, *515*, 143–146. [CrossRef]
161. Ayadi, L.; Galvanin, A.; Pichot, F.; Marchand, V.; Motorin, Y. RNA ribose methylation (2′-O-methylation): Occurrence, biosynthesis and biological functions. *Biochim. Biophys. Acta Gene Regul. Mech.* **2018**. [CrossRef] [PubMed]
162. Dimitrova, D.G.; Teysset, L.; Carre, C. RNA 2′-O-Methylation (Nm) Modification in Human Diseases. *Genes* **2019**, *10*, 117. [CrossRef] [PubMed]
163. Bachellerie, J.P.; Cavaille, J.; Huttenhofer, A. The expanding snoRNA world. *Biochimie* **2002**, *84*, 775–790. [CrossRef]
164. Cavaille, J.; Buiting, K.; Kiefmann, M.; Lalande, M.; Brannan, C.I.; Horsthemke, B.; Bachellerie, J.P.; Brosius, J.; Huttenhofer, A. Identification of brain-specific and imprinted small nucleolar RNA genes exhibiting an unusual genomic organization. *Proc. Natl. Acad. Sci. USA* **2000**, *97*, 14311–14316. [CrossRef]
165. Vitali, P.; Basyuk, E.; Le, M.E.; Bertrand, E.; Muscatelli, F.; Cavaille, J.; Huttenhofer, A. ADAR2-mediated editing of RNA substrates in the nucleolus is inhibited by C/D small nucleolar RNAs. *J. Cell Biol.* **2005**, *169*, 745–753. [CrossRef]
166. Yi-Brunozzi, H.Y.; Easterwood, L.M.; Kamilar, G.M.; Beal, P.A. Synthetic substrate analogs for the RNA-editing adenosine deaminase ADAR-2. *Nucleic Acids Res.* **1999**, *27*, 2912–2917. [CrossRef]
167. Mizrahi, R.A.; Phelps, K.J.; Ching, A.Y.; Beal, P.A. Nucleoside analog studies indicate mechanistic differences between RNA-editing adenosine deaminases. *Nucleic Acids Res.* **2012**, *40*, 9825–9835. [CrossRef]
168. Inoue, H.; Hayase, Y.; Imura, A.; Iwai, S.; Miura, K.; Ohtsuka, E. Synthesis and hybridization studies on two complementary nona(2′-O-methyl)ribonucleotides. *Nucleic Acids Res.* **1987**, *15*, 6131–6148. [CrossRef]
169. Majlessi, M.; Nelson, N.C.; Becker, M.M. Advantages of 2′-O-methyl oligoribonucleotide probes for detecting RNA targets. *Nucleic Acids Res.* **1998**, *26*, 2224–2229. [CrossRef]
170. Tsourkas, A.; Behlke, M.A.; Bao, G. Hybridization of 2′-O-methyl and 2′-deoxy molecular beacons to RNA and DNA targets. *Nucleic Acids Res.* **2002**, *30*, 5168–5174. [CrossRef]
171. Yu, B.; Yang, Z.; Li, J.; Minakhina, S.; Yang, M.; Padgett, R.W.; Steward, R.; Chen, X. Methylation as a crucial step in plant microRNA biogenesis. *Science* **2005**, *307*, 932–935. [CrossRef] [PubMed]
172. Dominissini, D.; Nachtergaele, S.; Moshitch-Moshkovitz, S.; Peer, E.; Kol, N.; Ben-Haim, M.S.; Dai, Q.; Di Segni, A.; Salmon-Divon, M.; Clark, W.C.; et al. The dynamic N1-methyladenosine methylome in eukaryotic messenger RNA. *Nature* **2016**, *530*, 441–446. [CrossRef] [PubMed]
173. Li, X.; Xiong, X.; Wang, K.; Wang, L.; Shu, X.; Ma, S.; Yi, C. Transcriptome-wide mapping reveals reversible and dynamic N(1)-methyladenosine methylome. *Nat. Chem. Biol.* **2016**, *12*, 311–316. [CrossRef] [PubMed]
174. Zhang, C.; Jia, G. Reversible RNA Modification N(1)-methyladenosine (m(1)A) in mRNA and tRNA. *Genom. Proteom. Bioinform.* **2018**, *16*, 155–161. [CrossRef]
175. Liu, F.; Clark, W.; Luo, G.; Wang, X.; Fu, Y.; Wei, J.; Wang, X.; Hao, Z.; Dai, Q.; Zheng, G.; et al. ALKBH1-Mediated tRNA Demethylation Regulates Translation. *Cell* **2016**, *167*, 816–828. [CrossRef]

176. Zhou, H.; Kimsey, I.J.; Nikolova, E.N.; Sathyamoorthy, B.; Grazioli, G.; McSally, J.; Bai, T.; Wunderlich, C.H.; Kreutz, C.; Andricioaei, I.; et al. m(1)A and m(1)G disrupt A-RNA structure through the intrinsic instability of Hoogsteen base pairs. *Nat. Struct. Mol. Biol.* **2016**, *23*, 803–810. [CrossRef]
177. Squires, J.E.; Patel, H.R.; Nousch, M.; Sibbritt, T.; Humphreys, D.T.; Parker, B.J.; Suter, C.M.; Preiss, T. Widespread occurrence of 5-methylcytosine in human coding and non-coding RNA. *Nucleic Acids Res.* **2012**, *40*, 5023–5033. [CrossRef]
178. Van Haute, L.; Dietmann, S.; Kremer, L.; Hussain, S.; Pearce, S.F.; Powell, C.A.; Rorbach, J.; Lantaff, R.; Blanco, S.; Sauer, S.; et al. Deficient methylation and formylation of mt-tRNA(Met) wobble cytosine in a patient carrying mutations in NSUN3. *Nat. Commun.* **2016**, *7*, 12039. [CrossRef]
179. Nakano, S.; Suzuki, T.; Kawarada, L.; Iwata, H.; Asano, K.; Suzuki, T. NSUN3 methylase initiates 5-formylcytidine biogenesis in human mitochondrial tRNA(Met). *Nat. Chem. Biol.* **2016**, *12*, 546–551. [CrossRef]
180. Goll, M.G.; Kirpekar, F.; Maggert, K.A.; Yoder, J.A.; Hsieh, C.L.; Zhang, X.; Golic, K.G.; Jacobsen, S.E.; Bestor, T.H. Methylation of tRNAAsp by the DNA methyltransferase homolog Dnmt2. *Science* **2006**, *311*, 395–398. [CrossRef]
181. Trixl, L.; Lusser, A. The dynamic RNA modification 5-methylcytosine and its emerging role as an epitranscriptomic mark. *Wiley Interdiscip. Rev. RNA* **2019**, *10*, e1510. [CrossRef] [PubMed]
182. Hussain, S.; Sajini, A.A.; Blanco, S.; Dietmann, S.; Lombard, P.; Sugimoto, Y.; Paramor, M.; Gleeson, J.G.; Odom, D.T.; Ule, J.; et al. NSun2-mediated cytosine-5 methylation of vault noncoding RNA determines its processing into regulatory small RNAs. *Cell Rep.* **2013**, *4*, 255–261. [CrossRef] [PubMed]
183. Khoddami, V.; Cairns, B.R. Identification of direct targets and modified bases of RNA cytosine methyltransferases. *Nat. Biotechnol.* **2013**, *31*, 458–464. [CrossRef] [PubMed]
184. Jurkowski, T.P.; Meusburger, M.; Phalke, S.; Helm, M.; Nellen, W.; Reuter, G.; Jeltsch, A. Human DNMT2 methylates tRNA(Asp) molecules using a DNA methyltransferase-like catalytic mechanism. *RNA* **2008**, *14*, 1663–1670. [CrossRef] [PubMed]
185. Schaefer, M.; Pollex, T.; Hanna, K.; Tuorto, F.; Meusburger, M.; Helm, M.; Lyko, F. RNA methylation by Dnmt2 protects transfer RNAs against stress-induced cleavage. *Genes Dev.* **2010**, *24*, 1590–1595. [CrossRef]
186. Aguilo, F.; Li, S.; Balasubramaniyan, N.; Sancho, A.; Benko, S.; Zhang, F.; Vashisht, A.; Rengasamy, M.; Andino, B.; Chen, C.H.; et al. Deposition of 5-Methylcytosine on Enhancer RNAs Enables the Coactivator Function of PGC-1alpha. *Cell Rep.* **2016**, *14*, 479–492. [CrossRef]
187. Sergiev, P.V.; Bogdanov, A.A.; Dontsova, O.A. Ribosomal RNA guanine-(N2)-methyltransferases and their targets. *Nucleic Acids Res.* **2007**, *35*, 2295–2301. [CrossRef]
188. Chen, W.; Song, X.; Lv, H.; Lin, H. iRNA-m2G: Identifying N(2)-methylguanosine Sites Based on Sequence-Derived Information. *Mol. Ther. Nucleic Acids* **2019**, *18*, 253–258. [CrossRef]
189. Bavi, R.S.; Kamble, A.D.; Kumbhar, N.M.; Kumbhar, B.V.; Sonawane, K.D. Conformational preferences of modified nucleoside N(2)-methylguanosine (m(2)G) and its derivative N(2), N(2)-dimethylguanosine (m(2)(2)G) occur at 26th position (hinge region) in tRNA. *Cell Biochem. Biophys.* **2011**, *61*, 507–521. [CrossRef]
190. Bavi, R.S.; Sambhare, S.B.; Sonawane, K.D. MD simulation studies to investigate iso-energetic conformational behaviour of modified nucleosides m(2)G and m(2) 2G present in tRNA. *Comput. Struct. Biotechnol. J.* **2013**, *5*, e201302015. [CrossRef]
191. Pinto, Y.; Buchumenski, I.; Levanon, E.Y.; Eisenberg, E. Human cancer tissues exhibit reduced A-to-I editing of miRNAs coupled with elevated editing of their targets. *Nucleic Acids Res.* **2018**, *46*, 71–82. [CrossRef] [PubMed]
192. Esteller, M.; Pandolfi, P.P. The Epitranscriptome of Noncoding RNAs in Cancer. *Cancer Discov.* **2017**, *7*, 359–368. [CrossRef] [PubMed]
193. Meyer, K.D.; Patil, D.P.; Zhou, J.; Zinoviev, A.; Skabkin, M.A.; Elemento, O.; Pestova, T.V.; Qian, S.B.; Jaffrey, S.R. 5′ UTR m(6)A Promotes Cap-Independent Translation. *Cell* **2015**, *163*, 999–1010. [CrossRef] [PubMed]
194. Xiang, Y.; Laurent, B.; Hsu, C.H.; Nachtergaele, S.; Lu, Z.; Sheng, W.; Xu, C.; Chen, H.; Ouyang, J.; Wang, S.; et al. RNA m(6)A methylation regulates the ultraviolet-induced DNA damage response. *Nature* **2017**, *543*, 573–576. [CrossRef]
195. Zhou, J.; Wan, J.; Gao, X.; Zhang, X.; Jaffrey, S.R.; Qian, S.B. Dynamic m(6)A mRNA methylation directs translational control of heat shock response. *Nature* **2015**, *526*, 591–594. [CrossRef]

196. Blanco, S.; Bandiera, R.; Popis, M.; Hussain, S.; Lombard, P.; Aleksic, J.; Sajini, A.; Tanna, H.; Cortes-Garrido, R.; Gkatza, N.; et al. Stem cell function and stress response are controlled by protein synthesis. *Nature* **2016**, *534*, 335–340. [CrossRef]
197. Blanco, S.; Dietmann, S.; Flores, J.V.; Hussain, S.; Kutter, C.; Humphreys, P.; Lukk, M.; Lombard, P.; Treps, L.; Popis, M.; et al. Aberrant methylation of tRNAs links cellular stress to neuro-developmental disorders. *EMBO J.* **2014**, *33*, 2020–2039. [CrossRef]
198. Krogh, N.; Jansson, M.D.; Hafner, S.J.; Tehler, D.; Birkedal, U.; Christensen-Dalsgaard, M.; Lund, A.H.; Nielsen, H. Profiling of 2′-O-Me in human rRNA reveals a subset of fractionally modified positions and provides evidence for ribosome heterogeneity. *Nucleic Acids Res.* **2016**, *44*, 7884–7895. [CrossRef]
199. Marcel, V.; Ghayad, S.E.; Belin, S.; Therizols, G.; Morel, A.P.; Solano-Gonzalez, E.; Vendrell, J.A.; Hacot, S.; Mertani, H.C.; Albaret, M.A.; et al. p53 acts as a safeguard of translational control by regulating fibrillarin and rRNA methylation in cancer. *Cancer Cell* **2013**, *24*, 318–330. [CrossRef]
200. Gatsiou, A.; Stellos, K. Dawn of Epitranscriptomic Medicine. *Circ. Genom. Precis. Med.* **2018**, *11*, e001927. [CrossRef]
201. Stellos, K.; Gatsiou, A.; Stamatelopoulos, K.; Perisic Matic, L.; John, D.; Lunella, F.F.; Jae, N.; Rossbach, O.; Amrhein, C.; Sigala, F.; et al. Adenosine-to-inosine RNA editing controls cathepsin S expression in atherosclerosis by enabling HuR-mediated post-transcriptional regulation. *Nat. Med.* **2016**, *22*, 1140–1150. [CrossRef] [PubMed]
202. Veliz, E.A.; Easterwood, L.M.; Beal, P.A. Substrate analogues for an RNA-editing adenosine deaminase: Mechanistic investigation and inhibitor design. *J. Am. Chem. Soc.* **2003**, *125*, 10867–10876. [CrossRef] [PubMed]
203. Xiang, J.F.; Yang, Q.; Liu, C.X.; Wu, M.; Chen, L.L.; Yang, L. N(6)-Methyladenosines Modulate A-to-I RNA Editing. *Mol. Cell* **2018**, *69*, 126–135.e126. [CrossRef] [PubMed]
204. Rupaimoole, R.; Slack, F.J. MicroRNA therapeutics: Towards a new era for the management of cancer and other diseases. *Nat. Rev. Drug Discov.* **2017**, *16*, 203–222. [CrossRef]
205. Telonis, A.G.; Magee, R.; Loher, P.; Chervoneva, I.; Londin, E.; Rigoutsos, I. Knowledge about the presence or absence of miRNA isoforms (isomiRs) can successfully discriminate amongst 32 TCGA cancer types. *Nucleic Acids Res.* **2017**, *45*, 2973–2985. [CrossRef]
206. Schaefer, M.; Kapoor, U.; Jantsch, M.F. Understanding RNA modifications: The promises and technological bottlenecks of the 'epitranscriptome'. *Open Biol.* **2017**, *7*, 170077. [CrossRef]

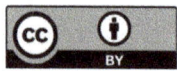

© 2019 by the authors. Licensee MDPI, Basel, Switzerland. This article is an open access article distributed under the terms and conditions of the Creative Commons Attribution (CC BY) license (http://creativecommons.org/licenses/by/4.0/).

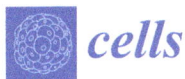

Article

Prolonged Hyperoxygenation Treatment Improves Vein Graft Patency and Decreases Macrophage Content in Atherosclerotic Lesions in ApoE3*Leiden Mice

Laura Parma [1,2], Hendrika A. B. Peters [1,2], Fabiana Baganha [1,2], Judith C. Sluimer [3,4], Margreet R. de Vries [1,2,†] and Paul H. A. Quax [1,2,*,†]

1. Department of surgery; Leiden University Medical Center, 2300 RC Leiden, The Netherlands; l.parma@lumc.nl (L.P.); H.A.B.Peters@lumc.nl (H.A.B.P.); F.Baganha_Carreiras@lumc.nl (F.B.); M.R.de_Vries@lumc.nl (M.R.d.V.)
2. Einthoven laboratory for experimental vascular medicine, Leiden University Medical Center, 2300 RC Leiden, The Netherlands
3. Cardiovascular Research Institute Maastricht, Department of Pathology, Maastricht University Medical Center, 6200 MD Maastricht, The Netherlands; judith.sluimer@maastrichtuniversity.nl
4. Centre for Cardiovascular Science, University of Edinburgh, Edinburgh EH16 4SA, UK
* Correspondence: p.h.a.quax@lumc.nl
† Shared last author.

Received: 20 January 2020; Accepted: 30 January 2020; Published: 1 February 2020

Abstract: Unstable atherosclerotic plaques frequently show plaque angiogenesis which increases the chance of rupture and thrombus formation leading to infarctions. Hypoxia plays a role in angiogenesis and inflammation, two processes involved in the pathogenesis of atherosclerosis. We aim to study the effect of resolution of hypoxia using carbogen gas (95% O_2, 5% CO_2) on the remodeling of vein graft accelerated atherosclerotic lesions in ApoE3*Leiden mice which harbor plaque angiogenesis. Single treatment resulted in a drastic decrease of intraplaque hypoxia, without affecting plaque composition. Daily treatment for three weeks resulted in 34.5% increase in vein graft patency and increased lumen size. However, after three weeks intraplaque hypoxia was comparable to the controls, as were the number of neovessels and the degree of intraplaque hemorrhage. To our surprise we found that three weeks of treatment triggered ROS accumulation and subsequent Hif1a induction, paralleled with a reduction in the macrophage content, pointing to an increase in lesion stability. Similar to what we observed in vivo, in vitro induction of ROS in bone marrow derived macrophages lead to increased Hif1a expression and extensive DNA damage and apoptosis. Our study demonstrates that carbogen treatment did improve vein graft patency and plaque stability and reduced intraplaque macrophage accumulation via ROS mediated DNA damage and apoptosis but failed to have long term effects on hypoxia and intraplaque angiogenesis.

Keywords: hyperoxygenation; vein graft disease; atherosclerosis; macrophages; vascular biology

---

1. Introduction

The (in)stability of atherosclerotic plaques determines the incidence of major cardiovascular events such as myocardial infarction and stroke [1]. Lack of oxygen within the plaque, or intraplaque hypoxia, has been identified as one of the major contributors to plaque instability [2,3]. It has been detected in advanced human atherosclerotic lesions [4] as well as in murine atherosclerotic lesions [5,6].

The intraplaque lack of oxygen is provoked by progressive thickening of the neointimal layer [7] and overconsumption of O_2 by plaque inflammatory cells [4]. The key regulator of hypoxia is the transcription factor Hif1a [8]. Low oxygen levels, or hypoxia, prevents degradation of Hif1a, promoting its dimerization with the Hif1b subunit. This complex activates the transcription of multiple genes, the most important being Vegfa, that triggers the formation of neovessels in the plaque. Intraplaque neovessels are often immature and therefore leaky, leading to intraplaque hemorrhage, a phenomenon characterized by extravasation of inflammatory cells and red blood cells inside the plaque. Hypoxia also upregulates the expression of transcription factors that cause vascular calcification in vascular smooth muscle cells [9], a characteristic feature of atherosclerosis. Both intraplaque neovessels and vascular calcification are regulated by hypoxia [9] and contribute to plaque instability. The combination of those processes results in a larger plaque which is more unstable and prone to rupture [10,11]. Hif1a was shown to be present in macrophage-rich and foam cell-rich areas and its expression in macrophages was correlated with accelerated atherosclerosis development in LDLR$^{-/-}$ mice [12]. Moreover, it has been shown that hypoxia can influence gene expression in macrophages, leading to an inflammatory response with increased production of pro-inflammatory cytokines [13,14].

Thus, the reoxygenation of the atherosclerotic plaque would be expected to prevent intraplaque hypoxia and atherosclerotic plaque progression. Previously, Marsch et al. showed that plaque reoxygenation in LDLR$^{-/-}$ mice via breathing of the hyperoxic gas carbogen, composed of 95% O_2 and 5% CO_2, prevented necrotic core expansion by enhancing efferocytosis [15]. The response of intraplaque angiogenesis to reoxygenation could not be studied in this model, as intraplaque angiogenesis is virtually nonexistent in plaques of LDLR$^{-/-}$ mice. To examine the effect of carbogen treatment on intraplaque angiogenesis we used vein grafts in hypercholesterolemic ApoE3*Leiden mice that do harbor extensive intraplaque angiogenesis, and have been shown to be morphologically similar to rupture-prone plaques in humans. The lesions in this model have the typical characteristics of late stage atherosclerosis, including the presence of foam cells, intraplaque neovascularization, calcification and cholesterol clefts [16] and eventually also occlusion of the graft.

We hypothesized that carbogen gas exposure would reduce hypoxia in vein grafts in the ApoE3* Leiden mice and consequently would reduce intraplaque angiogenesis and increase lesion stability. Thus, we used this model to study plaque reoxygenation and its effect on vein graft remodeling, intraplaque neovascularization, inflammation and vein graft patency. Moreover, since prolonged hyperoxia has the risk of introducing reactive oxygen species [17], we investigated the effect of reactive oxygen species in vitro on bone marrow derived macrophages and in vivo in the atherosclerotic lesions and their effect on the plaque environment.

2. Materials and Methods

2.1. Mice

This study was performed in compliance with Dutch government guidelines and the Directive 2010/63/EU of the European Parliament. All animal experiments were approved by the animal welfare committee of the Leiden University Medical Center. Male ApoE3*Leiden mice, crossbred in our own colony on a C57BL/background, 8 to 16 weeks old, were fed a diet containing 15% cacao butter, 1% cholesterol and 0.5% cholate (100193, Triple A Trading, Tiel, The Netherlands) for three weeks prior to surgery until sacrifice.

2.2. Vein Graft Surgery

Vein graft surgery was performed by donor mice caval vein interpositioning in the carotid artery of recipient mice as previously described [5,18]. Briefly, thoracic caval veins from donor mice were harvested. In recipient mice, the right carotid artery was dissected and cut in the middle. The artery was everted around the cuffs that were placed at both ends of the artery and ligated with 8.0 sutures. The caval vein was sleeved over the two cuffs, and ligated. On the day of surgery and on the day of sacrifice mice were anesthetized with midazolam (5 mg/kg, Roche Diagnostics, Basel, Switzerland), medetomidine (0.5 mg/kg, Orion, Espoo, Finland) and fentanyl (0.05 mg/kg, Janssen

Pharmaceutical Beerse, Belgium). The adequacy of the anesthesia was monitored by keeping track of the breathing frequency and the response to toe pinching of the mice. After surgery, mice were antagonized with atipamezol (2.5 mg/kg, Orion Espoo, Finland) and fluminasenil (0.5 mg/kg, Fresenius Kabi, Bad Homburg vor der Höhe, Germany). Buprenorphine (0.1 mg/kg, MSD Animal Health, Keniworth, NJ, USA) was given after surgery to relieve pain.

2.3. Carbogen Treatment

Acute reoxygenation was investigate in ApoE3*Leiden mice on day 28 after vein graft surgery. Mice were randomized in two groups, a control group ($n = 13$) and a carbogen treated group ($n = 12$) and exposed for 90 min to air (21% O_2) or carbogen gas (95% O_2, 5% CO_2) respectively. Halfway during the treatment, the mice received intraperitoneal injection of hypoxia specific marker pimonidazole (100 mg/kg, hypoxyprobe Omni kit, Hypoxyprobe Inc., Burlington, MA, USA) and anesthesia. Directly after the end of the treatment, mice were sacrificed after 5 min of in vivo perfusion-fixation under anesthesia. Vein grafts were harvested, fixated in 4% formaldehyde, dehydrated and paraffin-embedded for histology.

Chronic reoxygenation was investigated in ApoE3*Leiden mice starting on day 7 after vein graft surgery. The decision for this timepoint was based on our previous finding that intraplaque angiogenesis is detectable in ApoE3*Leiden mice starting from day 14 after vein graft surgery [5]. Mice were randomized based on their plasma cholesterol levels (Roche Diagnostics, kit 1489437, Basel, Switzerland) and body weight in two groups, a control group ($n = 16$) and a carbogen treated group ($n = 16$) and exposed daily for 90 min to air (21% O_2) or carbogen (95% O_2, 5% CO_2) respectively, until the day of sacrifice. On day 28 after surgery, mice received the last treatment and halfway during this last treatment they received intraperitoneal injection of hypoxia specific marker pimonidazole (100 mg/kg, hypoxyprobe Omni kit, Hypoxyprobe Inc., Burlington, MA, USA) and anesthesia. Immediately after the end of the treatment, mice were sacrificed as previously described for the acute reoxygenation experiment.

2.4. Histological and Immunohistochemical Assessment of Vein Grafts

Vein graft samples were embedded in paraffin, and sequential cross-sections (5 µm thick) were made throughout the embedded vein grafts. To quantify the vein graft thickening (vessel wall area), MOVAT pentachrome staining was performed. Total size of the vein graft and lumen were measured. Thickening of the vessel wall (measured as intimal thickening + media thickening) was defined as the area between lumen and adventitia and determined by subtracting the luminal area from the total vessel area. The optimal lumen area was calculated by converting the luminal circumference, measured as the luminal perimeter, into luminal area.

Intraplaque angiogenesis was measured as the amount of $CD31^+$ vessels in the vessel wall area and intraplaque hemorrhage (IPH) was monitored by the amount of erythrocytes outside the (neo)vessels and scored as either not present, low, moderate or high.

Antibodies directed at alpha smooth muscle cell actin (αSMActin, Sigma, Santa Clara, CA, USA), Mac-3 (BD Pharmingen, Franklin Lakes, NJ, USA), Pimonidazole (mouse IgG1 monoclonal antibody, clone 4.3.11.3, Hypoxyprobe Inc., Burlington, MA, USA), 8OHdG (bs-1278R, Bioss antibodies, Woburn, MA, USA), CD31 (sc-1506-r, Santa Cruz, Dallas, TX, USA), Ter119 (116202, Biolegend, San Diego, CA, USA), Ki67 (ab16667, Abcam, Cambridge, UK) and cleaved caspase 3 (9661-S, Cell SignalingDanvers, MA, USA) were used for immunohistochemical staining. Sirius red staining (80115, Klinipath, Amsterdam, The Netherlands) was performed to quantify the amount of collagen present in the vein grafts. The immuno-positive areas are expressed as a total area or percentage of the lesion area. Stained slides were photographed using microscope photography software (Axiovision, Carl Zeiss Microscopy, White Plains, NY, USA) or Ultrafast Digital Pathology Slide Scanner and associated software (Philips, Cambridge, MA, USA) and image analysis softwares were used to quantify the vein graft intimal hyperplasia and composition (Qwin, Leica, Wetzlar, Germany and Imagej, Bethesda, MD, USA).

2.5. RNA Isolation, cDNA Synthesis and qPCR

Total RNA was isolated from 10 (20 μm thick) paraffin sections (at least $n = 6$/group) following the manufacture's protocol (FFPE RNA isolation kit, Qiagen, Venlo, the Netherlands). cDNA was synthesized using the Superscript IV VILO kit according to the manufacture's protocol (TermoFisher, Waltham, MA, USA).

Commercially available TaqMan gene expression assays for the housekeeping gene hypoxanthine phosphoribosyl transferase (Hprt) (Mm01545399_m1), and selected genes were used (Applied Biosystems, Foster City, CA, USA); Vegfa (Mm03015193_m1), Hif1a (Mm00468869_m1), Cxcl12 (Mm00445553_m1), Epas1 (Mm01236112_m1), Il6 (Mm00446190_m1), Tnf (Mm00443258_m1) and Ccl2 (Mm00441242_m1). Q-PCRs were performed on the ABI 7500 Fast system (Applied Biosystems). The 2-ΔΔCt method was used to analyze the relative changes in gene expression.

2.6. Bone Marrow Derived Macrophages Isolation and In Vitro Experiments

Monocytes were isolated from bone marrow of tibias and femurs of male ApoE3*Leiden mice ($n = 4$) and cultured in RPMI 1640 medium (52400-025, ThermoFisher, GIBCO, Waltham, MA, USA,) supplemented with 25% heat inactivated fetal calf serum (Gibco® by Life Technologies), 100 U/mL Penicillin/Streptomycin (ThermoFisher, GIBCO, Waltham, MA, USA) and 0.1 mg/mL macrophage colony-stimulating factor (, 14-8983-80, ThermoFisher, E-Bioscience Waltham, MA, USA). After eight days the derived macrophages were seeded in a 12 wells plate for RNA isolation and in a chamber slide for immunocytochemistry (ICC) (NUNC LAB-TEK II, 154534, ThermoFisher, Waltham, MA, USA). 24 h later, when BMM were fully attached, BMM were stimulated with either 200 or 400 μm tert-butylhydroperoxide, t-BHP, (Luperox, 458139, Sigma Aldrich, St. Louis, Missouri, USA) as a ROS mimic for 6 h.

RNA was isolated according to standard protocol using TRIzol® (Ambion®, ThermoFisher,Waltham, MA, USA) after which sample concentration and purity were examined by nanodrop (Nanodrop Technologies, ThermoFisher, Waltham, MA, USA). Complementary DNA (cDNA) was prepared using the High Capacity cDNA Reverse Transcription Kit (Applied Biosystems, ThermoFisher, Waltham, MA, USA) according to manufacturer's protocol. For qPCR, commercially available TaqMan gene expression assays for the selected genes were used as explained above.

For ICC cells were fixated in 4% formaldehyde and antibodies directed at Mac-3 (BD Pharmingen, Franklin Lakes, NJ, USA), 8OHdG (bs-1278R, Bioss antibodies, Woburn, MA, USA) and cleaved caspase 3 (9661-S, Cell Signaling, Danvers, MA, USA) were used for immunocytochemical staining. Tile-scans of stained slides were photographed using a fluorescent microscope (Leica AF-6000, Leica, Wetzlar, Germany) and Fiji image analysis software was used to quantify the mean grey value expression of the targets (Imagej, Bethesda, MD, USA).

2.7. Statistical Analysis

Results are expressed as mean ± SEM. A 2-tailed Student's t-test was used to compare individual groups. Non-Gaussian distributed data were analyzed using a Mann-Whitney U test using GraphPad Prism version 6.00 for Windows (GraphPad Software). Probability-values < 0.05 were regarded significant.

3. Results

3.1. Acute Carbogen Exposure Reduces Intraplaque Hypoxia

To evaluate the effect of acute carbogen treatment on advanced atherosclerotic vein graft lesions, ApoE3*Leiden mice that underwent vein graft surgery were exposed for 90 min to carbogen gas or normal breathing air. Mice exposed to carbogen gas ($n = 8$) showed a significant reduction of intraplaque (IP) hypoxia in the vein graft lesion compared to the air breathing group ($n = 8$) as shown by a 84% decrease in the immuno-area positive for pimonidazole in the lesions of carbogen treated mice compared to the control (p-value = 0.027) (Figure 1A–C).

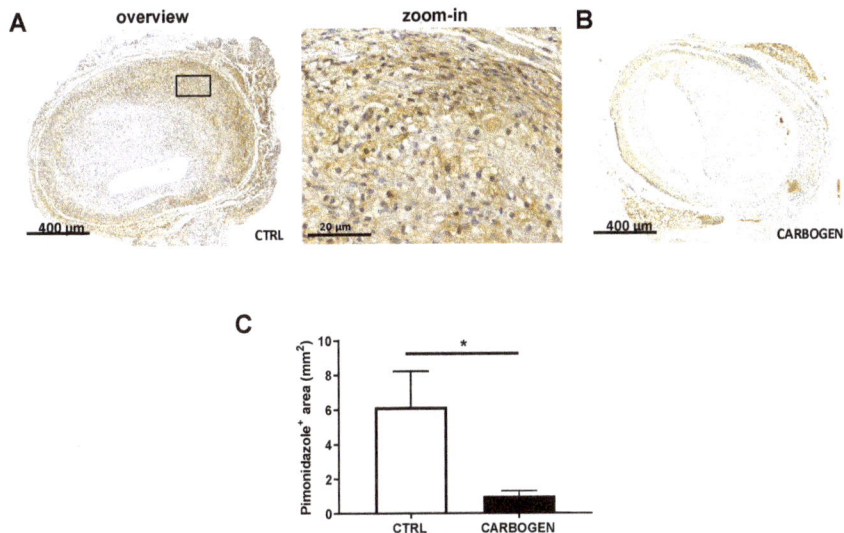

Figure 1. Short term carbogen exposure drastically reduces intraplaque hypoxia. (A) Representative pictures of sections from vein graft lesions in ApoE3* Leiden mice stained for pimonidazole in the control group (n = 8) and (B) one-time carbogen treated group (n = 8). (C) Quantification of pimonidazole positive area. Data are presented as mean ± SEM. * $p < 0.05$; by two-sided Student's t test.

Regarding the aspect of vein graft patency, single 90-min carbogen exposure directly before sacrifice did not affect vein graft patency (Figure 2A), vessel wall area, lumen perimeter, lumen area or optimal lumen area (Figure 2B,C). Furthermore, weight nor cholesterol levels were changed (Figure S1).

The percentage of collagen present in the lesion was comparable between the two groups (Figure 2D) and at a cellular level, the percentage of macrophages (Figure 2E) and SMCs (Figure 2F) were not altered by the acute exposure to carbogen.

3.2. Chronic Carbogen Exposure Does not Influence Intraplaque Hypoxia

To evaluate the effect of hyperoxic carbogen treatment on plaque composition and remodeling we performed a chronic carbogen treatment on ApoE3*Leiden mice with advanced atherosclerotic vein graft lesions. Mice were exposed for 90 min daily to carbogen gas (n = 13) or normal breathing air (n = 12) for 21 days. Neither weight or cholesterol levels were affected by the treatment (Figure S2).

Surprisingly chronic exposure to carbogen gas did not reduce intraplaque hypoxia in the treated group when compared to the air breathing group (Figure 3). In fact, the degree of pimonidazole staining in the vein graft area was not different between the two groups (Figure 3).

3.3. Chronic Exposure to Carbogen Plays a Protective Role Against Occlusions

Chronic carbogen treatment resulted in a beneficial effect on vein graft patency, increasing the rate of vein graft patency by 34.5% (Figure 4A). In fact, only 53% of the mice of the control group presented a patent vein graft (Figure 4A), while 87.5% of the mice exposed to carbogen gas had a patent vein graft.

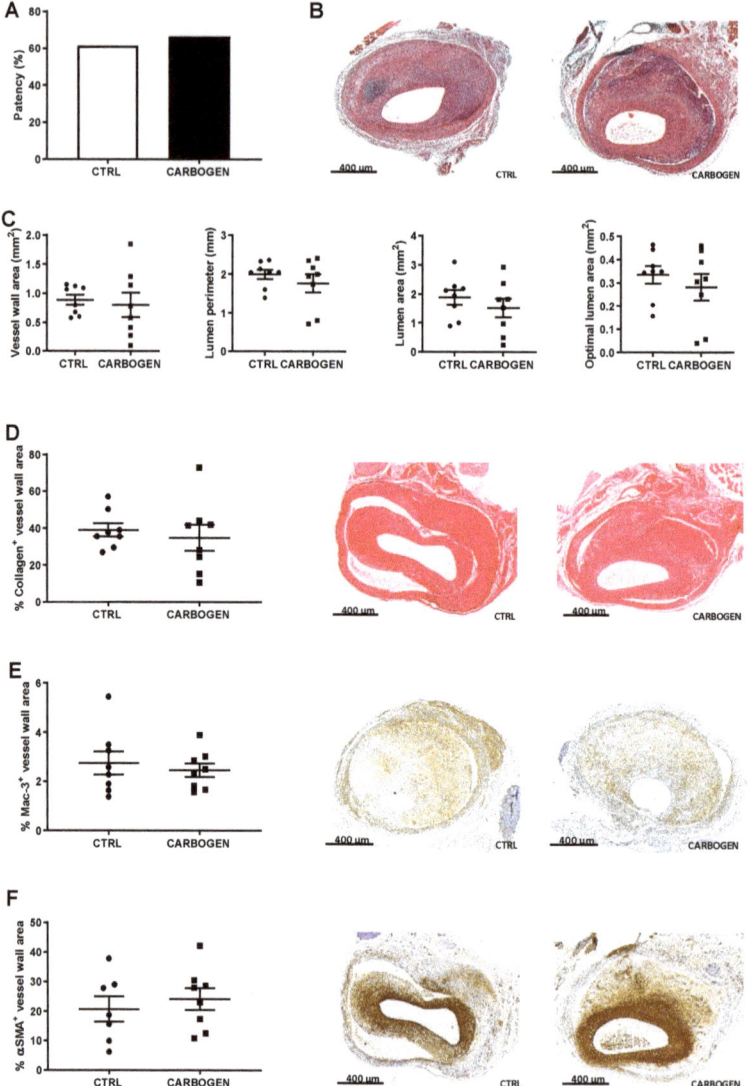

Figure 2. Short term exposure to carbogen gas does not influence plaque size nor composition. (**A**) Quantitative measurement of vein graft patency in ApoE3*Leiden mice from the control and one-time carbogen treated groups. Data are analyzed by Chi-square test (**B**) Representative pictures of MOVAT staining of vein graft sections from control ($n = 8$) and carbogen group ($n = 8$). (**C**) Quantification of vessel wall area, lumen perimeter, lumen area and optimal lumen area. Percentage of positive vessel wall area and representative pictures for (**D**) collagen ($n = 8$ for control and carbogen groups), (**E**) macrophages ($n = 8$ for control and carbogen groups) and (**F**) smooth muscle cells staining ($n = 8$ for control and $n = 7$ for carbogen groups). Data are presented as mean ± SEM.

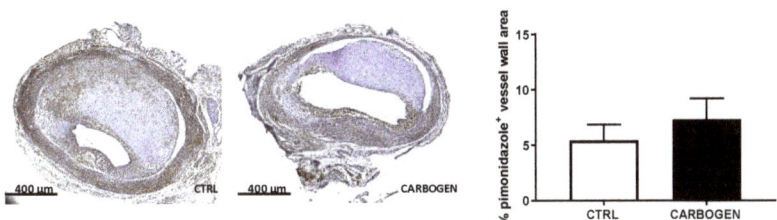

Figure 3. Chronic carbogen treatment does not affect intraplaque hypoxia. Representative pictures of vein graft cross sections stained for pimonidazole in control (n = 8) and chronic-treated carbogen groups (n = 13) and quantitative measurement of percentage of vessel wall area positive for pimonidazole staining. Data are presented as mean ± SEM.

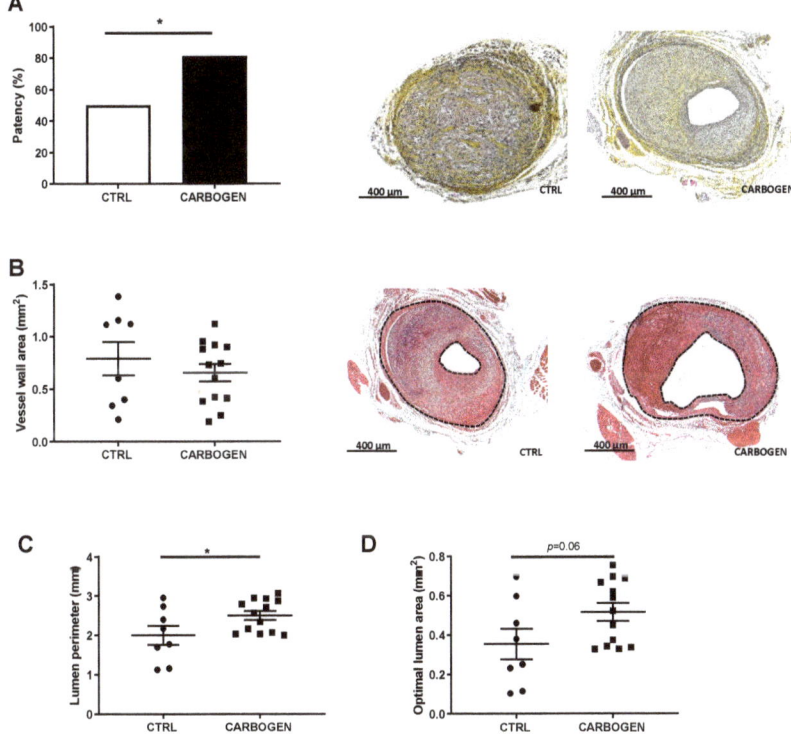

Figure 4. Chronic exposure to carbogen plays a protective role against vein graft occlusions. (**A**) Quantitative measurement of vein graft patency in ApoE3*Leiden mice from the control and prolonged carbogen treated groups. Data are analyzed by Chi-square test. * $p < 0.05$. Representative pictures of non-patent and patent vein grafts in ApoE3* Leiden mice at day 28 after surgery in the right panel. (**B**) Quantitative measurements of vein graft thickening. In the right panel, representative pictures of MOVAT staining in vein grafts from control (n = 8) and long term carbogen treated mice (n = 13), with vessel wall area as the area between the two dotted lines. (**C**) Quantification of lumen perimeter and (**D**) optimal lumen area. Data are presented as mean ± SEM. * $p < 0.05$; by two-sided Student's t test.

Vessel wall area thickening was not affected by exposure to carbogen gas since no differences could be detected between the two groups when taken only the patent grafts into account (Figure 4B). More importantly lumen size was affected by carbogen gas. In fact, carbogen treated mice presented a significant increase in the lumen perimeter when compared to control (Figure 4C,E, p-value = 0.048), and an increase in the optimal lumen area (Figure 4D, p-value = 0.067).

3.4. Chronic Carbogen Treatment Does Not Have an Effect on Intraplaque Angiogenesis and Intraplaque Hemorrhage

To see whether exposure to carbogen gas had an effect on the hypoxia triggered IP angiogenesis, the amount of $CD31^+$ vessels in the vein graft lesions (white arrows in Figure 5A zoom in) was evaluated and no difference in the number of neovessels in the carbogen group was observed when compared to the control group (p-value > 0.99).

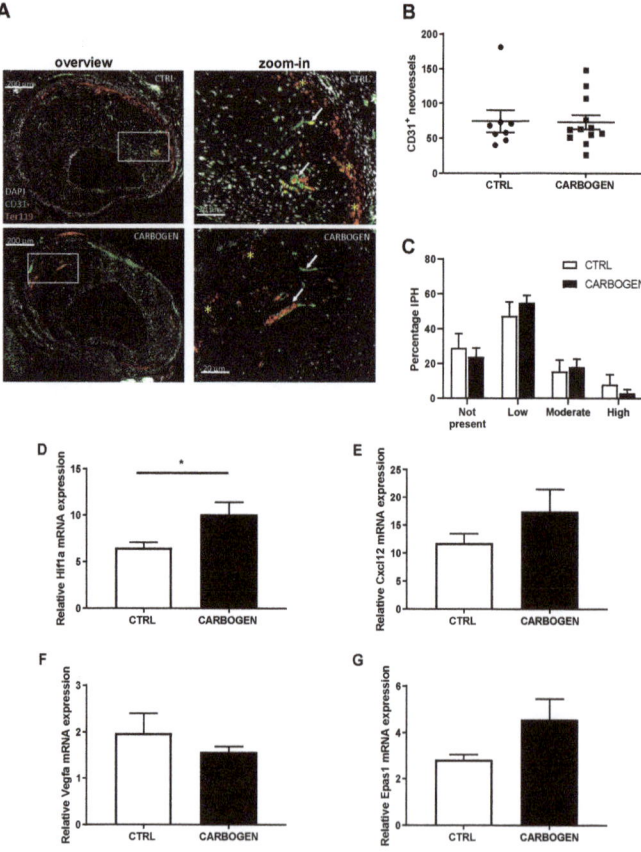

Figure 5. Chronic carbogen treatment does not affect intraplaque neovascularization. (**A**) Representative pictures of vein grafts lesions stained for DAPI (white), CD31 (green) and Ter119 (red). (**B**) Quantification of CD31 positive neovessels in the vessel wall area in the control group (n = 8) and in the carbogen treated group (n = 12). (**C**) Bar graphs representing the quantitative measurements for IPH in the control and long term carbogen treated groups. IPH was scored as not present, low, moderate or high. Total vessel wall gene expression of (**D**) Hif1a, (**E**) Cxcl12, (**F**) Vegfa and (**G**) Hif2a, relative to Hprt, was measured in the control and long term carbogen treated groups. Data are presented as mean ± SEM. * p < 0.05; by two-sided Student's t test.

In addition, when corrected for intimal thickness no differences were observed between the groups (*p*-value = 0.91) (Figure 5A,B). As a measure of the quality of the IP angiogenesis the degree of intraplaque hemorrhage was analyzed (yellow stars in Figure 5A zoom-in) as the amount of Ter119$^+$ cells found outside the neovessels and quantified as not present, low, moderate or high, and no differences could be seen when comparing the two groups (Figure 5C).

To determine the effects of hyperoxia on angiogenesis related genes the expression of Hif1a was analyzed. We surprisingly found a significant upregulation of Hif1a mRNA expression in the carbogen treated group when compared to the control (Figure 5D, *p*-value = 0.05), while mRNA expression of Cxcl12, Vegfa and Epas1 were not altered (Figure 5E–G). No differences between control and one-time carbogen treated group were found when analyzing gene expression in vein grafts from the acute carbogen treatment (Figure S3).

3.5. Chronic Carbogen Treatment Induces Accumulation of Reactive Oxygen Species and Apoptosis

Although an effect on Hif1a upregulation was observed, surprisingly no effect on angiogenesis could be seen. Therefore, we looked into other mechanisms that could possibly regulate Hif1a. We hypothesized that the mRNA upregulation of Hif1a in the carbogen treated group (Figure 5D) was caused by an accumulation of reactive oxygen species (ROS) induced by the carbogen treatment. ROS is known to be induced by prolonged hyperoxia [17] and to regulate the transcription of different genes involved in hypoxia and in inflammation such as Hif1a and Il6.

Il6 mRNA expression was studied as a representative for ROS induced factors and quantification of its expression showed a trend towards increased expression in the carbogen group of the chronic exposure study when compared to the control group (Figure 6A, *p*-value = 0.09).

Next the presence of ROS was studied in the vein graft lesions by quantifying the amount of ROS–mediated DNA damage, analyzed by 8-hydroxy-2′deoxy-guanosine (8OHdG) immunohistochemical staining. We determined the subcellular location of the staining of 8OHdG. As observed in Figure 6C, a strong 8OHdG positive staining was found in the nuclei of the cells, with an occasional staining outside of the nuclei in the mitochondria, seen as cytoplasmic staining (Figure 6C, right panel). This suggests that the main site of ROS induced DNA damage is nuclear, and not mitochondrial. 8OHdG positive staining could be seen as light blue staining in the nuclei of the cells as a results of co-localized DAPI and 8OHdG staining (Figure 6D zoom-in) and the quantification corrected for the vessel wall area resulted in an increase of DNA damage in the carbogen treated group when compared to the control group (Figure 6B,D), supporting the idea that ROS levels are increased.

ROS is known to induce apoptosis as a consequence of DNA damage. Therefore, the amount of cells positive for cleaved caspase 3 (CC3) in the atherosclerotic vein graft lesions was determined in the carbogen treated and in the control groups (Figure 6E). Due to their high oxygen consumption we hypothesized that macrophages could possibly be the main cell type affected by DNA damage induced by ROS and subsequent apoptosis. As shown in the bottom panel of Figure 6D, macrophages rich areas in the lesions of mice treated with carbogen were found to be strongly positive for CC3 when compared to control (Figure 6E bottom panel).

When looking at the total amount of cells positive for cleaved caspase 3 in the intimal area, an increase in apoptotic cells CC3$^+$ in the lesions of mice exposed to carbogen gas was found compared to the air breathing group (Figure 6E, *p*-value = 0.06).

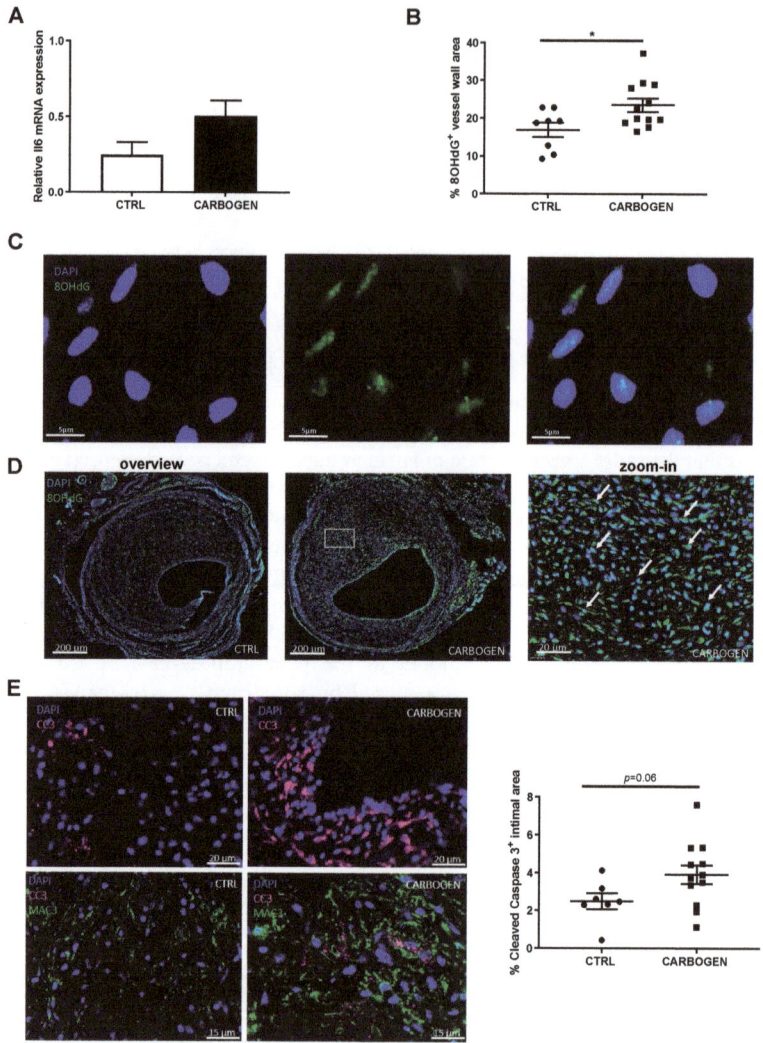

Figure 6. Chronic carbogen treatment induces accumulation of ROS. (**A**) Il6 gene expression relative to Hprt in the total vessel wall of control and chronic carbogen treated groups. (**B**) Quantification of the percentage of vessel wall area positive for 8OHdG. (**C**) Representative pictures of DAPI (in blue, left panel), 8OHdG (in green, central panel) and merged (right panel) staining in the vein graft lesions. (**D**) representative pictures of DAPI (blue) and 8OHdG (green) staining in vein graft lesions from control ($n = 8$) and carbogen treated ($n = 12$) mice. Light blue staining represents nuclei positive for 8OHdG and examples are indicated by white arrows. (**E**) In the top panels, representative pictures of DAPI (blue) and cleaved caspase 3 (CC3, in magenta) staining and in the bottom panels representative pictures of DAPI (blue), CC3 (magenta) and Mac3 (green) staining in control and carbogen groups respectively. In the right panel quantification of percentage of intimal area positive for cleaved caspase 3. Data are presented as mean ± SEM. * $p < 0.05$ by two-sided Student's t test.

3.6. Chronic Carbogen Exposure Reduces Inflammatory Cell Content

The effects of chronic carbogen gas treatment on intraplaque inflammation were studied on macrophages since they produce high amounts of ROS, consume elevate amounts of O_2 and are known to be hypoxic [6]. Interestingly, the group of mice exposed daily to carbogen for 21 days showed a significant reduction in macrophage content when compared to the control group breathing normal air (p-value = 0.0126).

When corrected for the differences in vein graft thickening, the relative percentage of macrophages was significantly decreased in the carbogen exposed group by the 15.2% (Figure 7A, p-value = 0.0044).

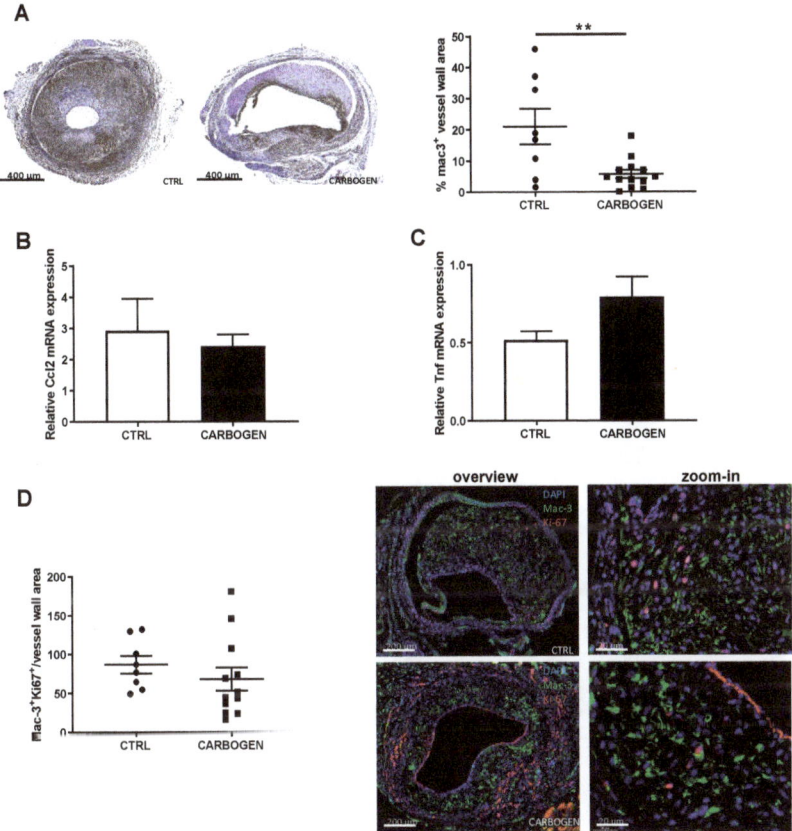

Figure 7. Chronic carbogen treatment reduces macrophages infiltration in the plaque. (**A**) Representative pictures of ApoE3* Leiden mice vein grafts from control (n = 8) and chronic carbogen treated (n = 13) groups stained for Mac-3. In the right panel quantitative measurements of the percentage of vessel wall area positive for Mac-3. Data are presented as mean ± SEM. ** $p < 0.01$; by two-sided Student's t test. Total wall gene expression of (**B**) Ccl2 and (**C**) Tnf relative to Hprt. (**D**) Quantification of the number of cells positive for Mac-3 and Ki67 in the vessel wall area of control (n = 8) and carbogen treated group (n = 13) and representative pictures of the staining with DAPI presented in blue, Mac-3 in green and Ki67 in red. Data are presented as mean ± SEM. ** $p < 0.01$ by 2-sided Student t test.

To study whether the decrease in macrophages was not due to a reduced infiltration of macrophages, nor a reduced proliferation of resident macrophages, local cytokines expression in the vein grafts was studied and the proliferation of macrophages was analyzed.

First, the mRNA expression levels of Ccl2 and Tnf in the vein graft atherosclerotic lesions were examined. The mRNA levels of Ccl2 and Tnf did not differ between the carbogen treated group and the control (Figure 7B,C).

Using a triple IHC staining for Mac-3, Ki-67 and DAPI the amount of proliferating macrophages was determined. As shown in Figure 7D and, there was no difference in the number of proliferative macrophages corrected for the vessel wall thickening (p-value = 0.16).

Thus, the data suggest that the reduction of plaque macrophages could be due to enhanced macrophage apoptosis.

3.7. Chronic Carbogen Treatment Does Not Affect Plaque Size but Increases Plaque Stability

To evaluate the effect of prolonged carbogen treatment and accumulation of ROS on plaque composition, the amount of collagen (positive collagen area in the total vessel wall) and smooth muscle cells (positive αSMA area in the total vessel wall) was analyzed, two main predictors of plaque stability.

The collagen content in the plaque was not affected by carbogen treatment, and was comparable between the two groups (Figure 8A). Similarly, SMCs content in the carbogen group was not different from the control group (Figure 8B). Interestingly, when calculating the plaque stability index, defined as the amount of collagen and SMCs divided by the vessel wall area, atherosclerotic plaques of the mice daily exposed to carbogen resulted to be more stable than the lesion of the control group (Figure 8C, p-value = 0.05).

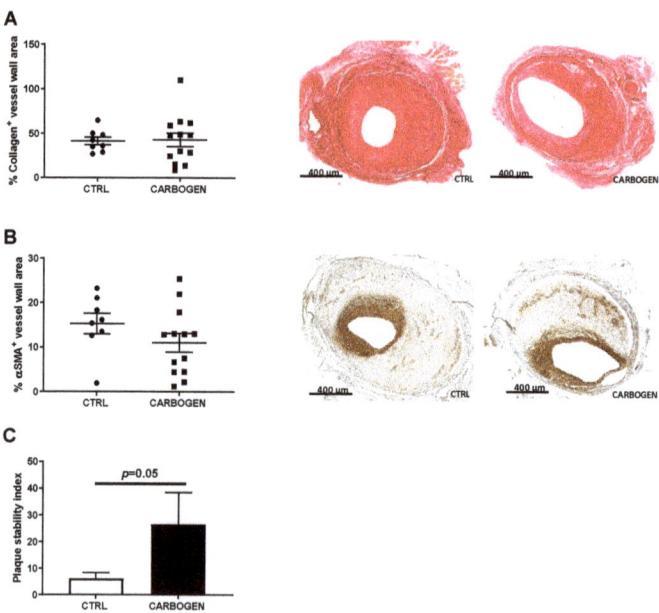

Figure 8. Chronic carbogen treatment does not affect collagen nor smooth muscle cells content in the lesion but increases plaque stability. (**A**) Quantitative measurement vessel wall area positive for collagen in ApoE3*Leiden mice from the control (n = 8) and carbogen treated (n = 13) groups. In the right panel representative pictures for collagen staining. (**B**) Quantification of percentage of vessel wall area positive for smooth muscle cell actin and representative pictures from the control (n = 8) and carbogen treated (n = 13) groups. (**C**) Quantification of plaque stability index. Data are presented as mean ± SEM.

3.8. ROS Increases DNA Damage and Apoptosis in Bone Marrow Derived Macrophages In Vitro

To unravel the molecular and cellular mechanism underlying the observed changes in macrophage content, in particular whether this could be due to hyperoxia induced ROS accumulation, we treated macrophages derived from bone marrow of APOE3*Leiden mice with t-BHP, a known ROS mimic [19]. t-BHP treatment increased the occurrence of DNA damage in BMM as measured by 8-OHdG immunocytochemical staining (Figure 9A), confirming its activity as a ROS mimic and the induction of DNA damage by ROS.

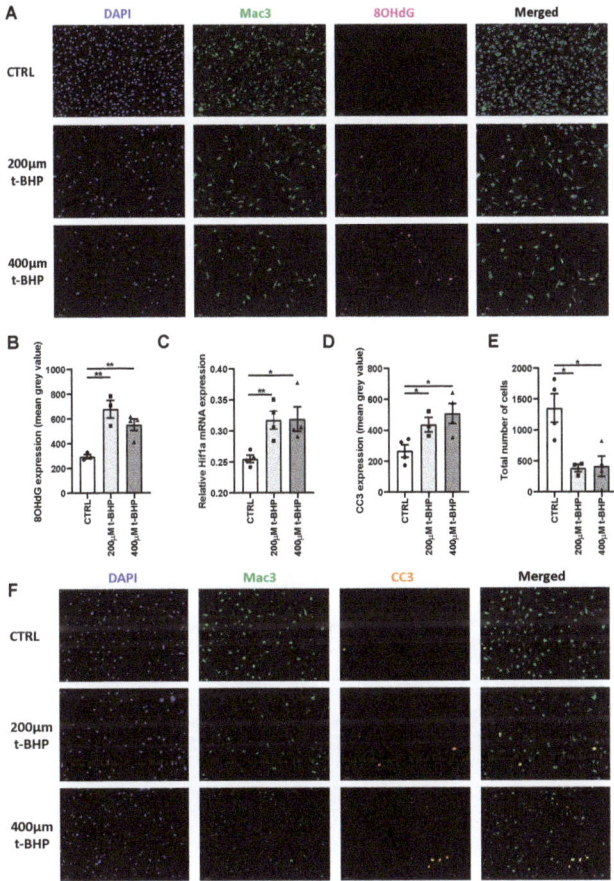

Figure 9. ROS induces DNA damage and apoptosis on in vitro bone marrow macrophages (BMM) (**A**) Representative pictures of CTRL BMM and BMM treated with 200 or 400 μm t-BHP respectively are shown. Examples images stained for DAPI (blue), Mac3 (green) and 8OHdG (magenta) as well as a merged image are shown per each condition tested. (**B**) Quantification of 8OHdG expression as mean intensity is shown. (**C**) Total mRNA expression of Hif1a relative to Hprt. (**D**) Quantification of CC3 expression as mean intensity is shown. (**E**) Quantification of total amount of cells per condition tested expressed as total amount of positive DAPI nuclei. (**F**) Representative pictures of CTRL BMM and BMM treated with 200 or 400 μm t-BHP respectively. Examples images stained for DAPI (blue), Mac3 (green) and cleaved caspase 3 (CC3) (orange) as well as a merged image are shown per each condition tested. Data are presented as mean ± SEM. * $p < 0.05$, ** $p < 0.01$; by two-sided Student's t test.

Quantification revealed a 2.2-fold increase in DNA damage in macrophages treated with 200 μm t-BHP (p-value = 0.006) and a two-fold increase in DNA damage in macrophages treated with 400 μm t-BHP (p-value = 0.006) when compared to control (Figure 9B).

We then evaluated the effect of the ROS mimic t-BHP on the expression of several genes. Similar to changes in expression in vivo, we found that t-BHP-induced ROS caused a significant increase of Hif1a mRNA expression (p-value = 0.007 and 0.02 respectively) when compared to control (Figure 9C). Interestingly, we also found that ROS caused an increase in the expression of pro-inflammatory genes Ccl2 and Tnf, but decreased Epas1 expression compared to control (Figure S4)

To assess if ROS ultimately causes apoptosis in cultured BMM, we examined the expression of CC3 and found a significant and dose dependent increase in CC3 expression, thus apoptosis, in t-BHP treated BMM when compared to control (Figure 9F). The group treated with 200 μm t-BHP showed a 10% increase (p-value = 0.03) and the group treated with 400 μm t-BHP a 27% increase (p-value = 0.01) in CC3 expression when compared to control (Figure 9D). Moreover, we observed a drastic reduction in the total number of cells by 72% and 70% in the groups treated with 200 and 400 μm t-BHP, respectively, when compared to control (Figure 9E, p-value = 0.01 for both groups). Combined these data demonstrate that ROS directly affects gene expression in macrophages and causes DNA damage and apoptosis.

4. Discussion

The results of the present study show that carbogen treatment in an acute short term setting resulted in a profound reduction of intraplaque hypoxia in murine vein grafts lesions in vivo. Long term treatment with carbogen resulted in a beneficial effect on vein graft patency in ApoE3*Leiden mice, but surprisingly, had no effect on hypoxia, intraplaque angiogenesis and intraplaque hemorrhage. On the other hand, long term carbogen treatment resulted in hyperoxia-induced ROS formation with consequent effects on HIF1a mRNA levels and macrophage apoptosis. A reduction in macrophage content in the vein graft lesions was observed, resulting in less unstable lesions. Moreover, comparable to what was observed in vivo, in vitro induction of ROS using the ROS mimic t-BHP in BMM resulted in a strong increment in DNA damage and apoptosis.

Carbogen inhalation is widely used in the oncological field [20,21]. It has been shown that the time to achieve a maximal increase in tumor oxygenation with carbogen inhalation depends on various factors such as the type of cell involved, the location, and the size of the tumor [22,23]. Moreover, Hou et al. observed an effect of carbogen treatment comparable to what was observed in the present study, both in the short and the long term experiments. Single carbogen inhalation significantly increased tumor oxygenation, while during multiple administrations of carbogen the effect was reduced, indicating that the response to chronic carbogen is not consistent over days [22]. Nevertheless, we showed that prolonged carbogen treatment has a protective role against vein graft occlusions. Vein graft occlusion is a phenomenon often seen after vein grafting in which the vessel lumen is narrowed due to extensive intimal hyperplasia that progress to stenosis and occlusion [24]. This phenomenon is also observed in ApoE3*Leiden mice that undergo vein graft surgery. Besides the reduction in vein graft occlusions, an increase in vein graft patency due to an increase in lumen perimeter and optimal lumen area of the hyperoxic vein grafts was observed, similar to the study by Fowler et al. [25]. In that study carbogen is used in the treatment of central retinal artery occlusion to increase blood oxygen maintaining oxygenation of the retina [25]. This effect of hyperoxygenation on retinal artery remodeling can be related to the effect of carbogen on patency and increase in lumen perimeter and increase in the optimal lumen found in the present study.

We did not observe a reduction in hypoxia nor an effect on intraplaque angiogenesis in the prolonged carbogen study. Furthermore, no changes in local gene expression of Vegfa were observed in the vein grafts, but interestingly Hif1a was upregulated in the prolonged carbogen exposure study and not downregulated as expected. In fact following our initial hypothesis we would have expected a reduction in intraplaque angiogenesis in parallel with a reduction in Hif1a and Vegfa expression.

For this reason, we studied other known processes that regulate Hif1a and observed an accumulation of ROS in the carbogen exposed group when compared to the control group. Repeated exposure to hyperoxia is known to be associated at a cellular level with an accumulation of ROS [26,27]. When the exposure is repeated too often, the oxidant insult is no longer compensated by the host's antioxidant defense mechanisms and therefore cell injury and death ensue [28]. Cell injury induced by ROS comprises lipid peroxidation, protein oxidation and DNA damage [29,30]. We observed an increase in DNA damage measured as an augmented presence of 8OHdG staining in the long term carbogen treated group when compared to the control group, indicating that a daily long term treatment with carbogen gas results in accumulation of ROS that in turns induces DNA damage in the atherosclerotic lesions. Moreover, we also observed an increase in DNA damage in bone marrow macrophages in vitro under ROS stimulation. It is known that DNA damage can be found in the nuclei and in the mitochondria [31,32]. Both in the vein graft lesions in vivo and in the cultured t-BHP treated macrophages in vitro, a strong 8OHdG positive staining in the nuclei of the cells, with an occasional cytoplasmic staining could be seen. The subcellular location of the staining of 8OHdG suggests that the main site of ROS induced DNA damage is nuclear, and not mitochondrial. ROS generated by repeated hyperoxia treatment can alter gene expression by modulating transcription factor activation, like NF-kβ, which then impact downstream targets [33]. It has been shown that hyperoxia also results in nuclear translocation of NF-kβ and NF-kβ activation in several cell types [34]. Our results show that long term carbogen treatment result in Hif1a gene expression upregulation. In addition, in vitro BMM treated with the ROS mimic t-BHP also showed an upregulation of Hif1a gene expression. Interestingly, the transcription of this gene is known to be regulated by NF-kβ transcription factor. In fact, Bonello et al., demonstrated that ROS induced Hif1a transcription via binding of NF-kβ to a specific site in the Hif1a promoter [35]. Those findings could be further investigated in future experiments using antioxidants such as NAC to see whether it can reverse the carbogen treatment.

We showed that the accumulation of ROS in the carbogen treated group caused an increase in apoptosis, accumulated in macrophages rich areas, and resulted in a decrease in the amount of macrophages. Even though we cannot exclude that the association of macrophages with cleaved caspase 3 could be due to efferocytosis of apoptotic cells, macrophage efferocytosis is frequently hampered in atherosclerotic lesions, therefore it is likely that these macrophages are apoptotic. Previously, in contrast with our findings, a strong correlation between macrophage content and hypoxia was shown by Marsch et al. [15]. Moreover, hypoxia potentiates macrophage glycolytic flux in a Hif1a dependent manner [36] in order to fulfill the need of ATP for protein production and migration. Taken together, this points to a high request and high use of O_2 by plaque macrophages and a consequent high exposure of these inflammatory cells to ROS accumulated during hyperoxia. We demonstrated that ROS causes accumulation of DNA damage and subsequently an increase in apoptosis and cell death in BMM in vitro. The link between ROS induced DNA damage and apoptosis detected in vitro might explain the observed apoptosis in macrophages in vivo. Moreover, a reduction in the number of macrophages is associated with plaque stability and plaque stability is reflected in an increase in vein graft patency as observed in the present study.

Previously Marsch et al. showed that repeated carbogen treatment in LDLR$^{-/-}$ mice lead to reduction in intraplaque hypoxia, necrotic core size and apoptosis [15]. In the present study we showed that repeated carbogen treatment in accelerated vein graft atherosclerotic lesions in ApoE3* Leiden mice resulted in increased apoptosis and unaltered intraplaque hypoxia when compared to controls. Accelerated atherosclerotic lesions in ApoE3*Leiden mice highly resemble human atherosclerotic lesions and, differently from LDLR$^{-/-}$ mice, do present intraplaque angiogenesis. Our results show that although we did not observe reduced intraplaque angiogenesis and IPH daily hyperoxia treatment with carbogen gas in this murine model lead to accumulation of ROS that could not be cleared by anti-oxidant agents and the ROS build-up lead to DNA damage and induced apoptosis. In fact, differently from Marsch et al., who treated mice daily for five days, followed by two days of no carbogen exposure we performed the treatment daily and started our treatment seven days after mice underwent vein graft surgery, when the atherosclerotic lesions already started forming. This starting time point was based on our previous findings [5] in which we found that intraplaque neovascularization in ApoE3*Leiden mice that underwent vein graft surgery is visible 14 days after surgery. Therefore, we were able to study the effect of carbogen treatment on lesion stabilization rather than on lesion formation.

One of the limitations of the current study may be the choice of the model used, the ApoE3*Leiden mice vein grafts. However, since in most mouse models for spontaneous atherosclerosis intraplaque angiogenesis is absent, and the lesions observed in the ApoE3*Leiden mice vein grafts show many features that can also be observed in advanced human lesions, including intraplaque hypoxia, angiogenesis and intraplaque hemorrhage, we believe this model is suitable for the current studies. The fact that the most prominent effects observed relate to hyperoxygenation induced ROS production, macrophage apoptosis and vein graft patency, whereas the experimental set-up was initially designed to identify effects on intraplaque angiogenesis, might indicate another limitation in our study set-up.

Based on the results obtained in the present study we can conclude that although short term carbogen gas treatment leads to a profound reduction in intraplaque hypoxia, the treatment has mixed effects. Despite the beneficial effects of the hyperoxygenation treatment on vein grafts, i.e., improved vein graft patency and a strong trend towards an increased plaque stability index, chronic hyperoxygenation also induced Hif1a mRNA expression, ROS accumulation and apoptosis. That all will harm the vein grafts in the current model under the current conditions. This indicates that in order to define potential therapeutic benefits of hyperoxygenation treatment further research is needed to define optimal conditions for this treatment in vein graft disease.

Supplementary Materials: The following are available online at http://www.mdpi.com/2073-4409/9/2/336/s1, Figure S1: Bodyweight and cholesterol levels acute carbogen exposure, Figure S2: Bodyweight and cholesterol levels chronic carbogen exposure, Figure S3: Total wall gene expression, Figure S4: inflammatory gene expression in cultured BMM, Figure S5: BMM 8OHdG IHC.

Author Contributions: Conceptualization, L.P., M.R.d.V. and P.H.A.Q.; formal analysis, L.P. and M.R.d.V.; investigation, L.P., H.A.B.P., F.B. and M.R.d.V.; resources, M.R.d.V. and P.H.A.Q.; supervision, M.R.d.V. and P.H.A.Q.; visualization, L.P., M.R.d.V. and P.H.A.Q.; writing—original draft, L.P.; writing—review and editing, L.P., J.C.S., M.R.d.V. and P.H.A.Q. All authors have read and agreed to the published version of the manuscript.

Funding: This research was funded by a grant from the European Union, Horizon 2020 MSCA joint doctoral project, MOGLYNET [Project number 675527].

Conflicts of Interest: The authors declare no conflict of interest.

References

1. Bentzon, J.F.; Otsuka, F.; Virmani, R.; Falk, E. Mechanisms of plaque formation and rupture. *Circ. Res.* **2014**, *114*, 1852–1866. [CrossRef]
2. de Vries, M.R.; Quax, P.H. Plaque angiogenesis and its relation to inflammation and atherosclerotic plaque destabilization. *Curr. Opin. Lipidol.* **2016**, *27*, 499–506. [CrossRef] [PubMed]
3. Lee, E.S.; Bauer, G.E.; Caldwell, M.P.; Santilli, S.M. Association of artery wall hypoxia and cellular proliferation at a vascular anastomosis. *J. Surg. Res.* **2000**, *91*, 32–37. [CrossRef] [PubMed]
4. Sluimer, J.C.; Gasc, J.M.; van Wanroij, J.L.; Kisters, N.; Groeneweg, M.; Sollewijn Gelpke, M.D.; Cleutjens, J.P.; van den Akker, L.H.; Corvol, P.; Wouters, B.G.; et al. Hypoxia, hypoxia-inducible transcription factor, and macrophages in human atherosclerotic plaques are correlated with intraplaque angiogenesis. *J. Am. Coll. Cardiol.* **2008**, *51*, 1258–1265. [CrossRef] [PubMed]
5. de Vries, M.R.; Parma, L.; Peters, H.A.B.; Schepers, A.; Hamming, J.F.; Jukema, J.W.; Goumans, M.; Guo, L.; Finn, A.V.; Virmani, R.; et al. Blockade of vascular endothelial growth factor receptor 2 inhibits intraplaque haemorrhage by normalization of plaque neovessels. *J. Intern. Med.* **2019**, *285*, 59–74. [CrossRef]
6. Marsch, E.; Sluimer, J.C.; Daemen, M.J. Hypoxia in atherosclerosis and inflammation. *Curr. Opin. Lipidol.* **2013**, *24*, 393–400. [CrossRef]
7. Subbotin, V.M. Excessive intimal hyperplasia in human coronary arteries before intimal lipid depositions is the initiation of coronary atherosclerosis and constitutes a therapeutic target. *Drug Discov. Today* **2016**, *21*, 1578–1595. [CrossRef]

8. Jain, T.; Nikolopoulou, E.A.; Xu, Q.; Qu, A. Hypoxia inducible factor as a therapeutic target for atherosclerosis. *Pharmacol. Ther.* **2018**, *183*, 22–33. [CrossRef]
9. Balogh, E.; Toth, A.; Mehes, G.; Trencsenyi, G.; Paragh, G.; Jeney, V. Hypoxia Triggers Osteochondrogenic Differentiation of Vascular Smooth Muscle Cells in an HIF-1 (Hypoxia-Inducible Factor 1)-Dependent and Reactive Oxygen Species-Dependent Manner. *Arter. Thromb. Vasc. Biol.* **2019**, *39*, 1088–1099. [CrossRef]
10. Parma, L.; Baganha, F.; Quax, P.H.A.; de Vries, M.R. Plaque angiogenesis and intraplaque hemorrhage in atherosclerosis. *Eur. J. Pharm.* **2017**, *816*, 107–115. [CrossRef]
11. Sluimer, J.C.; Kolodgie, F.D.; Bijnens, A.P.; Maxfield, K.; Pacheco, E.; Kutys, B.; Duimel, H.; Frederik, P.M.; van Hinsbergh, V.W.; Virmani, R.; et al. Thin-walled microvessels in human coronary atherosclerotic plaques show incomplete endothelial junctions relevance of compromised structural integrity for intraplaque microvascular leakage. *J. Am. Coll. Cardiol.* **2009**, *53*, 1517–1527. [CrossRef] [PubMed]
12. Aarup, A.; Pedersen, T.X.; Junker, N.; Christoffersen, C.; Bartels, E.D.; Madsen, M.; Nielsen, C.H.; Nielsen, L.B. Hypoxia-Inducible Factor-1alpha Expression in Macrophages Promotes Development of Atherosclerosis. *Arter. Thromb. Vasc. Biol.* **2016**, *36*, 1782–1790. [CrossRef] [PubMed]
13. Hultén, L.M.; Levin, M. The role of hypoxia in atherosclerosis. *Curr. Opin. Lipidol.* **2009**, *20*, 409–414. [CrossRef] [PubMed]
14. Abe, H.; Semba, H.; Takeda, N. The Roles of Hypoxia Signaling in the Pathogenesis of Cardiovascular Diseases. *J. Atheroscler. Thromb.* **2017**, *24*, 884–894. [CrossRef] [PubMed]
15. Marsch, E.; Theelen, T.L.; Demandt, J.A.; Jeurissen, M.; van Gink, M.; Verjans, R.; Janssen, A.; Cleutjens, J.P.; Meex, S.J.; Donners, M.M.; et al. Reversal of hypoxia in murine atherosclerosis prevents necrotic core expansion by enhancing efferocytosis. *Arter. Thromb. Vasc. Biol.* **2014**, *34*, 2545–2553. [CrossRef] [PubMed]
16. de Vries, M.R.; Niessen, H.W.; Lowik, C.W.; Hamming, J.F.; Jukema, J.W.; Quax, P.H. Plaque rupture complications in murine atherosclerotic vein grafts can be prevented by TIMP-1 overexpression. *PLoS ONE* **2012**, *7*, e47134. [CrossRef] [PubMed]
17. Jamieson, D.; Chance, B.; Cadenas, E.; Boveris, A. The relation of free radical production to hyperoxia. *Annu. Rev. Physiol.* **1986**, *48*, 703–719. [CrossRef]
18. Simons, K.H.; de Vries, M.R.; Peters, H.A.B.; Hamming, J.F.; Jukema, J.W.; Quax, P.H.A. The protective role of Toll-like receptor 3 and type-I interferons in the pathophysiology of vein graft disease. *J. Mol. Cell. Cardiol.* **2018**, *121*, 16–24. [CrossRef]
19. Han, L.; Wang, Y.L.; Sun, Y.C.; Hu, Z.Y.; Hu, K.; Du, L.B. tert-Butylhydroperoxide induces apoptosis in RAW264.7 macrophages via a mitochondria-mediated signaling pathway. *Toxicol. Res.* **2018**, *7*, 970–976. [CrossRef]
20. Yip, K.; Alonzi, R. Carbogen gas and radiotherapy outcomes in prostate cancer. *Ther. Adv. Urol.* **2013**, *5*, 25–34. [CrossRef]
21. Zhang, L.J.; Zhang, Z.; Xu, J.; Jin, N.; Luo, S.; Larson, A.C.; Lu, G.M. Carbogen gas-challenge blood oxygen level-dependent magnetic resonance imaging in hepatocellular carcinoma: Initial results. *Oncol. Lett.* **2015**, *10*, 2009–2014. [CrossRef] [PubMed]
22. Hou, H.G.; Khan, N.; Du, G.X.; Hodge, S.; Swartz, H.M. Temporal variation in the response of tumors to hyperoxia with breathing carbogen and oxygen. *Med. Gas. Res.* **2016**, *6*, 138–146. [CrossRef] [PubMed]
23. Chakhoyan, A.; Corroyer-Dulmont, A.; Leblond, M.M.; Gerault, A.; Toutain, J.; Chazaviel, L.; Divoux, D.; Petit, E.; MacKenzie, E.T.; Kauffmann, F.; et al. Carbogen-induced increases in tumor oxygenation depend on the vascular status of the tumor: A multiparametric MRI study in two rat glioblastoma models. *J. Cereb. Blood Flow Metab.* **2017**, *37*, 2270–2282. [CrossRef]
24. de Vries, M.R.; Simons, K.H.; Jukema, J.W.; Braun, J.; Quax, P.H. Vein graft failure: From pathophysiology to clinical outcomes. *Nat. Rev. Cardiol.* **2016**, *13*, 451–470. [CrossRef] [PubMed]
25. Fowler, S.B. Carbogen in the management of a central retinal artery occlusion. *Insight (Am. Soc. Ophthalmic Regist. Nurses)* **2012**, *37*, 10–11.
26. Gore, A.; Muralidhar, M.; Espey, M.G.; Degenhardt, K.; Mantell, L.L. Hyperoxia sensing: From molecular mechanisms to significance in disease. *J. Immunotoxicol.* **2010**, *7*, 239–254. [CrossRef] [PubMed]
27. Zhao, M.; Tang, S.; Xin, J.; Wei, Y.; Liu, D. Reactive oxygen species induce injury of the intestinal epithelium during hyperoxia. *Int. J. Mol. Med.* **2018**, *41*, 322–330. [CrossRef]

28. Petrache, I.; Choi, M.E.; Otterbein, L.E.; Chin, B.Y.; Mantell, L.L.; Horowitz, S.; Choi, A.M. Mitogen-activated protein kinase pathway mediates hyperoxia-induced apoptosis in cultured macrophage cells. *Am. J. Physiol.* **1999**, *277*, L589–L595. [CrossRef]
29. Halliwell, B.; Chirico, S. Lipid peroxidation: Its mechanism, measurement, and significance. *Am. J. Clin. Nutr.* **1993**, *57*, 715S–724S, discussion 724S-725S. [CrossRef]
30. Evans, M.D.; Dizdaroglu, M.; Cooke, M.S. Oxidative DNA damage and disease: Induction, repair and significance. *Mutat. Res.* **2004**, *567*, 1–61. [CrossRef]
31. Santulli, G.; Xie, W.; Reiken, S.R.; Marks, A.R. Mitochondrial calcium overload is a key determinant in heart failure. *Proc. Natl. Acad. Sci. USA* **2015**, *112*, 11389–11394. [CrossRef] [PubMed]
32. Xie, W.; Santulli, G.; Reiken, S.R.; Yuan, Q.; Osborne, B.W.; Chen, B.X.; Marks, A.R. Mitochondrial oxidative stress promotes atrial fibrillation. *Sci. Rep.* **2015**, *5*, 11427. [CrossRef] [PubMed]
33. Traenckner, E.B.; Pahl, H.L.; Henkel, T.; Schmidt, K.N.; Wilk, S.; Baeuerle, P.A. Phosphorylation of human I kappa B-alpha on serines 32 and 36 controls I kappa B-alpha proteolysis and NF-kappa B activation in response to diverse stimuli. *EMBO J.* **1995**, *14*, 2876–2883. [CrossRef] [PubMed]
34. Michiels, C.; Minet, E.; Mottet, D.; Raes, M. Regulation of gene expression by oxygen: NF-kappaB and HIF-1, two extremes. *Free Radic. Biol. Med.* **2002**, *33*, 1231–1242. [CrossRef]
35. Bonello, S.; Zahringer, C.; BelAiba, R.S.; Djordjevic, T.; Hess, J.; Michiels, C.; Kietzmann, T.; Gorlach, A. Reactive oxygen species activate the HIF-1alpha promoter via a functional NFkappaB site. *Arter. Thromb. Vasc. Biol.* **2007**, *27*, 755–761. [CrossRef]
36. Tawakol, A.; Singh, P.; Mojena, M.; Pimentel-Santillana, M.; Emami, H.; MacNabb, M.; Rudd, J.H.; Narula, J.; Enriquez, J.A.; Traves, P.G.; et al. HIF-1alpha and PFKFB3 Mediate a Tight Relationship Between Proinflammatory Activation and Anaerobic Metabolism in Atherosclerotic Macrophages. *Arter. Thromb. Vasc. Biol.* **2015**, *35*, 1463–1471. [CrossRef]

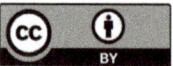

© 2020 by the authors. Licensee MDPI, Basel, Switzerland. This article is an open access article distributed under the terms and conditions of the Creative Commons Attribution (CC BY) license (http://creativecommons.org/licenses/by/4.0/).

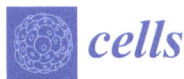

Review

Atherosclerosis and the Capillary Network; Pathophysiology and Potential Therapeutic Strategies

Tilman Ziegler [1,2], Farah Abdel Rahman [1], Victoria Jurisch [1] and Christian Kupatt [1,2,*]

[1] Klinik & Poliklinik für Innere Medizin I, Klinikum rechts der Isar, Technical University of Munich, 81675 Munich, Germany; tilman.ziegler@tum.de (T.Z.); farah.abdel-rahman@tum.de (F.A.R.); victoria.jurisch@googlemail.com (V.J.)
[2] DZHK (German Center for Cardiovascular Research), Partner Site Munich Heart Alliance, 80802 Munich, Germany
[*] Correspondence: christian.kupatt@tum.de; Tel.: +49-89-4140-9410

Received: 30 November 2019; Accepted: 21 December 2019; Published: 24 December 2019

Abstract: Atherosclerosis and associated ischemic organ dysfunction represent the number one cause of mortality worldwide. While the key drivers of atherosclerosis, arterial hypertension, hypercholesterolemia and diabetes mellitus, are well known disease entities and their contribution to the formation of atherosclerotic plaques are intensively studied and well understood, less effort is put on the effect of these disease states on microvascular structure an integrity. In this review we summarize the pathological changes occurring in the vascular system in response to prolonged exposure to these major risk factors, with a particular focus on the differences between these pathological alterations of the vessel wall in larger arteries as compared to the microcirculation. Furthermore, we intend to highlight potential therapeutic strategies to improve microvascular function during atherosclerotic vessel disease.

Keywords: atherosclerosis; pericyte; rAAV; capillary; endothelial cells

1. Introduction

Atherosclerosis remains an entity with continually growing incidence associated with a variety of disease states, which include ischemic stroke, peripheral artery disease and coronary artery disease. Taken together, cardiovascular disease, which can be seen as an expression of advanced atherosclerosis, account for 17.9 million deaths or 31% of all deaths per year globally, thus ranking it the number one cause of mortality today [1]. Multiple risk factors contributing to atherosclerosis have been identified and well-studied, mainly arterial hypertension, hypercholesterolemia, nicotine abuse and diabetes.

Atherosclerosis describes a pathological remodeling of the arterial wall initiated by the accumulation of lipids in the sub-endothelial layer of arteries. The retention of lipids triggers an inflammatory reaction leading to the invasion of multiple classes of leukocytes. This inflammatory state facilitates further endothelial dysfunction and remodeling of the extracellular matrix (ECM), ultimately leading to the formation of calcified, vulnerable plaques prone to rupture, which can lead to complete vessel occlusion via platelet activation and thrombosis.

This process of increasing vascular remodeling manifests initially as diffuse thickening of the Tunica intima, the innermost vascular layer, and an increase of intima thickness relative to the underlying Tunica media. Interestingly, these early stages in remodeling have been observed already at early ages, starting in the second decade of life [2]. The diffuse intimal thickening is mainly driven by the accumulation of lipids [3]. As proposed by Williams and Tabas in their response-to-retention hypothesis in 1995 [4,5], this accumulation of ECM-associated lipoproteins constitutes the initial step in the formation of an atherosclerotic lesion. The ECM-protein class of proteoglycans in particular has been identified as a key binding partner for lipid-complexes owing to their high affinity for lipoproteins [6,7].

Subsequently, the lipoprotein-proteoglycan complexes, which are prone to oxidation and aggregation, represent a source of oxidative stress on the surrounding endothelial cells and vascular smooth muscle cells (vSMC). This process induces the recruitment of macrophages, in part due to the increase in SMC-derived Monocyte chemoattractant protein-1 [8], which phagocytose the lipoprotein-proteoglycan complexes, leading to the accumulation of foam cells in the atherosclerotic plaque [9,10]. Owing to the increased number of macrophages and the subsequent release of inflammatory cytokines, vascular smooth muscle cells change from their resting state into a more fibroproliferative condition, e.g. they display a drastic increase in activation and expansion. They simultaneously demonstrate a heightened susceptibility to apoptosis, mediated by the induced expression of the pro-apoptotic regulator BAX (Bcl-2-associated X protein) [11]. In addition, activated vSMCs produce transforming growth factor β (TGF-β), tissue factor (TF) and further proteoglycans, thus attracting more lipoproteins and additional macrophages, which further worsens the progression of the atherosclerotic lesion [12–14]. In the later stages of atherosclerotic plaque formation, atherosclerotic lesions can transform into thin cap fibroatheromas, characterized by a thin fibrous cap containing calcifications covering a necrotic lipid core. These atherosclerotic lesions are prone to rupture, exposing the blood stream to the underlying extracellular matrix, containing Von Willebrand factor, collagen and fibrin. These ECM-proteins subsequently bind to platelets and lead to their activation and subsequent organization into a thrombus, resulting in the occlusion of the vessel [15–17].

In clinical practice, strategies for the treatment of atherosclerosis focus on the reduction of the risk factors of this pathological condition and on interventional or surgical revascularization. However, atherosclerosis is generally seen as a predominant problem of the macrocirculation with a focus on the formation of atherosclerotic plaques, rather than a disease affecting the whole circulatory system. In this review we discuss the impact of the known predominant risk factors—arterial hypertension, hypercholesterolemia and diabetes—on the development and progression of atherosclerosis with a focus on their influence on the microcirculation, e.g., arterioles, capillaries and venules. Furthermore, we highlight potential therapeutic strategies that might improve overall vascular function in atherosclerotic patients.

2. Cardiovascular Risk Factors Contributing to Atherosclerosis: The Macro

Arterial Hypertension represents a key driver in the development of atherosclerosis, and thus, cardiovascular disease. The prevalence of hypertension in ischemic stroke, coronary or peripheral artery disease lies reportedly around 60–90% depending on the localization of the atherosclerotic lesion [18,19]. Arterial hypertension can be divided into two classes: primary or essential hypertension, triggered by an interplay of underlying causes as well as secondary hypertension, caused by either endocrinological disorders or stenosis of the renal arteries. While the causes of arterial hypertension vary, the effect on the vascular system remains the same. It is currently unclear whether arterial hypertension represents the cause of vascular dysfunction or the result of it; however, a bidirectional interaction between hypertension and atherosclerosis appears the most likely explanation. Initial evidence that endothelial dysfunction causes hypertension stems from early observations that the inhibition of the endothelial nitric oxide synthase, which produces the potent vasodilator NO, leads to hypertension in human subjects [20]. One key regulator of arterial blood pressure is identified in the Renin-Angiotensin-Aldosterone system (RAAS), also regulating fluid and electrolyte homeostasis. Here, Angiotensin II, the main effector peptide of this system, has been demonstrated to directly induce endothelial dysfunction via the recruitment of macrophages to the vascular wall in a CCR2/MCP-1 dependent manner. Angiotensin II furthermore increases endothelial oxidative stress via NADPH oxidase–derived superoxide anion production, predominantly by interacting with the endothelial AT_{1A} receptor [21–23].

Hypercholesterolemia represents an additional risk factor with increasing prevalence in the development of cardiovascular disease [24,25]. Particularly, western style diets (high-fat and cholesterol, high-protein, high-sugar) lead to an increase in cholesterol, LDL-levels and LDL/HDL ratios [26].

Low density lipoproteins enter the vascular wall at predilection sites characterized by disturbed blood flow and preexisting endothelial dysfunction [27]. Once LDLs enter the vascular wall, they form complexes with proteoglycans (with versican, decorin, syndecan-4, biglycan and perlecan being the predominant proteoglycans in the vascular wall [28]) via the interaction of the LDL-component Apolipoprotein B [29]. This interaction facilitates changes to the lipid composition and the configuration of Apolipoprotein B [30], which enhances the oxidation of LDL to oxidized LDL (oxLDL) via reactive oxygen species generated by the activated endothelium and vascular smooth muscle cells [31]. This oxidation step represents a prerequisite for the detection and phagocytosis of LDL-particles by macrophages [32], leading to the formation of foam cells. This transformation increases the expression of inflammatory cytokines and oxidative stress markers in those macrophages [33]. Furthermore, oxLDL facilitates endothelial expression of leucocyte adhesion molecules (vacular cell adhesion protein 1, P-Selectin [34,35]) and cytokines [36], attracting additional macrophages, thus, enhancing the inflammatory state of the atherosclerotic lesion.

The last main contributor to the development of atherosclerosis can be identified in diabetes mellitus (DM). The hallmark feature of diabetes is the elevation of blood glucose levels (hyperglycemia). One key effect of hyperglycemia lies in the increased formation of superoxides, which enhances the oxidative stress of the vascular wall further. This process is partly mediated by the increased formation of advanced glycation end products (AGEs). Advanced glycation end products occur when excess glucose forms dicarbonyl compounds, which react spontaneously with amino groups of proteins [37]. These AGEs then bind to their respective receptor (RAGE), expressed on endothelial cells, macrophages and vascular smooth muscle cells. Particularly in endothelial cells, AGEs induce the activation of the NAD(P)H-oxidase [38] and also the expression of adhesion proteins and cytokines via the nuclear translocation of NFκB [39,40]. In macrophages, AGE-signaling enhances oxLDL uptake via an upregulation of CD36 and Macrophage Scavenger Receptor Class A [41]. Additionally, RAGE itself acts as an endothelial adhesion protein in concert with ICAM-1 [42], necessary for the adhesion of leukocytes. Further mechanisms enhancing ROS production upon hyperglycemic conditions are to be found in the Lipoxygenase pathway [43] and the Polypol pathway, respectively [44].

As discussed in the previous paragraphs, the formation of atherosclerotic lesions can be driven by multiple interdependent risk factors. However, arterial hypertension, diabetes mellitus and hypercholesterolemia also drastically change the functionality of the microcirculatory vessels, a fact rarely pointed out as compared to classical large-vessel pathologies. Therefore, in the following paragraphs we focus on the pathologies elicited by these risk factors in small vessels.

3. Hypertension, Hypercholesterolemia and Diabetes Mellitus in Capillaries: The Micro

Unlike larger vessels (arteries and veins), the smaller units of the vascular system lose their classical three layered structure consisting of Tunica intima, Tunica media and Tunica adventitia. While arterioles still contain a covering sheet of vascular smooth muscle cells throughout, capillaries are only sporadically covered in pericytes, a sort of mural cell closely related to vascular smooth muscle cells, but often lacking their contractile phenotype [45–47]. Venules on the other hand generally lack a complete cover of vSMCs. In their biological function, pericytes further differ from vascular smooth muscle cell layers due to their close interaction with endothelial cells. In the microcirculation, pericytes represent key regulators of endothelial quiescence, predominantly by secreting the growth factor Angiopoietin-1, which binds to the endothelial Tie-2 receptor [48]. Activation of this receptor tyrosine kinase facilitates the expression of survival factors, such as Survivin, and suppressing the expression of pro-apoptotic signaling molecules, like procaspase-9 and BAD (BCL2 Associated Agonist Of Cell Death) in endothelial cells [49,50]. Furthermore, Angiopoietin-1 enhances the recruitment of additional pericytes to the endothelial monolayer in a HB-EGF (heparin binding EGF like growth factor) and HGF (hepatocyte growth factor) dependent positive feedback loop [51,52]. In addition to Ang-1, pericytes regulate endothelial proliferation rates via TGF-β (transforming growth factor β) [53,54], bFGF (basic fibroblast growth factor) [55] and VEGF (vascular endothelial growth factor) [56]. Of note, pathological stimuli such as inflammation, hypoxia and neoplasia generally do not manifest themselves in a proliferation of mural cells in the microcirculation but, rather, a decrease in endothelial pericyte coverage. While this loss in pericytes has been widely reported, their fate remains unknown. Speculations range from de-differentiation to migration or apoptosis, depending on the particular vascular bed and stimulus [57–60]. Furthermore, the influx of macrophages into the vessel wall and subsequent transition into foam cells, one key driver in the development of atherosclerosis, does not occur in the same way in capillaries, since there is no comparable structure – e.g., tunica media – in these smallest vessels. These differences in morphology and in the reaction of pericytes to pathological stimuli also have an impact on the functional and morphological changes of capillaries exposed to those stimuli. However, while some reactions of the vascular system to the exposure to risk factors still remain in effect in capillaries (increased expression of endothelial adhesion molecules and of reactive oxygen species leading to a state of endothelial dysfunction), the following paragraphs will focus on the specific differences between the microcirculation and larger vessels in response to pro-atherosclerotic stimuli.

Arterial hypertension leads to an increase in the vascular pericyte coverage. Apart from this enhancement of the number of pericytes, this cell type also undergoes a transformation into a more vascular smooth muscle cell like phenotype, indicated by an increase in the expression of contractile proteins [61,62]. This effect is in part mediated by an upregulation of the endothelial-derived growth factor FGF-2 and interleukin-6 [63]. Interestingly, this increase is not accompanied by a gain in capillary density, but rather the opposite. Capillary rarefication is routinely seen both in human as well as in animal studies during arterial hypertension [64,65]. The growing number of pericytes and endothelial coverage with pericytes during arterial hypertension however appears to be unique to the hypertensive stimulus, since hypercholesterolemia, hyperglycemia and the subsequent inflammation elicited generally leads to a drastic decrease in pericyte coverage. To this end, hypercholesterolemia leads to a decrease in endothelial pericyte coverage in part via the downregulation of the endothelial NO synthase, a potent driver of microvascular mural cell recruitment [66–68]. In addition, hypercholesterolemia facilitates the above mentioned accumulation of reactive oxygen species and the increased recruitment of leukocytes [69]. Other effects seen during states of increased lipid deposition are the reduction of angiogenic sprouting via a downregulation of vascular endothelial growth factor (VEGF-A) and an additional reduction of endothelial N-Cadherin, the key anchoring protein with which endothelial cells and pericytes interact [70,71]. Diabetes as well seems to be associated with a drastic loss in pericytes. In this context, pericyte loss represents a key feature in the case of diabetic retinopathy. This complication of end-stage diabetes constitutes a well-studied phenomenon, due to the accessibility of the vascular bed to investigation both in human specimens as well as animal models. In both, capillary rarefication as well as a loss in pericytes is observed during diabetic retinopathy [72,73], while this process has also been demonstrated in additional vascular beds [74], mediated in part by advanced glycation end product accumulation [75].

4. Current and Future Treatment Strategies

Multiple therapies have been in clinical use to treat atherosclerotic lesions and the underlying cardiovascular risk factors. Two treatment options can be destinguished: firstly, the treatment of the predisposing factors causing atherosclerosis in order to reduce the progression of the disease once diagnosed. For primary arterial hypertension a host of antihypertensive drugs are available with varying efficacies and substance-class specific secondary effects. Notably, ACE-inhibitors and angiotensin 2 receptor antagonists not only lower the blood pressure but also reduce the degree of endothelial dysfunction by reducing leukocyte recruitment and the production of reactive oxygen species [76], an effect also demonstrated for calcium channel blockers [77]. Antidiabetic drugs too display pleiotropic effects beneficial for cardiovascular mortality. To this end, metformin and the novel class of PCSK9 inhibitors additionally reduce reactive oxygen species production [78,79]. Lastly, the pleiotropic effects of statins, the first line treatment option for hypercholesterolemia, have been well documented throughout the last decades. These drugs reduce endothelial cytokine production [80], production of reactive oxygen species [81] and vascular smooth muscle cell proliferation [82].

Mechanical revascularization, either via bypass surgery or percutaneous angioplasty, represents the second category in the treatment of atherosclerosis. These methods have demonstrated their merit over time for both coronary as well as peripheral artery disease. However, while extensive research has been undertaken to optimize surgery procedures and percutaneous vascular intervention strategies, no-reflow phenomena routinely occur in patients undergoing revascularization both in acute ischemic events as well as chronic vascular occlusion with rates varying from 2% up to 25%, depending on the vascular bed and the abruptness of occlusion [83,84]. In the case of acute myocardial or limb ischemia, these events can be attributed to a high thrombotic burden in the occluded vessel. However, the predominant vascular risk factors for the development of atherosclerotic lesions can have additional effects in the microcirculation as described above. In particular, the rarefication of capillaries and the dysfunctionality of the remaining capillaries, leading to a dysfunctional downstream vessels system, resulting in a drastic decrease in overall capillary diameter. This reduction in available runoff contributes to low-flow phenomena through recently implanted stents and increase the risk of stent thrombosis (see Figure 1).

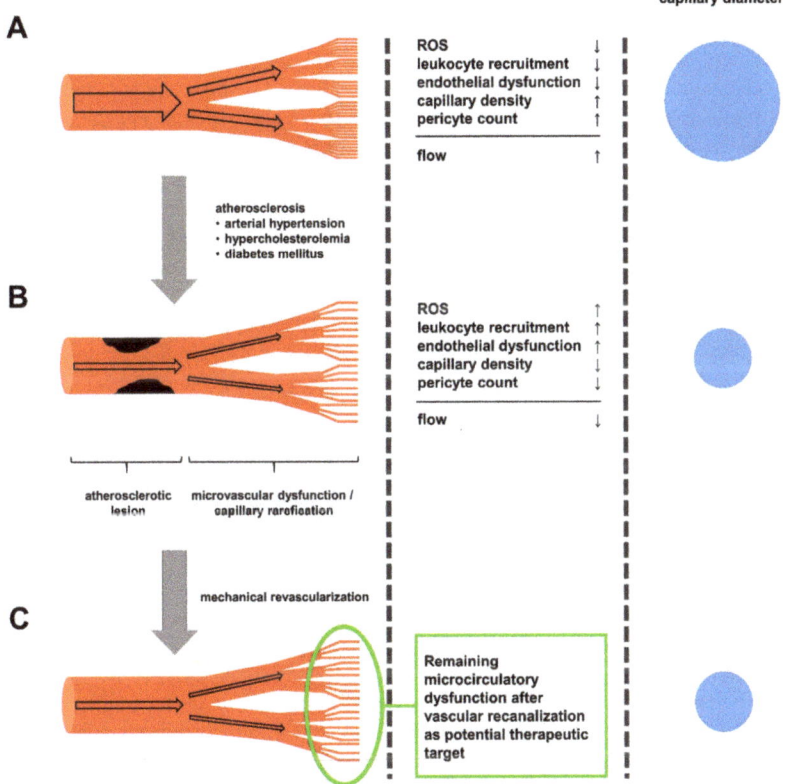

Figure 1. (**A**) The healthy circulatory system is characterized by minimal lipid accumulation in larger arteries and an overall low state of endothelial activation, leading to low levels of ROS production and leukocyte recruitment. (**B**) Upon prolonged exposure to the atherosclerotic risk factors arterial hypertension, hypercholesterolemia and diabetes, endothelial cells experience constant activation enhancing leukocyte recruitment, oxidative stress and loss of pericytes in the microcirculation, leading

to capillary rarefication, limiting the potential blood flow through the now sparse capillary network. (C) Even after mechanical revascularization, via bypass operations or percutaneous angioplasty, the capillary rarefication remains, continuously limiting blood flow, thus hindering the recovery of the ischemic tissue and leaving newly opened vessels susceptible for restenosis and stent thrombosis. Here, strategies to improve capillary density, and thus, microcirculatory flow, appear to be worthwhile therapeutic targets in the treatment of atherosclerosis currently not yet addresses.

Consequently, therapeutic strategies to ameliorate capillary rarefication and improve the functionality of the downstream capillary network need to be established. Since capillary stability crucially relies on proper pericyte adhesion to the endothelial tube, factors increasing pericyte abundance, as well as promoting angiogenic sprouting appear to be among the most promising targets to reduce the loss in capillaries during chronic.

One such agent can be found in the small peptide Thymosin β4. Thymosin β4 was first identified as an actin sequestering peptide binding G-actin in competition with Myocardin-related transcription factor A (MRTF-A) [85]. MRTF-A in its unbound form, i.e., free of G-actin binding, is capable to translocate into the nucleus, where it regulates the expression of SRF (serum response factor) target genes, in particular *CCN1* and *CCN2* [86]. CCN1 and CCN2 have been shown to promote angiogenic sprouting and vascular maturation via the recruitment of pericytes to newly formed vessels [87,88]. Increasing either the availability of Thymosin β4 or MRTF-A can promote MRTF-A nuclear translocation during chronic ischemia, as demonstrated in mouse and pig models of chronic limb ischemia as well as myocardial ischemia and reperfusion and hibernating myocardium [74,86,89]. Interestingly, Thymosin β4 has proven successful in improving myocardial perfusion in a model of chronic myocardial ischemia in otherwise healthy pigs and also hypercholesterolemic pigs and transgenic diabetic pigs [74,89], indicating its potential in the treatment of patients with underlying risk factors. Since arterial hypertension, hypercholesterolemia and diabetes mellitus are chronic disease states, a long term treatment seems preferable under these conditions. Thus, recombinant adeno-associated viral vectors (rAAV), as used in these studies, appear a favorable option, given their ability to facilitate long-term transgene expression with minimal genomic integration and low levels of host immune responses [90,91]. Another key regulator of angiogenic sprouting ameliorating capillary rarefication can be identified in vascular endothelial growth factor A (VEGF-A). VEGF-A promotes endothelial proliferation and tip-cell formation. However, long-term overexpression of VEGF-A leads to the formation of hemangioma-like structures with poor perfusion [92]. This effect can be prevented, when VEGF-A is administered as a combination treatment with a pericyte recruiting agent, such as PDGF-B, which stabilize newly formed vessels via the integration of pericytes into the sprouting vascular network [93]. Thus, a cotransfection of rabbits undergoing chronic hind limb ischemia with both rAAV.PDGF-B as well as rAAV. VEGF-A can induce collateral growth, increases capillary density and enhances the perfusion of the chronically occluded hind limb. Seeing as increased VEGF-A levels over prolonged periods of time lead to the formation of dysfunctional vessel, other modes of delivery might be advantageous. Overexpression of target genes in short bursts can be achieved via the transfection of modified RNA, which contains alternative nucleotides (pseudouridine, methylpseudouridine or 5-methyl-cytosine) to prevent TLR7/8 mediated host immune responses [94]. Using modRNA encoding for VEGF-A in mouse and pig models of chronic coronary occlusion, Carlsson et al. demonstrated a robust and short term VEGF-A expression, leading to an increase in both capillary and arteriole density. After proving the efficacy of an intramyocardial injection of VEGF-A modRNA, Gan et al. demonstrated in a recent phase Ia/b clinical study in diabetic patients, that localized injection of VEGF-A modRNA leads to a robust short term transgene expression without the induction of a significant immunresponse while locally improving perfusion [95]. Thus, capillary rarefication and loss of pericytes are treatment targets accessible for gene therapy approaches in vascular disease. However, other disease states accompanied by capillary rarefication might profit from similar gene therapy approaches, such as Duchenne muscular dystrophy (DMD). DMD is caused by mutations in the dystrophin gene, leading to the production of unstable, truncated and dysfunctional proteins [96,97]. While Duchenne muscular dystrophy is mostly recognized as a disease of the peripheral muscle and myocardium, it is also accompanied by capillary rarefication. This process contributes to the dire health status of patients afflicted by this genetic disorder by aggravating tissue ischemia [98]. In this context, our group was able to demonstrate that pigs lacking the exon 52 of the dystrophin gene (DMDΔ52), which leads to the expression of a similarly shortened and unstable dystrophin protein [99], also display a decrease in tissue capillary density and pericyte coverage. Once treated with rAAV containing a split Cas9 protein and guide RNAs targeting Exon 51, these animals not only regained expression of a functional dystrophin gene, but also showed a drastic improvement of tissue capillarization, a process accompanied by a reduction in CD68 positive macrophages (Figure 2, Moretti et al., Nature Medicine, accepted for publishing).

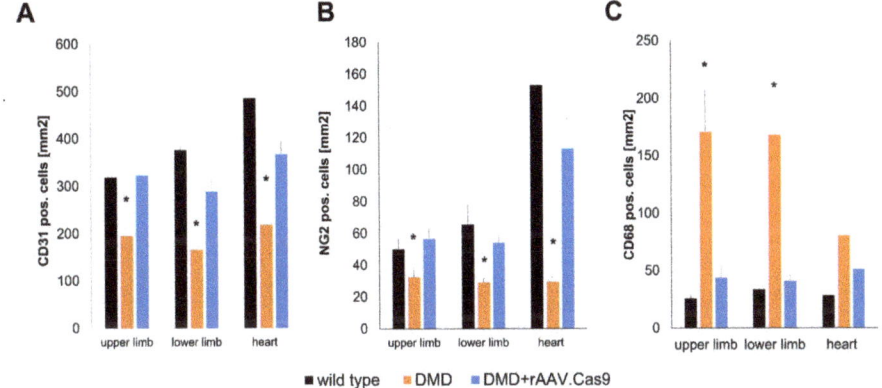

Figure 2. Effect of in vivo genome editing via rAAV and Cas9 mediated deletion of exon 51 of Duchenne muscular dystrophy on the vascularization and macrophage recruitment in the heart and upper and lower hind limb in DMDΔ52 pigs. (**A**) staining for CD31 positive endothelial cells highlights a significant decrease in capillary density in pigs suffering from Duchenne muscular dystrophy which ins ameliorated in pigs receiving Cas9 mediated Exon 51 deletion thus restoring dystrophin expression. (**B**) Similarly, edited DMD pigs display an amelioration of pericyte loss seen in dystrophin deficient pigs. (**C**) Lastly, the reduction in both endothelial cells as well as pericytes in dystrophin deficient pigs is accompanied by an increased recruitment of CD68 positive macrophages into the tissue, similarly to the recruitment seen in atherosclerotic states, which is again reversed upon normalization of dystrophin expression (*$p < 0.05$ versus wild type and DMD+rAAV.Cas9, error bars are given as SEM).

Interestingly, these findings combined highlight potential therapeutic strategies to target the rather neglected pathophysiological changes mediated by atherosclerotic risk factors in the microcirculation and represent a potential addition to the classical treatment strategies to ameliorate the disease burden of vascular occlusive disease.

5. Conclusions

Atherosclerosis represents a multifactorial disease mainly driven by arterial hypertension, hypercholesterolemia and diabetes mellitus, which, through the stenosis and occlusion of arteries, leads to organ ischemia and thus constitutes a main driver of mortality worldwide. The three main contributors to the development of atherosclerosis can originate from similar sources, such as sedentary lifestyle, western diet and obesity and exerted damage to the vessel wall via distinct but overlapping pathomechanisms. The hallmark of vascular alterations elicited by all three disease entities lies in the endothelial dysfunction seen in atherosclerosis, which is largely driven by an increase in endothelial activation with an elevated uptake of lipids, namely low-density lipoproteins, into the vascular wall.

This process triggers the production of reactive oxygen species as well as the attraction of macrophages to the site of plaque formation, leading to their transformation into foam cells. All of those pathological alterations can enter into a positive feedback loop aggravating the development of plaque formation. One additional component in this disease progression is the proliferation of vascular smooth muscle cells, which can participate in the uptake of oxidized LDL and can also transform into foam cells, which serve as a source for inflammatory cytokines, attracting more macrophages. Herein lies one key difference between the macrocirculation (e.g., larger arteries) and the microcirculation exemplified by capillaries. Capillaries are surrounded not by vascular smooth muscle cells but by pericytes, a cell type related to vascular smooth muscle cells but with distinct functions in the vascular unit. Unlike vSMCs, pericytes react to the pathological stimuli elicited by hyperglycemia and hypercholesterolemia with a detachment from the underlying endothelium, resulting in further endothelial activation and apoptosis. This leads to capillary rarefaction and reduced blood flow due to a decrease in capillary surface area.

Here, we highlighted potential therapeutic targets to improve microvascular dysfunction, namely by expressing proangiogenic growth factors and pericyte chemoattractants, either combined in one signaling molecule (as is the case for Thymosin β4) or in a cooperative fashion (such as the combined overexpression of VEGF-A and PDGF-B), all of which are mediated by a recombinant adeno-associated viral vector mediated overexpression, or the short-term burst expression of VEGF-A alone in the form of VEGF-A encoding modified RNA.

Taken together, the microcirculatory changes during atherosclerosis warrant further investigation and represent a worthwhile topic for additional studies.

Funding: This research received no external funding.

Conflicts of Interest: The authors declare no conflict of interest.

References

1. World Health Organization. *Cardiovascular Disease (CVDs)*; World Health Organization: Geneva, Switzerland, 2017.
2. Nakashima, Y.; Chen, Y.X.; Kinukawa, N.; Sueishi, K. Distributions of diffuse intimal thickening in human arteries: Preferential expression in atherosclerosis-prone arteries from an early age. *Virchows Arch.* **2002**, *441*, 279–288. [CrossRef]
3. Guyton, J.R.; Bocan, T.M.; Schifani, T.A. Quantitative ultrastructural analysis of perifibrous lipid and its association with elastin in nonatherosclerotic human aorta. *Arteriosclerosis* **1985**, *5*, 644–652. [CrossRef]
4. Tabas, I.; Williams, K.J.; Boren, J. Subendothelial lipoprotein retention as the initiating process in atherosclerosis: Update and therapeutic implications. *Circulation* **2007**, *116*, 1832–1844. [CrossRef]
5. Williams, K.J.; Tabas, I. The response-to-retention hypothesis of early atherogenesis. *Arterioscler. Thromb. Vasc. Biol.* **1995**, *15*, 551–561. [CrossRef]
6. Lee, R.T.; Yamamoto, C.; Feng, Y.; Potter-Perigo, S.; Briggs, W.H.; Landschulz, K.T.; Turi, T.G.; Thompson, J.F.; Libby, P.; Wight, T.N. Mechanical strain induces specific changes in the synthesis and organization of proteoglycans by vascular smooth muscle cells. *J. Biol. Chem.* **2001**, *276*, 13847–13851. [CrossRef]
7. Little, P.J.; Tannock, L.; Olin, K.L.; Chait, A.; Wight, T.N. Proteoglycans synthesized by arterial smooth muscle cells in the presence of transforming growth factor-beta1 exhibit increased binding to LDLs. *Arterioscler. Thromb. Vasc. Biol.* **2002**, *22*, 55–60. [CrossRef]
8. Cushing, S.D.; Berliner, J.A.; Valente, A.J.; Territo, M.C.; Navab, M.; Parhami, F.; Gerrity, R.; Schwartz, C.J.; Fogelman, A.M. Minimally modified low density lipoprotein induces monocyte chemotactic protein 1 in human endothelial cells and smooth muscle cells. *Proc. Natl. Acad. Sci. USA* **1990**, *87*, 5134–5138. [CrossRef]
9. Hurt-Camejo, E.; Camejo, G.; Rosengren, B.; Lopez, F.; Ahlstrom, C.; Fager, G.; Bondjers, G. Effect of arterial proteoglycans and glycosaminoglycans on low density lipoprotein oxidation and its uptake by human macrophages and arterial smooth muscle cells. *Arterioscler. Thromb.* **1992**, *12*, 569–583. [CrossRef]

10. Karakikes, I.; Chaanine, A.H.; Kang, S.; Mukete, B.N.; Jeong, D.; Zhang, S.; Hajjar, R.J.; Lebeche, D. Therapeutic cardiac-targeted delivery of miR-1 reverses pressure overload-induced cardiac hypertrophy and attenuates pathological remodeling. *J. Am. Heart Assoc.* **2013**, *2*, e000078. [CrossRef]
11. Kockx, M.M.; De Meyer, G.R.; Muhring, J.; Jacob, W.; Bult, H.; Herman, A.G. Apoptosis and related proteins in different stages of human atherosclerotic plaques. *Circulation* **1998**, *97*, 2307–2315. [CrossRef]
12. Merrilees, M.J.; Beaumont, B. Structural heterogeneity of the diffuse intimal thickening and correlation with distribution of TGF-beta 1. *J. Vasc. Res.* **1993**, *30*, 293–302. [CrossRef]
13. Murry, C.E.; Gipaya, C.T.; Bartosek, T.; Benditt, E.P.; Schwartz, S.M. Monoclonality of smooth muscle cells in human atherosclerosis. *Am. J. Pathol.* **1997**, *151*, 697–705.
14. Nakata, A.; Miyagawa, J.; Yamashita, S.; Nishida, M.; Tamura, R.; Yamamori, K.; Nakamura, T.; Nozaki, S.; Kameda-Takemura, K.; Kawata, S.; et al. Localization of heparin-binding epidermal growth factor-like growth factor in human coronary arteries. Possible roles of HB-EGF in the formation of coronary atherosclerosis. *Circulation* **1996**, *94*, 2778–2786. [CrossRef]
15. Alshehri, O.M.; Hughes, C.E.; Montague, S.; Watson, S.K.; Frampton, J.; Bender, M.; Watson, S.P. Fibrin activates GPVI in human and mouse platelets. *Blood* **2015**, *126*, 1601–1608. [CrossRef]
16. Naimushin, Y.A.; Mazurov, A.V. Von Willebrand factor can support platelet aggregation via interaction with activated GPIIb-IIIa and GPIb. *Platelets* **2004**, *15*, 419–425. [CrossRef]
17. Sarratt, K.L.; Chen, H.; Zutter, M.M.; Santoro, S.A.; Hammer, D.A.; Kahn, M.L. GPVI and alpha2beta1 play independent critical roles during platelet adhesion and aggregate formation to collagen under flow. *Blood* **2005**, *106*, 1268–1277. [CrossRef]
18. Cassese, S.; Byrne, R.A.; Tada, T.; Pinieck, S.; Joner, M.; Ibrahim, T.; King, L.A.; Fusaro, M.; Laugwitz, K.L.; Kastrati, A. Incidence and predictors of restenosis after coronary stenting in 10 004 patients with surveillance angiography. *Heart* **2014**, *100*, 153–159. [CrossRef]
19. Gray, W.A.; Keirse, K.; Soga, Y.; Benko, A.; Babaev, A.; Yokoi, Y.; Schroeder, H.; Prem, J.T.; Holden, A.; Popma, J.; et al. A polymer-coated, paclitaxel-eluting stent (Eluvia) versus a polymer-free, paclitaxel-coated stent (Zilver PTX) for endovascular femoropopliteal intervention (IMPERIAL): A randomised, non-inferiority trial. *Lancet* **2018**, *392*, 1541–1551. [CrossRef]
20. Sander, M.; Chavoshan, B.; Victor, R.G. A large blood pressure-raising effect of nitric oxide synthase inhibition in humans. *Hypertension* **1999**, *33*, 937–942. [CrossRef]
21. Bush, E.; Maeda, N.; Kuziel, W.A.; Dawson, T.C.; Wilcox, J.N.; DeLeon, H.; Taylor, W.R. CC chemokine receptor 2 is required for macrophage infiltration and vascular hypertrophy in angiotensin II-induced hypertension. *Hypertension* **2000**, *36*, 360–363. [CrossRef]
22. Ryan, M.J.; Didion, S.P.; Mathur, S.; Faraci, F.M.; Sigmund, C.D. Angiotensin II-induced vascular dysfunction is mediated by the AT1A receptor in mice. *Hypertension* **2004**, *43*, 1074–1079. [CrossRef]
23. Wang, H.D.; Xu, S.; Johns, D.G.; Du, Y.; Quinn, M.T.; Cayatte, A.J.; Cohen, R.A. Role of NADPH oxidase in the vascular hypertrophic and oxidative stress response to angiotensin II in mice. *Circ. Res.* **2001**, *88*, 947–953. [CrossRef]
24. World Health Organization. *Global Health Observatory*; World Health Organization: Geneva, Switzerland, 2018.
25. Landsberg, L.; Aronne, L.J.; Beilin, L.J.; Burke, V.; Igel, L.I.; Lloyd-Jones, D.; Sowers, J. Obesity-related hypertension: Pathogenesis, cardiovascular risk, and treatment—A position paper of the The Obesity Society and The American Society of Hypertension. *Obesity* **2013**, *21*, 8–24. [CrossRef]
26. Nahrendorf, M.; Swirski, F.K. Lifestyle effects on hematopoiesis and atherosclerosis. *Circ. Res.* **2015**, *116*, 884–894. [CrossRef]
27. Gimbrone, M.A., Jr.; Garcia-Cardena, G. Vascular endothelium, hemodynamics, and the pathobiology of atherosclerosis. *Cardiovasc. Pathol.* **2013**, *22*, 9–15. [CrossRef]
28. Fogelstrand, P.; Boren, J. Retention of atherogenic lipoproteins in the artery wall and its role in atherogenesis. *Nutr. Metab. Cardiovasc. Dis.* **2012**, *22*, 1–7. [CrossRef]
29. Iverius, P.H. The interaction between human plasma lipoproteins and connective tissue glycosaminoglycans. *J. Biol. Chem.* **1972**, *247*, 2607–2613.
30. Flood, C.; Gustafsson, M.; Pitas, R.E.; Arnaboldi, L.; Walzem, R.L.; Boren, J. Molecular mechanism for changes in proteoglycan binding on compositional changes of the core and the surface of low-density lipoprotein-containing human apolipoprotein B100. *Arterioscler. Thromb. Vasc. Biol.* **2004**, *24*, 564–570. [CrossRef]

31. Ungvari, Z.; Wolin, M.S.; Csiszar, A. Mechanosensitive production of reactive oxygen species in endothelial and smooth muscle cells: Role in microvascular remodeling? *Antioxid. Redox Signal.* **2006**, *8*, 1121–1129. [CrossRef]
32. Krieger, M. Scavenger receptor class B type I is a multiligand HDL receptor that influences diverse physiologic systems. *J. Clin. Investig.* **2001**, *108*, 793–797. [CrossRef]
33. Lara-Guzman, O.J.; Gil-Izquierdo, A.; Medina, S.; Osorio, E.; Alvarez-Quintero, R.; Zuluaga, N.; Oger, C.; Galano, J.M.; Durand, T.; Munoz-Durango, K. Oxidized LDL triggers changes in oxidative stress and inflammatory biomarkers in human macrophages. *Redox Biol.* **2018**, *15*, 1–11. [CrossRef]
34. Khan, B.V.; Parthasarathy, S.S.; Alexander, R.W.; Medford, R.M. Modified low density lipoprotein and its constituents augment cytokine-activated vascular cell adhesion molecule-1 gene expression in human vascular endothelial cells. *J. Clin. Investig.* **1995**, *95*, 1262–1270. [CrossRef]
35. Vora, D.K.; Fang, Z.T.; Liva, S.M.; Tyner, T.R.; Parhami, F.; Watson, A.D.; Drake, T.A.; Territo, M.C.; Berliner, J.A. Induction of P-selectin by oxidized lipoproteins. Separate effects on synthesis and surface expression. *Circ. Res.* **1997**, *80*, 810–818. [CrossRef]
36. Berliner, J.A.; Schwartz, D.S.; Territo, M.C.; Andalibi, A.; Almada, L.; Lusis, A.J.; Quismorio, D.; Fang, Z.P.; Fogelman, A.M. Induction of chemotactic cytokines by minimally oxidized LDL. *Adv. Exp. Med. Biol.* **1993**, *351*, 13–18. [CrossRef]
37. Brownlee, M. Biochemistry and molecular cell biology of diabetic complications. *Nature* **2001**, *414*, 813–820. [CrossRef]
38. Wautier, M.P.; Chappey, O.; Corda, S.; Stern, D.M.; Schmidt, A.M.; Wautier, J.L. Activation of NADPH oxidase by AGE links oxidant stress to altered gene expression via RAGE. *Am. J. Physiol. Endocrinol. Metab.* **2001**, *280*, E685–E694. [CrossRef]
39. Basta, G.; Schmidt, A.M.; De Caterina, R. Advanced glycation end products and vascular inflammation: Implications for accelerated atherosclerosis in diabetes. *Cardiovasc. Res.* **2004**, *63*, 582–592. [CrossRef]
40. Neumann, A.; Schinzel, R.; Palm, D.; Riederer, P.; Munch, G. High molecular weight hyaluronic acid inhibits advanced glycation endproduct-induced NF-kappaB activation and cytokine expression. *FEBS Lett.* **1999**, *453*, 283–287. [CrossRef]
41. Iwashima, Y.; Eto, M.; Hata, A.; Kaku, K.; Horiuchi, S.; Ushikubi, F.; Sano, H. Advanced glycation end products-induced gene expression of scavenger receptors in cultured human monocyte-derived macrophages. *Biochem. Biophys. Res. Commun.* **2000**, *277*, 368–380. [CrossRef]
42. Ziegler, T.; Horstkotte, M.; Lange, P.; Ng, J.; Bongiovanni, D.; Hinkel, R.; Laugwitz, K.L.; Sperandio, M.; Horstkotte, J.; Kupatt, C. Endothelial RAGE exacerbates acute postischaemic cardiac inflammation. *Thromb. Haemost.* **2016**, *116*, 300–308. [CrossRef]
43. Natarajan, R.; Gerrity, R.G.; Gu, J.L.; Lanting, L.; Thomas, L.; Nadler, J.L. Role of 12-lipoxygenase and oxidant stress in hyperglycaemia-induced acceleration of atherosclerosis in a diabetic pig model. *Diabetologia* **2002**, *45*, 125–133. [CrossRef]
44. Wu, L.; Vikramadithyan, R.; Yu, S.; Pau, C.; Hu, Y.; Goldberg, I.J.; Dansky, H.M. Addition of dietary fat to cholesterol in the diets of LDL receptor knockout mice: Effects on plasma insulin, lipoproteins, and atherosclerosis. *J. Lipid Res.* **2006**, *47*, 2215–2222. [CrossRef]
45. Ho, K.L. Ultrastructure of cerebellar capillary hemangioblastoma. IV. Pericytes and their relationship to endothelial cells. *Acta Neuropathol.* **1985**, *67*, 254–264. [CrossRef]
46. Larson, D.M.; Carson, M.P.; Haudenschild, C.C. Junctional transfer of small molecules in cultured bovine brain microvascular endothelial cells and pericytes. *Microvasc. Res.* **1987**, *34*, 184–199. [CrossRef]
47. Rucker, H.K.; Wynder, H.J.; Thomas, W.E. Cellular mechanisms of CNS pericytes. *Brain Res. Bull.* **2000**, *51*, 363–369. [CrossRef]
48. Davis, S.; Aldrich, T.H.; Jones, P.F.; Acheson, A.; Compton, D.L.; Jain, V.; Ryan, T.E.; Bruno, J.; Radziejewski, C.; Maisonpierre, P.C.; et al. Isolation of angiopoietin-1, a ligand for the TIE2 receptor, by secretion-trap expression cloning. *Cell* **1996**, *87*, 1161–1169. [CrossRef]
49. Cardone, M.H.; Roy, N.; Stennicke, H.R.; Salvesen, G.S.; Franke, T.F.; Stanbridge, E.; Frisch, S.; Reed, J.C. Regulation of cell death protease caspase-9 by phosphorylation. *Science* **1998**, *282*, 1318–1321. [CrossRef]
50. Papapetropoulos, A.; Fulton, D.; Mahboubi, K.; Kalb, R.G.; O'Connor, D.S.; Li, F.; Altieri, D.C.; Sessa, W.C. Angiopoietin-1 inhibits endothelial cell apoptosis via the Akt/survivin pathway. *J. Biol. Chem.* **2000**, *275*, 9102–9105. [CrossRef]

51. Kobayashi, H.; DeBusk, L.M.; Babichev, Y.O.; Dumont, D.J.; Lin, P.C. Hepatocyte growth factor mediates angiopoietin-induced smooth muscle cell recruitment. *Blood* **2006**, *108*, 1260–1266. [CrossRef]
52. Iivanainen, E.; Nelimarkka, L.; Elenius, V.; Heikkinen, S.M.; Junttila, T.T.; Sihombing, L.; Sundvall, M.; Maatta, J.A.; Laine, V.J.; Yla-Herttuala, S.; et al. Angiopoietin-regulated recruitment of vascular smooth muscle cells by endothelial-derived heparin binding EGF-like growth factor. *FASEB J. Off. Publ. Fed. Am. Soc. Exp. Biol.* **2003**, *17*, 1609–1621. [CrossRef]
53. Orlidge, A.; D'Amore, P.A. Inhibition of capillary endothelial cell growth by pericytes and smooth muscle cells. *J. Cell Biol.* **1987**, *105*, 1455–1462. [CrossRef] [PubMed]
54. Marra, F.; Bonewald, L.F.; Park-Snyder, S.; Park, I.S.; Woodruff, K.A.; Abboud, H.E. Characterization and regulation of the latent transforming growth factor-beta complex secreted by vascular pericytes. *J. Cell. Physiol.* **1996**, *166*, 537–546. [CrossRef]
55. Watanabe, S.; Morisaki, N.; Tezuka, M.; Fukuda, K.; Ueda, S.; Koyama, N.; Yokote, K.; Kanzaki, T.; Yoshida, S.; Saito, Y. Cultured retinal pericytes stimulate in vitro angiogenesis of endothelial cells through secretion of a fibroblast growth factor-like molecule. *Atherosclerosis* **1997**, *130*, 101–107. [CrossRef]
56. Takagi, H.; King, G.L.; Robinson, G.S.; Ferrara, N.; Aiello, L.P. Adenosine mediates hypoxic induction of vascular endothelial growth factor in retinal pericytes and endothelial cells. *Investig. Ophthalmol. Vis. Sci.* **1996**, *37*, 2165–2176.
57. Austin, K.M.; Nguyen, N.; Javid, G.; Covic, L.; Kuliopulos, A. Noncanonical matrix metalloprotease-1-protease-activated receptor-1 signaling triggers vascular smooth muscle cell dedifferentiation and arterial stenosis. *J. Biol. Chem.* **2013**, *288*, 23105–23115. [CrossRef] [PubMed]
58. Pfister, F.; Feng, Y.; vom Hagen, F.; Hoffmann, S.; Molema, G.; Hillebrands, J.L.; Shani, M.; Deutsch, U.; Hammes, H.P. Pericyte migration: A novel mechanism of pericyte loss in experimental diabetic retinopathy. *Diabetes* **2008**, *57*, 2495–2502. [CrossRef]
59. Zehendner, C.M.; Wedler, H.E.; Luhmann, H.J. A novel in vitro model to study pericytes in the neurovascular unit of the developing cortex. *PLoS ONE* **2013**, *8*, e81637. [CrossRef]
60. Ziegler, T.; Horstkotte, J.; Schwab, C.; Pfetsch, V.; Weinmann, K.; Dietzel, S.; Rohwedder, I.; Hinkel, R.; Gross, L.; Lee, S.; et al. Angiopoietin 2 mediates microvascular and hemodynamic alterations in sepsis. *J. Clin. Investig.* **2013**, *123*, 3436–3445. [CrossRef]
61. Herman, I.M.; Jacobson, S. In situ analysis of microvascular pericytes in hypertensive rat brains. *Tissue Cell* **1988**, *20*, 1–12. [CrossRef]
62. Wallow, I.H.; Bindley, C.D.; Reboussin, D.M.; Gange, S.J.; Fisher, M.R. Systemic hypertension produces pericyte changes in retinal capillaries. *Investig. Ophthalmol. Vis. Sci.* **1993**, *34*, 420–430.
63. Ricard, N.; Tu, L.; Le Hiress, M.; Huertas, A.; Phan, C.; Thuillet, R.; Sattler, C.; Fadel, E.; Seferian, A.; Montani, D.; et al. Increased pericyte coverage mediated by endothelial-derived fibroblast growth factor-2 and interleukin-6 is a source of smooth muscle-like cells in pulmonary hypertension. *Circulation* **2014**, *129*, 1586–1597. [CrossRef] [PubMed]
64. Chen, I.I.; Prewitt, R.L.; Dowell, R.F. Microvascular raretaction in spontaneously hypertensive rat cremaster muscle. *Am. J. Physiol.* **1981**, *241*, H306–H310. [CrossRef] [PubMed]
65. Cheng, C.; Daskalakis, C.; Falkner, B. Capillary rarefaction in treated and untreated hypertensive subjects. *Ther. Adv. Cardiovasc. Dis.* **2008**, *2*, 79–88. [CrossRef] [PubMed]
66. Wolfle, S.E.; de Wit, C. Intact endothelium-dependent dilation and conducted responses in resistance vessels of hypercholesterolemic mice in vivo. *J. Vasc. Res.* **2005**, *42*, 475–482. [CrossRef]
67. Steinberg, H.O.; Bayazeed, B.; Hook, G.; Johnson, A.; Cronin, J.; Baron, A.D. Endothelial dysfunction is associated with cholesterol levels in the high normal range in humans. *Circulation* **1997**, *96*, 3287–3293. [CrossRef]
68. Ha, J.M.; Jin, S.Y.; Lee, H.S.; Shin, H.K.; Lee, D.H.; Song, S.H.; Kim, C.D.; Bae, S.S. Regulation of retinal angiogenesis by endothelial nitric oxide synthase signaling pathway. *Korean J. Physiol. Pharmacol.* **2016**, *20*, 533–538. [CrossRef]
69. Garcia-Quintans, N.; Sanchez-Ramos, C.; Prieto, I.; Tierrez, A.; Arza, E.; Alfranca, A.; Redondo, J.M.; Monsalve, M. Oxidative stress induces loss of pericyte coverage and vascular instability in PGC-1alpha-deficient mice. *Angiogenesis* **2016**, *19*, 217–228. [CrossRef]
70. Radice, G.L. N-cadherin-mediated adhesion and signaling from development to disease: Lessons from mice. *Prog. Mol. Biol. Transl. Sci.* **2013**, *116*, 263–289. [CrossRef]

71. Zechariah, A.; ElAli, A.; Hagemann, N.; Jin, F.; Doeppner, T.R.; Helfrich, I.; Mies, G.; Hermann, D.M. Hyperlipidemia attenuates vascular endothelial growth factor-induced angiogenesis, impairs cerebral blood flow, and disturbs stroke recovery via decreased pericyte coverage of brain endothelial cells. *Arterioscler. Thromb. Vasc. Biol.* **2013**, *33*, 1561–1567. [CrossRef]
72. Beltramo, E.; Porta, M. Pericyte loss in diabetic retinopathy: Mechanisms and consequences. *Curr. Med. Chem.* **2013**, *20*, 3218–3225. [CrossRef]
73. Kim, Y.H.; Park, S.Y.; Park, J.; Kim, Y.S.; Hwang, E.M.; Park, J.Y.; Roh, G.S.; Kim, H.J.; Kang, S.S.; Cho, G.J.; et al. Reduction of experimental diabetic vascular leakage and pericyte apoptosis in mice by delivery of alphaA-crystallin with a recombinant adenovirus. *Diabetologia* **2012**, *55*, 2835–2844. [CrossRef] [PubMed]
74. Hinkel, R.; Howe, A.; Renner, S.; Ng, J.; Lee, S.; Klett, K.; Kaczmarek, V.; Moretti, A.; Laugwitz, K.L.; Skroblin, P.; et al. Diabetes Mellitus-Induced Microvascular Destabilization in the Myocardium. *J. Am. Coll. Cardiol.* **2017**, *69*, 131–143. [CrossRef] [PubMed]
75. Yamagishi, S.; Takeuchi, M.; Matsui, T.; Nakamura, K.; Imaizumi, T.; Inoue, H. Angiotensin II augments advanced glycation end product-induced pericyte apoptosis through RAGE overexpression. *FEBS Lett.* **2005**, *579*, 4265–4270. [CrossRef] [PubMed]
76. Fiordaliso, F.; Cuccovillo, I.; Bianchi, R.; Bai, A.; Doni, M.; Salio, M.; De Angelis, N.; Ghezzi, P.; Latini, R.; Masson, S. Cardiovascular oxidative stress is reduced by an ACE inhibitor in a rat model of streptozotocin-induced diabetes. *Life Sci.* **2006**, *79*, 121–129. [CrossRef]
77. Lupo, E.; Locher, R.; Weisser, B.; Vetter, W. In vitro antioxidant activity of calcium antagonists against LDL oxidation compared with alpha-tocopherol. *Biochem. Biophys. Res. Commun.* **1994**, *203*, 1803–1808. [CrossRef]
78. Algire, C.; Moiseeva, O.; Deschenes-Simard, X.; Amrein, L.; Petruccelli, L.; Birman, E.; Viollet, B.; Ferbeyre, G.; Pollak, M.N. Metformin reduces endogenous reactive oxygen species and associated DNA damage. *Cancer Prev. Res.* **2012**, *5*, 536–543. [CrossRef]
79. Sabatine, M.S.; Leiter, L.A.; Wiviott, S.D.; Giugliano, R.P.; Deedwania, P.; De Ferrari, G.M.; Murphy, S.A.; Kuder, J.F.; Gouni-Berthold, I.; Lewis, B.S.; et al. Cardiovascular safety and efficacy of the PCSK9 inhibitor evolocumab in patients with and without diabetes and the effect of evolocumab on glycaemia and risk of new-onset diabetes: A prespecified analysis of the FOURIER randomised controlled trial. *Lancet Diabetes Endocrinol.* **2017**, *5*, 941–950. [CrossRef]
80. Inoue, I.; Goto, S.; Mizotani, K.; Awata, T.; Mastunaga, T.; Kawai, S.; Nakajima, T.; Hokari, S.; Komoda, T.; Katayama, S. Lipophilic HMG-CoA reductase inhibitor has an anti-inflammatory effect: Reduction of MRNA levels for interleukin-1beta, interleukin-6, cyclooxygenase-2, and p22phox by regulation of peroxisome proliferator-activated receptor alpha (PPARalpha) in primary endothelial cells. *Life Sci.* **2000**, *67*, 863–876. [CrossRef]
81. Bouitbir, J.; Charles, A.L.; Echaniz-Laguna, A.; Kindo, M.; Daussin, F.; Auwerx, J.; Piquard, F.; Geny, B.; Zoll, J. Opposite effects of statins on mitochondria of cardiac and skeletal muscles: A 'mitohormesis' mechanism involving reactive oxygen species and PGC-1. *Eur. Heart J.* **2012**, *33*, 1397–1407. [CrossRef]
82. Raiteri, M.; Arnaboldi, L.; McGeady, P.; Gelb, M.H.; Verri, D.; Tagliabue, C.; Quarato, P.; Ferraboschi, P.; Santaniello, E.; Paoletti, R.; et al. Pharmacological control of the mevalonate pathway: Effect on arterial smooth muscle cell proliferation. *J. Pharmcol. Exp. Ther.* **1997**, *281*, 1144–1153.
83. Tokuda, T.; Hirano, K.; Sakamoto, Y.; Takimura, H.; Kobayashi, N.; Araki, M.; Yamawaki, M.; Ito, Y. Incidence and clinical outcomes of the slow-flow phenomenon after infrapopliteal balloon angioplasty. *J. Vasc. Surg.* **2017**, *65*, 1047–1054. [CrossRef] [PubMed]
84. Harrison, R.W.; Aggarwal, A.; Ou, F.S.; Klein, L.W.; Rumsfeld, J.S.; Roe, M.T.; Wang, T.Y.; American College of Cardiology National Cardiovascular Data, Registry. Incidence and outcomes of no-reflow phenomenon during percutaneous coronary intervention among patients with acute myocardial infarction. *Am. J. Cardiol.* **2013**, *111*, 178–184. [CrossRef] [PubMed]
85. Morita, T.; Hayashi, K. G-actin sequestering protein thymosin-beta4 regulates the activity of myocardin-related transcription factor. *Biochem. Biophys. Res. Commun.* **2013**, *437*, 331–335. [CrossRef] [PubMed]
86. Hinkel, R.; Trenkwalder, T.; Petersen, B.; Husada, W.; Gesenhues, F.; Lee, S.; Hannappel, E.; Bock-Marquette, I.; Theisen, D.; Leitner, L.; et al. MRTF-A controls vessel growth and maturation by increasing the expression of CCN1 and CCN2. *Nat. Commun.* **2014**, *5*, 3970. [CrossRef]

87. Hall-Glenn, F.; De Young, R.A.; Huang, B.L.; van Handel, B.; Hofmann, J.J.; Chen, T.T.; Choi, A.; Ong, J.R.; Benya, P.D.; Mikkola, H.; et al. CCN2/connective tissue growth factor is essential for pericyte adhesion and endothelial basement membrane formation during angiogenesis. *PLoS ONE* **2012**, *7*, e30562. [CrossRef]
88. Hanna, M.; Liu, H.; Amir, J.; Sun, Y.; Morris, S.W.; Siddiqui, M.A.; Lau, L.F.; Chaqour, B. Mechanical regulation of the proangiogenic factor CCN1/CYR61 gene requires the combined activities of MRTF-A and CREB-binding protein histone acetyltransferase. *J. Biol. Chem.* **2009**, *284*, 23125–23136. [CrossRef]
89. Ziegler, T.; Bahr, A.; Howe, A.; Klett, K.; Husada, W.; Weber, C.; Laugwitz, K.L.; Kupatt, C.; Hinkel, R. Tbeta4 Increases Neovascularization and Cardiac Function in Chronic Myocardial Ischemia of Normo- and Hypercholesterolemic Pigs. *Mol. Ther.* **2018**, *26*, 1706–1714. [CrossRef]
90. Chirmule, N.; Propert, K.; Magosin, S.; Qian, Y.; Qian, R.; Wilson, J. Immune responses to adenovirus and adeno-associated virus in humans. *Gene Ther.* **1999**, *6*, 1574–1583. [CrossRef]
91. Nowrouzi, A.; Penaud-Budloo, M.; Kaeppel, C.; Appelt, U.; Le Guiner, C.; Moullier, P.; von Kalle, C.; Snyder, R.O.; Schmidt, M. Integration frequency and intermolecular recombination of rAAV vectors in non-human primate skeletal muscle and liver. *Mol. Ther.* **2012**, *20*, 1177–1186. [CrossRef]
92. Yla-Herttuala, S.; Rissanen, T.T.; Vajanto, I.; Hartikainen, J. Vascular endothelial growth factors: Biology and current status of clinical applications in cardiovascular medicine. *J. Am. Coll. Cardiol.* **2007**, *49*, 1015–1026. [CrossRef]
93. Hellstrom, M.; Kalen, M.; Lindahl, P.; Abramsson, A.; Betsholtz, C. Role of PDGF-B and PDGFR-beta in recruitment of vascular smooth muscle cells and pericytes during embryonic blood vessel formation in the mouse. *Development* **1999**, *126*, 3047–3055. [PubMed]
94. Kariko, K.; Buckstein, M.; Ni, H.; Weissman, D. Suppression of RNA recognition by Toll-like receptors: The impact of nucleoside modification and the evolutionary origin of RNA. *Immunity* **2005**, *23*, 165–175. [CrossRef] [PubMed]
95. Gan, L.M.; Lagerstrom-Fermer, M.; Carlsson, L.G.; Arfvidsson, C.; Egnell, A.C.; Rudvik, A.; Kjaer, M.; Collen, A.; Thompson, J.D.; Joyal, J.; et al. Intradermal delivery of modified mRNA encoding VEGF-A in patients with type 2 diabetes. *Nat. Commun.* **2019**, *10*, 871. [CrossRef] [PubMed]
96. Aartsma-Rus, A.; Van Deutekom, J.C.; Fokkema, I.F.; Van Ommen, G.J.; Den Dunnen, J.T. Entries in the Leiden Duchenne muscular dystrophy mutation database: An overview of mutation types and paradoxical cases that confirm the reading-frame rule. *Muscle Nerve* **2006**, *34*, 135–144. [CrossRef] [PubMed]
97. White, S.; Kalf, M.; Liu, Q.; Villerius, M.; Engelsma, D.; Kriek, M.; Vollebregt, E.; Bakker, B.; van Ommen, G.J.; Breuning, M.H.; et al. Comprehensive detection of genomic duplications and deletions in the DMD gene, by use of multiplex amplifiable probe hybridization. *Am. J. Hum. Genet.* **2002**, *71*, 365–374. [CrossRef] [PubMed]
98. Shimizu-Motohashi, Y.; Asakura, A. Angiogenesis as a novel therapeutic strategy for Duchenne muscular dystrophy through decreased ischemia and increased satellite cells. *Front. Physiol.* **2014**, *5*, 50. [CrossRef]
99. Klymiuk, N.; Blutke, A.; Graf, A.; Krause, S.; Burkhardt, K.; Wuensch, A.; Krebs, S.; Kessler, B.; Zakhartchenko, V.; Kurome, M.; et al. Dystrophin-deficient pigs provide new insights into the hierarchy of physiological derangements of dystrophic muscle. *Hum. Mol. Genet.* **2013**, *22*, 4368–4382. [CrossRef]

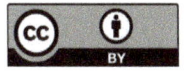

© 2019 by the authors. Licensee MDPI, Basel, Switzerland. This article is an open access article distributed under the terms and conditions of the Creative Commons Attribution (CC BY) license (http://creativecommons.org/licenses/by/4.0/).

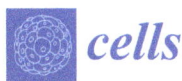

Review

Why Should Growth Hormone (GH) Be Considered a Promising Therapeutic Agent for Arteriogenesis? Insights from the GHAS Trial

Diego Caicedo [1,*], Pablo Devesa [2], Clara V. Alvarez [3] and Jesús Devesa [4,*]

1. Department of Angiology and Vascular Surgery, Complejo Hospitalario Universitario de Santiago de Compostela, 15706 Santiago de Compostela, Spain
2. Research and Development, The Medical Center Foltra, 15886 Teo, Spain; pdevesap@foltra.org
3. . Neoplasia and Endocrine Differentiation Research Group. Center for Research in Molecular Medicine and Chronic Diseases (CIMUS). University of Santiago de Compostela, 15782. Santiago de Compostela, Spain; clara.alvarez@usc.es
4. Scientific Direction, The Medical Center Foltra, 15886 Teo, Spain
* Correspondence: diego.caicedo.valdes@sergas.es (D.C.); devesa.jesus@gmail.com (J.D.); Tel.: +34-981-800-000 (D.C.); +34-981-802-928 (J.D.)

Received: 29 November 2019; Accepted: 25 March 2020; Published: 27 March 2020

Abstract: Despite the important role that the growth hormone (GH)/IGF-I axis plays in vascular homeostasis, these kind of growth factors barely appear in articles addressing the neovascularization process. Currently, the vascular endothelium is considered as an authentic gland of internal secretion due to the wide variety of released factors and functions with local effects, including the paracrine/autocrine production of GH or IGF-I, for which the endothelium has specific receptors. In this comprehensive review, the evidence involving these proangiogenic hormones in arteriogenesis dealing with the arterial occlusion and making of them a potential therapy is described. All the elements that trigger the local and systemic production of GH/IGF-I, as well as their possible roles both in physiological and pathological conditions are analyzed. All of the evidence is combined with important data from the GHAS trial, in which GH or a placebo were administrated to patients suffering from critical limb ischemia with no option for revascularization. We postulate that GH, alone or in combination, should be considered as a promising therapeutic agent for helping in the approach of ischemic disease.

Keywords: GH and eNOS; IGF-I; oxidative stress and arterial inflammation; vascular homeostasis; neovascularization; arteriogenesis; GHAS trial

---

1. Introduction

The fact that growth hormone (GH) is a necessary actor for many physiological processes and a real breakthrough for the treatment of many pathological situations beyond simple human longitudinal growth does not need justification [1]. Today, GH is considered a key hormone that acts in virtually all organs and tissues, in which it performs important specific functions. From the current knowledge of GH actions, it can be inferred that, overall, this hormone is a hormone for cell proliferation and survival. The persistent GH secretion out of the growth period is clear proof of the importance of the actions of this hormone at multiple levels, such as the gonads, liver, kidneys, nervous system, adipose tissue, skeletal muscle, and bone, as well as on the cardiovascular, hematopoietic, and immune systems [1].

In fact, virtually all organs and tissues have receptors for this endocrine hormone, and the hormone is also produced in practically all the cells of the organism, where it plays specific autocrine/paracrine roles [1]. However, the sometimes-contradictory results of the use of GH in clinical trials only reflect how little we know about how this hormone really works and how dependent it is on the physiological or pathological state and the microenvironment in which it is acting or the dose or time during which GH is administered. In this review, we analyze the effects of GH on the cardiovascular system, particularly on vascular homeostasis. Since IGF-I is an important mediator of GH actions, the role of IGF-I on vascular homeostasis is also analyzed.

Much evidence supports the participation of local or circulating GH in vascular homeostasis, because when a deficiency of this hormone is present, an endothelial dysfunction appears with serious consequences; this is most likely the reason by which untreated GH-deficiency (GHD) is associated with an increased risk of atherosclerosis and vascular mortality, while GH treatment may reverse early atherosclerosis [2–5]. A recent study in subjects without GHD or any cardiovascular disease (CVD) but with one or more CV risk factors (age, smoking, obesity, hypertension, dyslipidemia, and insulin resistance) demonstrated that GH and its mediator IGF-I play a protective role in arterial wall changes associated with vascular aging [6]. In fact, receptors for GH (GHR) and IGF-I (IGF-IR) are expressed in the vascular endothelium [7–9], and some studies have suggested that GH itself is expressed in this special gland of internal secretion [10,11]. These data indicate that GH and IGF-I have to play a very important role in the maintenance of normal endothelial function. Endothelial dysfunction in GHD has been demonstrated by an impaired flow-mediated dilation, which improved with GH treatment [12], indicating that GH played a role in vascular reactivity [13], as had been shown by the group of Napoli [14]. Additionally, GH treatment in GHD patients has also been found to lead to the normalization of high arterial wall thickness and arterial stiffness in these patients [5], and it normalizes a series of markers of endothelial dysfunction that are generally increased in untreated GHD patients [15].

This brief introduction allows us to understand the very important role that GH plays in the cardiovascular system, as it has been reviewed in several occasions [9,16,17]. Detrimental changes in aging arteries negatively influence the ability to compensate after arterial occlusion [18], something that has to be highlighted as occurring parallelly with the GH decline that is experienced as we get older [1,19,20]. As is known, redox imbalance during aging is responsible for this negative effect on arteries, and GH exerts many positive effects for counteracting it, as is demonstrated throughout the text.

Hence, we review here how GH and its mediator IGF-I can act in the arterial wall to favor normal physiological functioning, as well as how both molecules play an important role in collateral remodeling after arterial occlusion. In addition, we bring to light some surprising data that may have been overlooked so far in arteriogenesis with the aim of improving the understanding of, not only of the typical role attributed to GH in the induction of endothelial nitric oxide synthase (eNOS) and the production of NO, but also some ideas about the role of the redox system in the control of homeostasis and vascular remodeling and to clarify how the vessels respond to shear stress forces (SSF) to increase their final size with the participation of the GH/IGF-I system. Arteriogenesis will be described underlining those aspects in which GH could help. Finally, we present some molecular data obtained from the GHAS trial about the benefit of using GH as a rescue therapy in real patients with critical limb ischemia without options for conventional revascularization.

2. Vascular Homeostasis: Role of the GH/IGFI Axis

A normal embryonic development needs the formation of blood vessels [21]; after birth, there is also the need of the formation of new blood vessels while growing, as well as in some physiological processes such as the menstrual cycle in women and the development of the mammary gland during pregnancy [22]; however, apart from these situations, neovascularization rarely occurs in adulthood, and, when it occurs, it is associated with pathological settings such as wounds, muscle injuries, fractures, tumors and hypoxia/ischemia.

As seems logical, hypoxia is a very important stimulus for the growth of new blood vessels [23], triggering this growth through hypoxia-inducible factors (HIF) that act on the expression of pro-angiogenic factors but also of anti-angiogenic factors to achieve the perfect number and size of the vessels necessary to compensate for the lack of oxygen supply and to regenerate the tissue [23]. This is a clear and well-established fact of angiogenesis. However, when a progressive narrowing of the vascular lumen appears, preexisting collaterals have to grow to compensate for the lack of distal flow, which is triggered in a totally different way as described below. In any case, the stimulation of eNOS that leads to the production of nitric oxide (NO) from the vascular endothelium seems to be the key mediator for both kind of reparative processes. NO is a potent vasodilator, and it therefore increases blood supply to the zone affected by hypoxia/ischemia. This implies changes in the vascular tone, vasorelaxation, and vasopermeability, which are affected in arteries that suffer for atherosclerotic damage. Interestingly, GH activates the NO pathway [14,24] through direct mechanisms that seem to be specific and independent of the GH-mediator IGF-I [24], although initial studies had indicated that the elevated plasma levels of IGF-I increase NO release in cultured endothelial cells (ECs) [25,26], and more recent data have shown that both GH and IGF-I regulate the expression of eNOS in the aorta of hypophysectomized rats [27]. Moreover, IGF-I has been shown to decrease the release of pro-inflammatory cytokines, such as IL-1β and induce the release of anti-inflammatory cytokines such as IL-10, at least in a model of induced pancreatitis [28]. At this point, it seems to be of interest to indicate that the GH-secretagogue ghrelin also induces vasorelaxation by stimulating eNOS expression in GHD rats [29]. Many studies have clearly shown that members of what we might call the GH system (GH itself, IGF-I, GHR, IGF-IR, GH-secretagogues, and inhibitors of GH-signaling pathways) play a key role in vascular homeostasis.

The mechanism by which GH acts at this level is explained further in the text and is schematized in Figure 1. However, it is necessary to highlight that endocrine GH interacts with its membrane receptor GHR and activates the associated JAK2/STAT5 (Janus kinase 2/signal transducer and activator of transcription 5) and Src family kinases, leading to a cascade of tyrosine phosphorylation responsible for mediating most of the effects of GH at the genomic level; it is especially involved in GH-induced cell proliferation (for a more detailed explanation see [30,31]) and has been postulated as responsible of eNOS activation [32], although this has not been demonstrated. Another key signaling pathway activated by tyrosine phosphorylation after the interaction GH–GHR is that of PI3K/Akt (phosphoinositide 3-kinase/serine-threonine kinase), which is stimulated after activation by JAK2 of the insulin receptor substrate (IRS) and is an inducer of eNOS activation and NO production [32]. Activated extracellular signal-regulated kinase (ERK) translocates into the nucleus and regulates the expression of genes involved in cell proliferation, differentiation, and survival, but it also, and perhaps more significantly, regulates cell motility and migration [33], a mechanism that is very important for the formation of new vessels, as we describe later. The interaction GH–GHR also induces the activation of the focal adhesion kinase (FAK), which responsible for the reorganization of the cytoskeleton in many cell types [34,35], although its effects on vascular ECs have not yet been demonstrated.

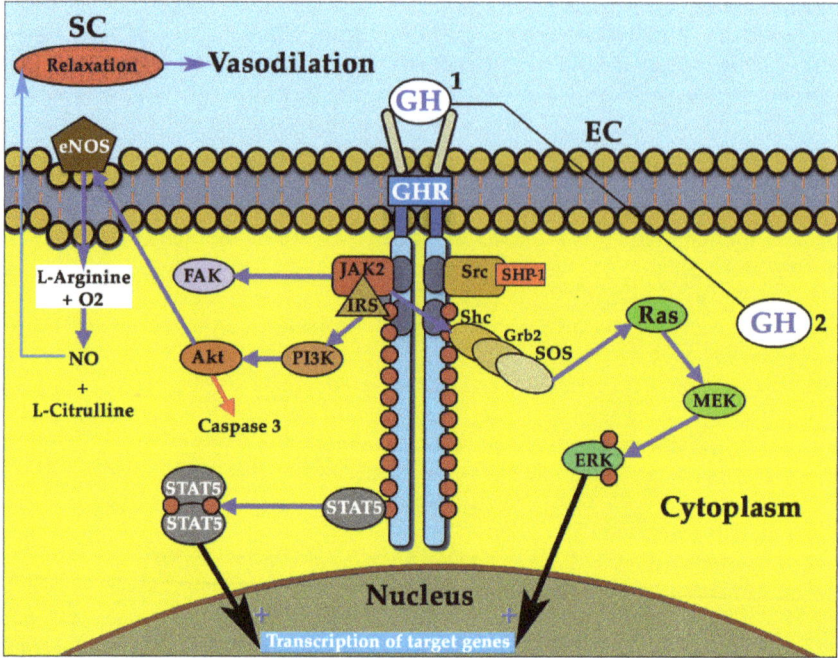

Figure 1. Effects of growth hormone (GH) on the vascular endothelium. The interaction GH–GHR (growth hormone receptor) produces the activation of the associated Janus kinase 2 (JAK2), which induces the phosphorylation (red circles) of tyrosine located in the cytoplasmic receptor domain, leading to the phosphorylation of GH-signaling pathways, such as signal transducers and activators of transcription (STATS). Among STATS (STATS 1 and 3 not shown in the Figure), STAT5 homodimerizes and is translocated to the nucleus, where it induces the transcription of a series of genes. Activated JAK2, acting on the insulin receptor substrate (IRS) induces the phosphorylation of phosphoinositide 3-kinase (PI3K) which, in turn, activates the cell survival factor serine-threonine kinase (Akt). This inhibits the proapoptotic enzyme Caspase 3 (red arrow), but it also activates endothelial nitric oxide synthase (eNOS) (blue arrow). Activated eNOS promotes the synthesis of nitric oxide (NO) (from L-Arginine and O2) and the formation of L-Citrulline. The formed NO flows from the cytoplasm to the muscle cell layer of the blood vessels, producing its relaxation and consequent vasodilation. The interaction GH–GHR also induces the activation of the Shc adapter proteins, which leads to the activation of the Grb2–SOS–Ras–Raf–MEK–ERK (extracellular signal-regulated kinase) pathway (Raf is not shown in the figure). Activated ERK translocates into the nucleus of the endothelial cells (ECs) and regulates the expression of genes involved in cell proliferation, differentiation, and survival, but it also regulates cell motility and migration (key for the formation of new vessels). The GH–GHR interaction also activates focal adhesion kinase (FAK). SHP: protein tyrosine phosphatase. Blue arrows: stimulation. Red arrow: inhibition. Black arrows: Translocation to the nucleus. 1: endocrine GH. 2: endothelial GH: plays and auto/paracrine role and in situations of the absence of endocrine GH perhaps plays the role of the former (black line).

Given the effects of GH on the production of endothelial NO, this GH-induced NO could be expected to produce a toxic effect on the vascular endothelium in situations of high levels of oxidative stress, since in these situations, NO can be transformed in superoxide ion (O_2^-) that leads to the production of peroxynitrite ($ONOO^-$) and the hydroxyl radical $OH^{\bullet}$), which have toxic effects in the endothelium [36,37]. Both molecules are encompassed into the term hROS or highly reactive oxygen species. As we see later in the text, the exact mechanism of the increase of NO bioavailability by GH, although not fully understood, could be mediated by modifying the action of prooxidative enzymes such as NOX4. This is in agreement with previous studies that have demonstrated that GH has a protective effect on mitochondria [38,39], which are the main source of oxidants within cells. This is the reason why mitochondrial dysfunction leads to a greater generation of hROS, which, in turn, contributes to the presentation of a senescent phenotype in ECs and to the activation of redox-sensitive transcription factor nuclear factor-kappa B (NF-κB) [40], which decreases endothelium-induced vasodilation and increases the expression of inflammatory genes in the vasculature of aged rats and elderly humans [41,42]. However, as indicated above, plasma physiological levels of GH and IGF-I modify the intracellular levels of oxidative stress [13,43,44]. These concepts are schematized in Figure 2.

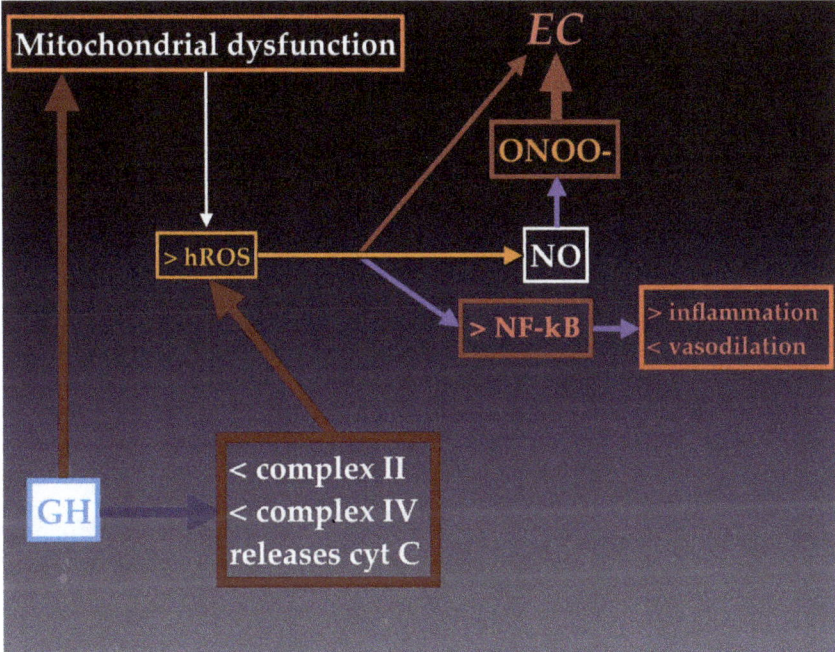

Figure 2. Mitochondrial dysfunction leads to vascular endothelium senescence. An excessive production of highly reactive oxygen species (hROS) by mitochondria induces the elimination of NO, because it is transformed into peroxynitrite (ONOO−), which is toxic for endothelial cells. Moreover, the excessive oxidative stress induces the activation of nuclear factor-kappa B (NF-kB), which increases the expression of inflammatory genes in the blood vessels and decreases vasodilation. These lead to the presentation of a senescent phenotype in the endothelial cells. GH administration corrects mitochondrial dysfunction, because GH is able to enter to mitochondria and decrease the activity of complexes II and IV of the mitochondrial respiratory chain. In addition, GH produces a decrease in the mitochondrial membrane potential which translates into the release of cytochrome C (cyt C) to the cytosol. Blue arrows: stimulation. Red arrows: inhibition or damage (in endothelial cells). Orange arrow: indicates that an increase in hROS induces the transformation of NO into ONOO−.

In vitro studies have shown that GH and GHR are capable of translocating to mitochondria through a pathway constituted by caveolae [45,46]. In isolated mitochondria, high concentrations of GH can decrease mitochondrial O_2^- production, most likely inducing a decrease in the activity of complexes II and IV of the mitochondrial respiratory chain [46] and modulating the mitochondrial membrane potential critical to maintain the physiological function of the respiratory chain to generate ATP, because when this membrane potential collapses, the cytochrome C is released in the cytosol, and, therefore, the mitochondrial respiratory chain is affected (Figure 2). In fact, in mice with decreased GH production, such as Ames dwarf mice, the production of hROS by mitochondria is increased in aortas and NO production is decreased in comparison to the oxidative stress observed in wild type animals with normal GH secretion; moreover, treatment with GH in cultured wild-type mice aortas and human coronary arterial endothelial cells has been found to significantly reduce mitochondrial hROS and to upregulate SOD (superoxide dismutase) genes and eNOS, providing an antioxidant phenotypic change [47]. This agrees with previous data showing that GH significantly reduces the intracellular production of hROS and increases NO release in cultures of a human endothelial cell line [8].

Therefore, it is clear that GH plays a positive role in the homeostasis of the vascular endothelium, not only by increasing NO production but also by protecting the endothelium, acting at the mitochondrial level, modulating oxidative stress. However, it has been described that this effect of GH does not occur acutely—rather, it occurs after a time, at least in studies performed in vitro [7,48]. Though this effect has not been properly studied in humans yet, we now provide some important insights from the GHAS trial that support this action.

Since, as indicated above, GH is expressed in ECs, where it plays an autocrine/paracrine role, one might think that the loss of the endocrine secretion of GH as we age could be compensated for by the cellular expression of this hormone, but this has been only seen in breast carcinomas [11], in which endothelial GH stimulates the proliferation, migration, survival, and capillary formation of ECs. Hence, there are no data to prove the possibility of an effect of autocrine/paracrine endothelial GH substituting the effects of endocrine GH in normal subjects. In addition, it is unknown how GH expression is regulated in vascular ECs and whether the decrease in the endocrine production of this hormone, in old people for instance, is accompanied by a deficit in its cellular production.

Another important effect of GH to explain its action on the vascular system is that exerted on mesenchymal stem cells (MSCs). These cells have been thought to proceed from the bone marrow, where they were identified in the past century [49], but we currently know that they can be found in virtually all adult tissues [50–52], particularly in adipose tissue, where they seem to be located in a perivascular zone close to pericytes and ECs [53,54]. This is very important because the external layer of blood vessels, also called tunica adventitia and being for long relegated as a mere support of the tunica media, is currently known to participate in vascular remodeling, since its cells can be activated in response to injuries [55–57], hypoxia [58], and hypertension [59]. Though the activation of adventitial progenitors mainly results in proliferation and differentiation into myofibroblasts that migrate into the inner layers of the vascular wall, they also release paracrine factors that regulate vascular remodeling [60]. MSCs also can differentiate into ECs in the presence of the vascular endothelial growth factor A (VEGF-A) [61,62], a factor that plays many roles in cell differentiation, proliferation, and angiogenesis. The relationships between GH and VEGF-A are not well known, but GH plays a pivotal role among the factors that regulate VEGF family expression in humans [63]. In addition, GH regulates the expression of different genes involved in Notch-1 signaling, at least at the ovarian level [63], and two Notch-1 ligands—delta-like protein Dl14 and Jagged 1—that directly regulate angiogenesis in the endothelium [64,65]. Therefore, given the relationships existing between Notch-1, VEGF-A, Notch-1, and GH, it is presumable that the differentiation of MSCs into ECs for neovascularization and endothelium repair may involve the participation of GH (for a more detailed explanation, see Figure 9 in reference [61]).

For vascular homeostasis to take place correctly, a negative regulation mechanism is also needed to prevent an excess of intracellular signaling by GH after its interaction with its membrane receptor. The negative regulation of GH signaling is mainly carried out by the intracellular protein tyrosine phosphatases 1B and H1, suppressors of cytokine signaling (SOCS, 1, 2, and 3), sirtuin 1, activated STAT protein inhibitors (1, 3, and 4), cytokine-induced SH2-containing protein (CIS), and tyrosine-protein phosphatase non-receptor type 6 (PTPN6 also called SHP-1) [66] (Figure 1). Given the different systems that act on the negative regulation of GH signaling pathways, there must be a perfect balance between them to prevent a pathological situation from occurring.

In summary, as we have just seen, GH plays a very important role in vascular homeostasis, acting on NO production, protecting from oxidative stress, regulating cell proliferation, differentiation and survival, regulating cell motility and migration, and inducing the differentiation of MSCs into vascular ECs. Since GH secretion decreases until it almost disappears as we age, it seems logical to assume that the loss of the hormone is one of the main causes of vascular problems that occur in old age.

3. Molecular Roles of GH/IGF-I in the Vascular Wall that Favor Arteriogenesis

3.1. GH/IGF-I Response to Shear Stress Forces (SSF): the Mechanosensing Pathway

In 2011, W. Schaper highlighted two key aspects of the arteriogenesis pathways: 1) only the inhibition of the total production of NO could inhibit collateral growth; 2) the mitogenic agent for the activation of smooth muscle cells (SMCs) from the vascular wall was still unknown. Though several candidates were given, mainly fibroblastic growth factor (FGF) and platelet-derived growth factor (PDGF), none met all the characteristics required [67]. However, considering the key role of the GH/IGF-I axis in the vascular homeostasis for regulating eNOS and NO, as stated above, and since both GH and IGF-I are potent mitogens [68] that are even stimulated by PDFG, perhaps both hormones should be considered candidates to be that unknown mitogenic agent or agents, because there might be more than one. Throughout this review, we try to present the evidence for this statement.

Since the discovery of the SSF as the main stimulator of collateral enlargement during arteriogenesis, many investigations trying to find the connection between mechanical and biological aspects have been developed. The genes involved in shear stress, activated by the stimulation of mechanical endothelial receptors, have been proposed as sensitive elements to increase the redirected flow through collaterals after arterial occlusion. However, some aspects have not yet been elucidated, as is the case of which molecules mediate the mechanical signaling pathway; in other words, are there factors involved in the arterial growth capable of being sensitive to mechanical forces? The answer to this question should be yes, and some of these factors could be locally produced hormones. Evidence accumulated in the last years has shown how the GH/IGF-I system can be regulated by multiple factors, such as growth factors, cytokines, lipoproteins, reactive oxygen species, hormones, neurotransmitters, and hemodynamic forces [69]. As is known, many patients with arterial hypertension develop left ventricle hypertrophy and aortic wall thickening, while patients suffering an aorto-cava fistula develop the hypertrophy of the right ventricle and an overload of the vena cava. Intuitively, one has to realize that something must orchestrate this adaptation to the pressure or the changes produced by volume. Given the strong mitogenic capacity of GH and IGF-I and the fact that there are many receptors for these hormones in large vessels, such as the aorta or vena cava [68,70,71], there should be a cross-talk between these hormones and hemodynamic forces. This hypothesis was demonstrated in an interesting study in which a volume or pressure overload was applied to rats to study the gene expression of GH receptors (GHR) and IGF-I mRNA in the vena cava and aorta. In the distended volume model of vena cava, 8-fold and 3.5-fold increases in IGF-I and GHR mRNA levels, respectively, were found compared to control animals, as early as day four. Additionally, the IGF-I protein was located in SMCs. In the aortic stress model, 4-fold and 5-fold increases in IGF-I and GHR mRNA, respectively, were found in aortas under pressure on day seven. Both vena cava and aorta showed structural adaptations with a growth response. This study was very important, since it represents a possible way of connection between the mechanical and biological pathways, with the autocrine/paracrine production of GH/IGF-I playing a major role. The increase in vascular wall stress, therefore, seems to trigger the overexpression of IGF-I and GHR mRNA in large vessels [71]. These data are consistent with the finding in a model of aortic coarctation in rats, in which an increase of more than double IGF-I levels was detected in blood vessels on day seven that was persistent on day 21 and was accompanied by a growth of SMCs and ECs [72]. Thus, in this model, IGF-I plays a pivotal role in the wall vessel remodeling of the aorta under high shear stress. Even more, the authors stated that IGF-I mRNA levels were also elevated in quiescent aortic SMCs, which underlines the role of IGF-I as an autocrine growth factor for dynamic changes in the vascular wall [73]. An earlier report also showed the same data but in a rat model of femoral artery overload, where a strong immunoreactivity for IGF-I was detected in the middle layer of the left femoral artery 24 hours after the right femoral ligation, along with a significant decrease in the expression of IGF-I in the occluded artery in the zone distal to the occlusion [74]. All these findings provide evidence for a major role of autocrine/paracrine GH/IGF-I system in mediating vessel wall growth during shear stress (Figure 3).

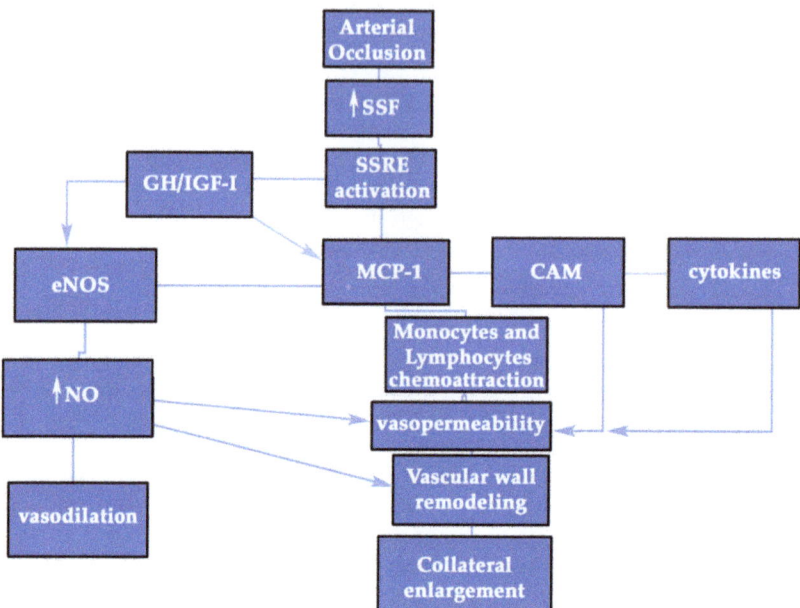

Figure 3. GH/IGF-I are also produced in response to shear stress forces (SSF) for collateral enlargement. Schematic representation of the activation of several molecules after the increase in SSF in which GH and IGF-1 have been added as new elements that enhance these mechanisms. Since GH and IGF-1 are potent mitogenic agents, they have to play a role in the translation of mechanosensing signals. The NO pathway not only is important for vasodilation, as it also has many actions in chemoattraction of inflammatory cells and vasopermeability. The local production of cytokines and hormones seems to be essential for collateral enlargement. SSF: shear stress forces; SSRE: shear stress response elements; eNOS: endothelial nitric oxide synthase; MCP-1: monocyte chemoattractant protein-1; CAM: cellular adhesion molecules; NO: nitric oxide.

To perform its mitogenic function, GH has been shown to directly stimulate Src family kinases (SFK), which in turn activate mitogen-activated protein kinase 1 (also known as extracellular signal-regulated kinase 2 (ERK2) and mitogen-activated protein kinase 3 (also known as ERK1) through a phospholipase Cγ–Ras pathway [75]. The prolactin (PRL) receptor similarly activates the same SFK signals [68], and it is well known that GH interacts with the PRL receptor with the same affinity that it does with its GHR [76].

All these adaptations in the vascular wall by GH/IGF-I may be supported by the fact that GH is capable of modifying the aortic content and composition of collagen and elastin, and even its mechanical behavior [77]. A decrease in collagen and elastin in the aorta wall can be detected in aged rats and humans in parallel to the decrease in GH/IGF-I levels, although plasma IGF-I is still maintained at lower levels, since its liver production does not exclusively depend on GH, which virtually disappears in the elderly [1]. In fact, the administration of GH to aged female rats was found to augment the collagen deposit by 300% and its turn-over in the media layer. It seems that the main mediator of this GH effect in the aorta is IGF-I, produced locally in SMCs. In the thoracic aorta of aged female rats, GH was found to increase the ratio of collagen I/III, improving both the stiffness in those areas under high overload and the extensibility in those with low overload, thus adjusting the aortic mechanical characteristics to the overload [77]. These studies shed some light on the idea that local hormone production participates in the regulation of structural adaptations of blood vessels under stress conditions; for this, the IGF-IR number plays a major role for SMCs response. On the one hand, the increase in the expression of IGF-IR by GH or other factors such as angiotensin II or FGF-2 is crucial for the mitogenic effects of IGF-I on SMCs. On the other hand, factors such as Tumor Necrosis Factor alpha (TNF-α) or ox-LDLc decrease IGF-IR, favoring SMCs apoptosis. Effectively, GH and IGF-I play a key role in vessels for the growth and survival of SMCs, inhibiting apoptosis produced by mitochondrial dysfunction induced by TNF-α and ox-LDLc [69].

3.2. GH and GHR: a Complex Regulation that Explains Different Results in the Studies Performed

Given the fact that many GHRs have been found in the vascular system, this organ must be a special target for GH. In addition, it seems to be clear that many of the effects of GH on the vascular wall are independent of IGF-I [7,8,76,78]. Indeed, although the GH/IGF-I axis is highly coordinated to act in different tissues, both GH and IGF-I may have independent actions [79]. The type of secretion of GH is another factor that influences the different actions of the hormone. That is, while pituitary GH is secreted in pulses, some of them of great amplitude, autocrine GH is produced in small quantities and almost continuously. These differences are responsible for the different effects that both types of GH induce. For example, the oncogenic potential of GH seems to be associated only with local secretion and not with the exogenously administered or pituitary hormone [11]. Effectively, both types of GH production regulate gene expression in different ways [80], a fact that also implies differences in the GHR-related signal transduction pathways [81].

Though GHRs have been found in different arterial layers, the endothelium seems to be the place where these receptors have been found in a greater concentration. Interestingly, the GHR gene is a hypoxia-inducible gene, since the overexpression of HIF-1α (hypoxia-inducible-factor-1-alpha) increases its expression, suggesting that GHR may be involved in hypoxia-induced processes, such as the generation of new vessels [82], although many factors can modulate the expression of the GHR gene [83]. However, many of the GH actions in the artery media layer are mediated by IGF-I, especially in SMCs [77], or they occur as a consequence of the diffusion of GH-generated signals from the endothelial layer, such as the diffusion of NO.

One of the most interesting locations of GHR that supports the role of the hormone in physiological arteriogenesis during adulthood is in the vessels of the endometrium, where GH seems to play an important role favoring the creation and maintenance of vessels during every sexual cycle in fertile women [63,84].

As widely described, GH induces eNOS expression and NO release in cultured human ECs [8]. When L-nitroarginine methyl ester (L-NAME) is administered, GH loses its action on NO, which confirms this main action on the endothelium [85]. To produce NO, eNOS has to be phosphorylated on serine 1177 via PI3K/Akt and activated by a calcium-calmodulin [86]. Diffusing NO triggers a soluble guanylyl cyclase into SMCs, increasing intracellular levels of cyclic GMP (cGMP) that activates protein kinase G1 via the phosphorylation of the inositol-triphosphate receptor-associated cGMP kinase and the sarcoplasmic reticulum ATPase. The consequence is that intracellular calcium decreases leading to vascular relaxation and modification of the arterial tone [86,87], one of the most important action of NO and GH, demonstrated after the arterial infusion of the hormone [14]. It has to be underlined that eNOS activity is highly regulated in cells at the transcriptional level and by other factors such as acylation and phosphorylation, or by protein–protein interactions [86]. However, vasodilation is not the only benefit of NO on the vascular wall, since it facilitates vasopermeability (by decreasing VE-cadherin activity) and the chemoattraction of monocytes, and it reduces lipoxygenase activity, ox-LDLc, platelet adhesion, and SMC proliferation and migration [13,88]. As described above, NO is the main route used by GH to contribute to vascular homeostasis.

A high concentration of GHRs has been detected in the aorta, femoral, and carotid arteries, where it mediates many GH effects by activating the JAK/STAT pathway, among others [68,70]. GH cannot induce the transcription of IGF-1 in ECs [76], but this does not mean that GH does not interact with IGF-I in the artery media layer as stated, where it precisely regulates the growth and survival of SMCs mediated by IGF-I, for which SMCs have many receptors [69]. GHR is crucial for the wide effects of GH, allowing the hormone to internalize in cells where GH triggers many signaling pathways and influencing gene transcription. This internalization is facilitated by GH-binding proteins (GHBP), the extracellular component of GHR. The concentration of GHRs determines the intensity of GH signals, mainly when considering the eNOS–NO pathway. The higher the number of GHRs, the greater the effect of GH. Nevertheless, there is a limit in which if more hormone is administered the effect not only does not increase but decreases. For instance, it has been shown that 1 nmol/L of GH produces 6.39 µmol/L NO, 10 nmol/L of GH produces 6.45 µmol/L NO, but 100 nmol/L of GH produces 6.38 µmol/L NO [89,90]. It is important to point out that GH itself controls the gene involved in the expression of its receptor and that this regulation depends on the time and dose of hormone administration. This fact is important to understand the reasons why GH has different effects depending on the dose and to understand why clinical trials with GH sometimes differ in their results. As explained before, the relationship between GHR and GH is bidirectional, and GHBP binds to the free hormone in the blood to control the amount of free GH that interacts with its receptor but also to regulate GH clearance. Even inside the cells, GH actions are exhaustively regulated. This is an important concept common to all the growth factors acting in the organism. The effects of GH on GHR gene expression seem to be dependent on the time/dose of exposure in addition to the cell type and whether the experiment is carried out in vivo or in vitro. However, GHR gene expression is even more complex, as it is also influenced by other factors such as nutritional intake, steroids, or diabetes mellitus. Furthermore, the GHR gene has multiple 5′ untranslated exons that are controlled by multiple promoters, thus showing the complexity and high quality regulation of the gene expression of this receptor [83].

3.3. GH/IGF-I may Favor Inflammation during Collateral Enlargement

During collateral enlargement, two types of cells are activated to achieve the great change, and both endothelial and SMCs acquire a proliferative and secretory phenotype after a previous phase of NO-dependent vasodilation because hemodynamic or short-term compensation always runs before than that originated by growth factors or long-term compensation. While flow and metabolism control is mainly carried out at the local level in physiological situations, when a pathological condition such as ischemia is present, a systemic response (centered on redistribution of flow and microvascular adaptations) is usually required [91]. That needs the neurohormonal axis effects. In both circumstances, local and systemic GH/IGF-I is important for regulating short and long-term adaptations.

The inflammation of the collateral wall aims to achieve vascular remodeling. To do this, two stages can be distinguished: First, ECs facilitate the inflammatory response in the vascular wall; second, SMCs proliferate to increase the vessel size. It is not the aim of this chapter to describe the whole process of arteriogenesis. However, it is necessary to highlight those aspects in which GH could participate. For example, it has been described how monocytes, monocyte chemoattractant protein-1 (MCP-1), and lymphocytes are crucial for vascular remodeling during arteriogenesis in the inflammatory phase [92], since this process is not complete or is delayed when all these factors are not present. It has been shown that GH strongly induces these cells and proteins [1,93,94], playing a pivotal role in the chemotaxis and migration of human monocytes.

MCP-1 has been found elevated in blood samples from the collateral network of coronary arteries [95], and it has been found to be transiently and selectively increased in the ischemic muscle during the first three days after ischemia [96], which underlines its importance in arteriogenesis.

The relationship between GH and MCP-1 has been conveniently studied and seems to be mediated by the activation of both JAK2 and p44/42 mitogen-activated protein kinase (MAPK), since MCP-1 significantly decreases in cells pretreated with the JAK2 inhibitor AG490 or MAPK inhibitor PD98050 [94]. In the referred experimental study, MCP-1 mRNA levels increased up to 8 times after the administration of a low dose of GH [94]. As is known, both MCP-1 and cell adhesion molecules (CAMs) play central roles in igniting the arteriogenic process. The former play roles in the attraction of inflammatory cells, and the latter play roles in the adhesion and invasion of the vascular wall by this type of cells.

CAMs are also related to GH, especially vascular cell adhesion molecule-1 (VCAM-1). GH significantly increases the expression of VCAM, as demonstrated when serum from healthy patients treated with the hormone is administered to cultured umbilical vein ECs [97]. An indirect mechanism has been proposed to explain this action, one perhaps mediated by VEGF, IGF-I, or SDF-1 [16,76,91,98], factors that upregulate CAMs [92]. This action has also been observed in adults with GHD, in which GH replacement therapy significantly increases VCAM-1. Therefore, both MCP-1 and VCAM could be modulated by GH, facilitating the first phase of arteriogenesis. In addition, CD34+ cells, also involved in arteriogenesis [99], are stimulated by GH, both in number and function. In fact, circulating CD34+ are decreased in adults with GHD, which contributes to the endothelial dysfunction detected in these patients. GH replacement therapy improves this dysfunction by correcting CD34+ cell depletion [100].

Almost all human immune cells express GHRs and produce its ligand that may act in an autocrine or paracrine manner [101,102]. GH produced by immune cells has the same structure as that GH found in the anterior pituitary gland [103]. In addition, immune cells have IGF-IRs and produce IGF-I. This also supports the fact that GH could mediate the arteriogenic process, since monocytes and T-lymphocytes are key cells for the inflammatory response needed for collateral enlargement [104,105] (Figures 3 and 4). GH can favor the migration and invasion of immune cells to the vascular wall, and once in the vascular wall, GH might directly or indirectly activate them to produce cytokines.

It is noteworthy that monocytes have to be activated to help in arteriogenesis, since when they are transplanted directly from the blood in animal models of ischemia, they do not influence this process. However, when these cells are previously activated by the monocyte colony stimulating factor (M-CSF), collateral growth begins [108]. Thus, M-CSF favors a suitable environment for stable monocytic function [18]. It has to be highlighted that GH is strongly related to M-CSF and that in vitro and in vivo studies have shown that GH activates monocytes to produce cytokines and stimulates the chemoattraction and random migration of the same even at picomolar concentrations of the hormone [109]. The cellular pathway involved was demonstrated many years ago [110], as GH stimulates the tyrosine phosphorylation of two proteins, p130Cas and CrkII, their association and the association of other multiple tyrosine-phosphorylated proteins that end up activating the c-Jun N-terminal kinase/stress-activated protein kinase (JNK/SAPK) [111]. Such a large multiprotein signaling complex is not only the basis for activating monocytes but is also essential for other effects such as cytoskeletal reorganization, cell migration, chemotaxis, mitogenesis, and/or the prevention of apoptosis and gene transcription [110].

Monocytes can also have trophic effects on homeostasis, e.g., secreting CSF during growth [112], suggesting that this factor interacts with the GH/IGF-I axis. Macrophages also produce IGF-I in response to CSF-1 or GM-CSF, and IGF-IRs are highly expressed in macrophages stimulated by the M-CSF family [105,113,114]. Despite this, the specific link between M-CSF family and GH has not yet been properly studied, although it has been seen that many CSF-1-dependent macrophages are present in the pituitary gland in the course of somatotropic cell development [115].

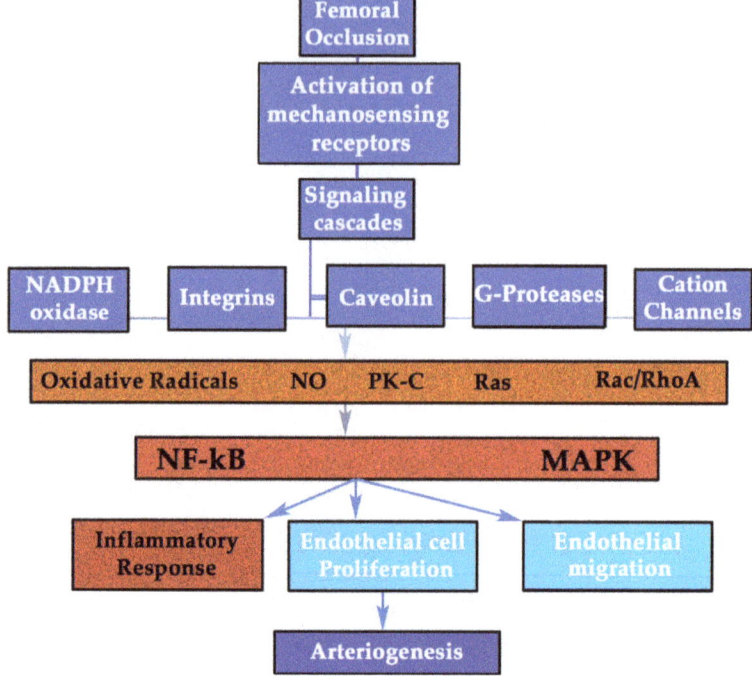

Figure 4. Signaling cascades for collateral growth: The redox system can play a very important role. Schematic representation of signaling cascades after an arterial occlusion, triggering both the inflammatory response and the phenomena of the proliferation and migration of endothelial cells into the artery media layer. Several pathways have been highlighted: Rho, involved in endothelial cells proliferation; Ras, for endothelial cells migration; and NO, for endothelial function and monocytes adhesion. The oxidative radicals produced in cellular metabolism are currently considered very important in the stimulation of the NO pathway for vascular homeostasis. They control NO bioavailability. The Rho pathway has been advocated as crucial for sensing of SSF. Caveolins: family of integral membrane proteins that play a role in the signaling of integrins and in the migration of endothelial cells. Cation channels, mainly the Ca^{2+} ion, are also related to the activation of Protein kinase C (PKC) and the RAS/RAC (rats' sarcoma-extracellular signal-regulated kinases/Ras-related C3 botulinum toxin substrate). All signaling cascades are activated by SSF. For more details, see reference [106,107]. NADPH oxidase: nicotinamide adenine dinucleotide phosphate oxidase; NO: nitric oxide; PK-C: protein kinase C, Ras: rats' sarcoma-extracellular signal-regulated kinases (currently known as GTPase Ras); Rho, hexameric protein found in prokaryotes, necessary for the process of terminating the transcription of some genes, Rac: Ras-related C3 botulinum toxin substrate (subfamily of the Rho family); NF-kB: nuclear factor-kappa B. MAPK: mitogen-activated protein kinase.

3.4. GH/IGF-I and eNOS in Arteriogenesis. Insights from the GHAS Trial: is Redox Balance the Main Actor?

As described above, several signaling pathways work together to grow the collateral arteries, and one of the most relevant, although with some contradictory results, is the NO pathway. This pathway has been considered crucial for many years for collateral enlargement, both during the early and late stages of arteriogenesis. Measuring several variables such as perfusion of the limb, the diameter of the collateral artery, and the number and location of pericytes within the ischemic hindlimb, less recovery of blood flow and a smaller collateral artery diameter have been demonstrated in the group of eNOS$^{-/-}$ and L-NAME mice than in the wild-type. The pericytes barely appeared, and they did so in a random pattern in the former groups compared to the wild-type [116]. Another fact that supports the role of this pathway in arteriogenesis is the finding of a lower eNOS expression both in the thigh and in the gastrocnemius muscles in diabetic mice, which leads to reduced collateral enlargement. The reduced expression of eNOS in diabetic mice (types 1 or 2) may contribute to the deficient arteriogenesis and angiogenesis seen in these animals, while the treatment with thiazolidinediones, that increases eNOS activity through the peroxisome proliferator-activated receptor gamma (PPARg) [117], restores these deficient responses [116]. Animal models of ischemia after training support the important role of eNOS and NO in arteriogenesis, with a greater effect than that induced by VEGF, because the latter is a secondary factor for collateral growth and eNOS a primary factor. Conversely, the role of eNOS in angiogenesis is less relevant, but VEGF also needs it to carry out its actions [118]. Therefore, the difference in NO dependence is the key factor that distinguishes between both processes.

However, not all authors agree completely, since it seems that eNOS and NO could be of great importance for the NO-mediated vasodilation of peripheral collateral vessels after arterial occlusion, but their relevance seems to be minor for collateral enlargement. Tissue perfusion and collateral-dependent blood flow was found significantly increased in mice overexpressing eNOS compared to wild-type mice, but only immediately after ligation. In eNOS$^{-/-}$ mice, collateral-dependent blood flow was found to remain poor until day seven, after which it recovered, thus suggesting a delay but not a complete impairment of collateral growth. Besides, no differences in collateral arteries between the three groups of mice were histologically confirmed at the end of the study, and the administration of a NO donor induced vasodilation in the collateral arteries of eNOS$^{-/-}$ mice, but it does not so in wild-type mice [119]. Interestingly, eNOS deficiency may be compensated for by iNOS activity [67], and this might be the explanation of this finding and other different results. That is, the exact role of eNOS is not fully understood. Nevertheless, some insights from the GHAS trial (Eudract 2012-002228-34), performed by our group, could be useful to clarify the activity of eNOS in humans. In this randomized, controlled, phase III trial, recombinant human growth hormone (rhGH) (0.4 mg/day for eight weeks) or a placebo was administered to patients with critical limb ischemia without revascularization options. The main characteristics of the patients studied are outlined in Table 1, while Table 2 shows the specific characteristics of the patients once distributed in each treatment group.

Table 1. Main characteristics of the patients recruited in the GHAS trial. Enrolled patients: patients with informed consent; age: years old ± standard deviation; ABI: ankle–brachial index; CRF: chronic renal failure; DM: diabetes mellitus; and rhGH: recombinant human growth hormone.

Enrolled Patients	Sex	Age (Mean ± SD)	Comorbidity	Baseline ABI (Mean)	Rutherford class 5–6
36	Male: 28 Female: 8	71 ± 12.7	Heart disease: 47% DM: 59% Neuropathy: 57.6% CRF: 26.5%	0.19	70.6%
Therapy	**Dose**	**Duration of treatment**	**Follow-up**	**Follow-up Periods**	
rhGH vs. Placebo	0.4 mg/day	8 weeks	12 months	0–2; 3–6; 7–12 months	

Muscle samples from the calf of the ischemic limb were taken at baseline and just after finishing the treatment of the patients. After analyzing mRNA expression of angiogenesis-related genes, the molecular data showed us a surprising finding: In the group treated with GH (group A, green bars), there was an increase in the level of eNOS mRNA compared to baseline, but this increase was significantly lower than that detected in the placebo-treated patients (group B, blue bars). Parallelly, a significant and strong decrease in NOX4 levels was only observed in the GH group (Figure 5); this means that the activity of eNOS depends largely on the redox balance in the ischemic muscle, or, even more, that the arteriogenic growth of the vessels depends largely on the redox imbalance and that GH, by correcting this stress, also reduces the signal that stimulates eNOS.

Table 2. Specific characteristics of the patients distributed by treatment groups studied in the GHAS trial. A homogeneous distribution can be seen, except for tobacco consumption. HT: arterial hypertension; DM: diabetes mellitus; CRF: chronic renal failure; HD: heart disease; n = sample size; y = year. Note that in this table, we show data of 34 of 36 patients enrolled, because two patients died after the signing of the informed consent.

		Total		GH Group		Placebo Group		p Value
		n	%	n	%	n	%	p
Age	< 65	14	41.18	6	33.33	8	50	
	65–80	8	23.53	3	16.67	5	31.25	0.1211
	> 80	12	35.29	9	50	3	18.75	
Gender	Male	27	79.41	13	72.22	14	87.5	0.2715
	Female	7	20.59	5	27.78	2	12.5	
Etiology	Atherosclerosis	24	70.59	11	61.11	13	81.25	
	Buerger	3	8.82	1	5.56	2	12.5	
	Scleroderma	1	2.94	1	5.56	-	-	
	Mix	6	17.65	5	27.78	1	6.25	
HT	No	12	35.29	4	22.22	8	50	0.0907
	Yes	22	64.71	14	77.78	8	50	
DM	No	14	41.18	6	33.33	8	50	0.3243
	Yes	20	58.82	12	66.67	8	50	
CRF	No	25	73.53	13	72.22	12	75	0.8546
	Yes	9	26.47	5	27.78	4	25	
HD	No	18	52.94	8	44.44	10	62.5	0.2924
	Yes	16	47.06	10	55.56	6	37.5	
Dialysis	No	33	97.06	17	94.44	16	100	0.3386
	Yes	1	2.94	1	5.56	-	-	
Tobacco	No	24	70.59	16	88.89	8	50	
	Ex-smoker <1y	2	5.88	1	5.56	1	6.25	0.0107
	Smoker	8	23.53	1	5.56	7	43.75	
Rutherford	3	5	14.71	3	16.67	2	12.5	
	4	5	14.71	-	-	5	31.25	0.188
	5	15	44.12	9	50	6	37.5	
	6	9	26.47	6	33.33	3	18.75	
Rest Pain	No	8	23.53	5	27.78	3	18.75	0.5356
	Yes	26	76.47	13	72.22	13	81.25	
Trophic Lesion	No	11	32.35	3	16.67	8	50	0.0381
	Yes	23	67.65	15	83.33	8	50	
Neuropathy	No	14	42.42	7	41.18	7	43.75	0.8812
	Yes	19	57.58	10	58.82	9	56.25	

This is an important concept because it indicates that there is an insensitivity to NO rather than a real depletion of it or eNOS in patients with peripheral ischemia [120], and this finding matches perfectly with the high redox stress and insensitivity to NO found by other authors in humans and animals with peripheral arterial disease [121–123]. This is also consistent with the fact that an increased oxidation can be seen in GHD-adults, secondary to an elevated activity of lipoxygenase activity and ox-LDLc (the main source of atherosclerotic lesion of the arteries) as a consequence of NO depletion. After GH replacement therapy, this redox alteration can be significantly reduced, together with the recovery of a normal flow mediated dilation test, compared to pre-GH administration and control patients [13]. At this point, it is of interest to remark that senescence, frequent in patients with peripheral arterial disease, is like a GHD state.

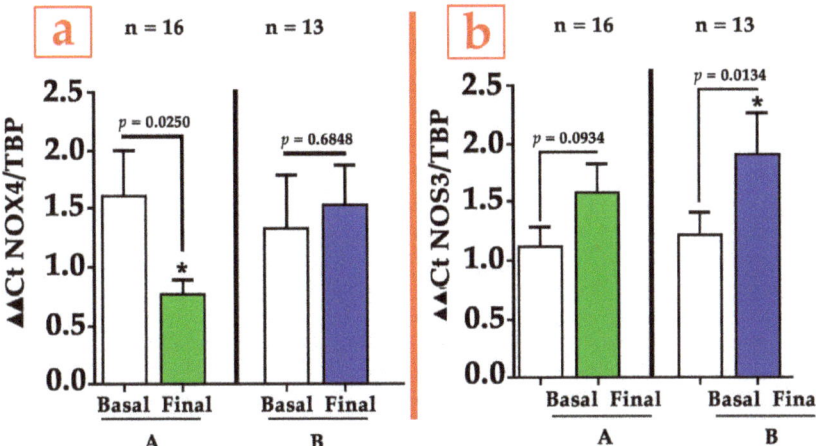

Figure 5. GH decreases the redox stress in ischemic muscles from the calf of patients with critical limb ischemia. Insights from the GHAS trial. (**a**): shows the significant decrease in NOX4 mRNA levels only seen in the GH-treated group (**A**, green bars) and not in Placebo-treated group (**B**, blue bars). (**b**): depicts the significant increase in the levels of NOS3 (eNOS) mRNA during the period of treatment in patients with placebo related to its baseline levels, while in the GH group (**A**), although there was also an increase in NOS3 mRNA levels after the treatment, this increase was not significant. Samples from soleus muscle. Group A: GH; Group B: placebo. Basal: baseline mRNA levels before treatment; final: final mRNA levels after 8 weeks of treatment. Statistics: non-parametric test. Note that of the 36 patients initially recruited for the study, complete muscle samples (basal and final) were only obtained from 28 of them as a result of deaths, limb amputations, or the patient´s refusal to allow for the second biopsy. * indicates statistically significant.

Therefore, the important message here is the relevance that redox balance exerts on collateral enlargement. As has been described, while small or acute redox stress, characterized by an elevated production of reactive oxygen species (ROS)/reactive nitrogen species (RNS), seems to positively influence neovascularization, a chronically high level of oxidation is detrimental for vascular remodeling [124]. In the GHAS trial, patients under placebo treatment maintained a high level of NOX4 and eNOS mRNAs in the calf muscle, trying to compensate for the decrease in NO bioavailability. The administration of GH stopped this vicious circus, lowering the redox imbalance and also increasing the bioavailability of NO without the need of an increase in the production of eNOS. Indeed, the bioavailability of NO depends largely on the production of ROS, since they react with NO to inactivate it, thus lowering its levels [32], which means that the negative regulation of redox stress by GH in patients with critical limb ischemia increases the bioavailability of NO without a significant elevation of eNOS in the ischemic skeletal muscle. This unexpected finding highlights the dynamic role of redox balance in vascular homeostasis. Typically, NOX4 is upregulated in cells by SSF, hypoxemia, or cytokines like TNF-α, and the latter is usually elevated in patients with ischemic process [125], favoring the inflammation and phosphorylation of eNOS, which reduces NO production [126].

In the GHAS trial, GH also significantly reduced the circulating levels of the inflammatory marker TNF-α in blood samples, which is consistent with other studies [127,128] and with the fact that GH improves redox balance (Table 3). The deleterious effects of TNF-α in these circumstances have been described, including the elevation of intracellular SOCS [91] and the diminishment of IGF-I and SMCs in the vascular wall [69]. GH, as seen, could correct these negative effects, decreasing TNF-α levels. Though proinflammatory activity has also been seen for GH, this is something that occurs when high levels of the hormone are considered, demonstrating, once again, that the role of GH depends on its physiological or pathological concentrations and on whether the morbid condition is stablished acutely or chronically [129]. However, C reactive protein (CRP) did not significantly change at the end of the treatment compared to the placebo. It has to be noted that this marker has a different meaning than TNF-α and that the levels of CRP were found to be significantly elevated in the GH group at baseline compared to the placebo group, which could have influenced the final results.

Table 3. GH decreases excess inflammation by lowering the circulating levels of TNF-α in patients with critical limb ischemia. Insights from the GHAS trial. Evolution of plasmatic levels of TNF-α and C reactive protein (CRP) in the GHAS trial after 8 weeks of treatment. TNF-α was significantly elevated in patients treated with GH compared to the placebo at baseline, which means that severe ischemia is accompanied by an increase in inflammation. In addition, inflammation was more severe in the group treated with GH, which was seen by the fact that levels of both TNF-α and CRP were significantly elevated at baseline in the GH group as compared to the placebo group. However, after 8 weeks of treatment, only patients receiving GH showed a significant decrease of circulating levels of TNF-α (TNF-α final), while CRP levels did not significantly change compared to baseline levels. TNF-α baseline: TNF-α levels at baseline (time before administering the treatment); TNF-α final: TNF-α levels after 8 weeks of treatment. Determination of TNF-α plasmatic levels: ELISA test (Quantikine, R&D Systems). Normal reference value for TNF-α levels: <8.1 pg/mL. Obs.: number of patients analyzed. SD: standard deviation. CRP: C-reactive protein (mg/L), normal values: < 1 mg/L. Note that only 32 of 36 patients in the GHAS trial had available baseline data of these markers. At the end of the treatment, there were some missed samples as a consequence of deaths or patient´s refusal to obtain the blood sample.

	GH-Treated			Placebo			
	Obs.	Mean	SD	Obs.	Mean	SD	p Value
TNF-α Baseline	16	12.35	5.2	16	8.78	3.94	0.018
TNF-α Final	15	10.92	5.12	14	8.04	3.6	0.046
CRP Baseline	16	2.07	2.86	16	0.78	0.69	0.045
CRP Final	15	1.1	1.34	14	3.42	7.51	0.218

Regarding ischemic disease, authors sometimes do not agree because they do not describe the same phenomenon, since an acute injury is normally produced in an animal model of ischemia, while a chronic process is usually developed in a human being with peripheral or coronary artery disease. In fact, in the human heart, after acute coronary occlusion, the arteriogenic phenomenon is very fast, just like in animal models, taking between one and two weeks for the great majority of patients [130]; meanwhile, in chronic ischemia, the collateral enlargement takes several months [131]. This is a concept that needs to be highlighted, as in the chronic ischemic state, due to the lower and slower activation of the physiological compensation that is impaired by age, GH could be useful by enhancing all these mechanisms and improving distal flow.

In a study in which animal models of acute and chronic ischemia were used simultaneously, it was shown that the mechanisms that regulate blood flow recovery, gene expression, macrophage infiltration, and hemangiocyte recruitment are critically different, since they depend on the arterial occlusion rate and the mechanisms that regulate the recovery of blood flow [132]. The most important finding in that study was that MCP-1 or shear stress-induced genes like eNOS or Egr-1 are not sufficiently activated to induce collateral artery enlargement in the model of gradual ischemia, since SSF through collaterals is weaker compared to that in an acute ischemia model; additionally eNOS or MCP-1 are less stimulated in gradual or chronic ischemia than in the acute process at the thigh, the place where collateral growth mainly takes place. Though the upregulation of VEGF and PlGF is found in acute models, particularly important are eNOS and KDR/Flk-1 in the remodeling of vessels [118], while in humans, as stated above, it seems that lowering the redox imbalance could be more profitable. Interestingly, in the GHAS trial, we also found a parallel and significant increase of VEGFA-R2 or

KDR/flk-1 mRNA levels from muscle samples in the GH group (group A) compared to the placebo group (group B) (Figure 6A), which confirmed the action of VEGFA, a finding consistent to that from animal models of hindlimb ischemia treated with the IGF-I plasmid [133]. This effect could be dependent of IGF-I, but we hypothesize that it is a direct action of GH on the muscle, because a parallel increase in IGF-I mRNA level has not been found, at least at the time in which muscle samples were obtained (Figure 6B). However, the elevation in KDR/flk-1 was not accompanied by a parallel significant increase of VEGFA mRNA levels after two months of treatment (Figure 6C). This fact could have an explanation. Knowing that VEGFA mRNA levels decrease after stimulation with very low levels within the fourth week [134,135], it is easy to understand that, muscle sample were obtained when the levels of this factor had already declined (at eight weeks), overlooking any possible elevation produced during the previous month.

This finding is also very important, as it has been advocated that the differences between VEGF action in different tissues might be determined by the number of its receptors rather than by the levels of VEGF [136]. VEGF receptors are usually normal in patients with peripheral arterial disease in the calf [137], albeit with controversial results; meanwhile in acute ischemia, VEGF and VEGFR-2 are diffusely expressed in the affected muscle, as in skeletal muscle that recovers from chronic ischemia, the former factors are restricted to atrophic and regenerating muscle areas [138]. This is consistent with the fact that KDR/Flk-1 expression appears in macrophages and fibroblast cells found in the necrotic area after myocardial infarction [139]. Here, we present clear evidence that VEGF is not normally augmented in distal limb muscles under chronic ischemia, as compared to control muscle samples obtained from limb amputations in non-ischemic patients, and that GH can increase VEGF actions through, at least, a raise of the KDR receptor, also favoring muscle regeneration accompanying vascular development. As is known, KDR mediates most VEGF actions on mitogenesis, survival, and permeability at the vascular wall, being mainly expressed in ECs but also in macrophages and SMCs. This receptor has also been found in myocytes from skeletal muscles, both in the membrane and in the cytoplasm [138], and KDR can be derived from myocytes; from this point of view, GH could act more at the muscular level rather than at the vascular one. However, recent experimental studies could support the fact that GH acts at the vascular level when the KDR receptor increases. First, this receptor appears to be a critical mediator for the action of extracellular RNA (eRNA) and the von Willebrand factor (VWF) released by ECs for the recruitment of leukocytes that initiate arteriogenesis in response to fluid shear stress [140]. Secondly, this receptor also seems to be important for the action of mast cells that, after activation, release VEGFA [141]. Therefore, the finding in our study of an increase in mRNA levels of VEGFA-R2 or KDR by GH must necessarily be related to the facilitation of the action of these molecules.

In any case, as is known, the increase in SSF after an arterial occlusion triggers the NO pathway, which inhibits the expression of VE-cadherin, which responsible for maintaining vascular membrane integrity and, therefore, increasing vascular permeability and the invasion by inflammatory cells of the vascular wall [142]. Both the disruption of endothelial junctions and the remodeling of the cytoskeleton are necessary factors for vascular permeability and the NO released by the endothelium is crucial. One approximation of the involved molecular mechanism has been shown in a study in which the lack of eNOS reduces VEGF-induced permeability that is mediated by an increase of the Rac GTPase activation. NO depletion impairs the recruitment of the guanine-nucleotide-exchange factor (GEF) TIAM1 to adherent junctions and VE-cadherin, and it reduces Rho activation. NO is crucial for the regulation of the Rho GTPase-dependent cytoskeleton architecture and its action leads to reversible changes in vascular permeability. It seems to be clear that when NO is inhibited, flow-induced arteriogenesis is also interrupted [118].

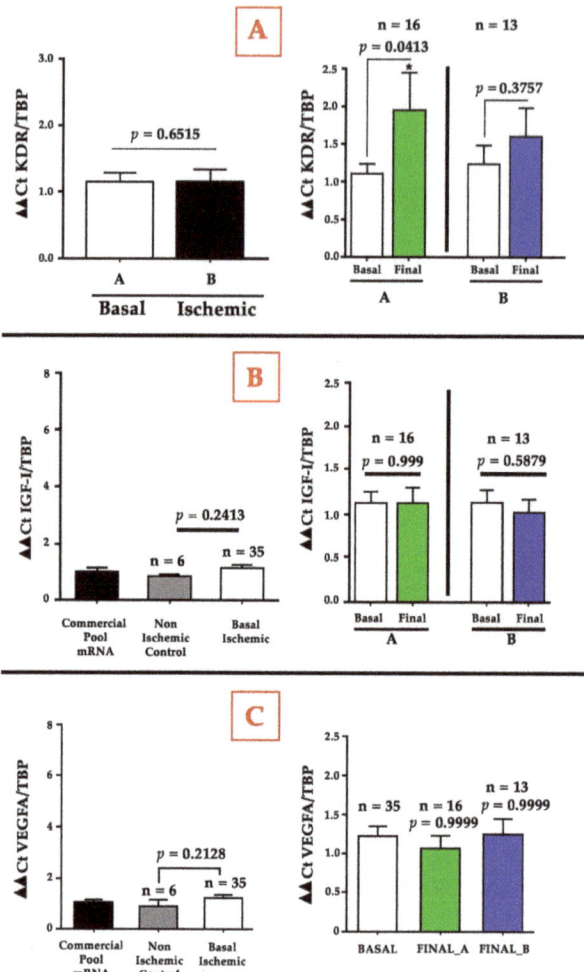

Figure 6. GH increases VEFGA-R2 or KDR/Flk-1 mRNA levels in ischemic muscles of patients with critical limb ischemia without apparent changes in IGF-I and vascular endothelial growth factor A (VEGFA) mRNA levels. Insights from the GHAS trial. (**A**). VEFG-R2 or KDR/Flk-1 mRNA levels in the GHAS trial. The left graph shows the baseline levels between both groups of treatment with no significant differences. In the right graph, a significant increase in KDR mRNA levels in the GH group compared to the placebo group were found during the period of treatment (8 weeks). (**B**). IGF-I mRNA levels in the GHAS trial. The graph on the left shows levels of IGF-I at baseline in ischemic vs non-ischemic muscle samples with no differences. The graph on the right shows the lack of changes in any group of treatment during the period of treatment. (**C**). VEGFA mRNA levels in the GHAS trial. The left graph depicts the comparison between VEGFA levels in ischemic vs non-ischemic muscle samples in the calf at baseline. The right graph depicts the lack of significant changes after 8 weeks of treatment. Group A, green bars: GH; Group B, blue bars: placebo. Non-ischemic muscle samples: sample of reference obtained from amputations in patients without limb ischemia. Commercial pool mRNA: a commercial mRNA from skeletal muscle used as a technical control for normalization of the different assays. A non-parametric test was used for the statistics. Note that although at the beginning of the study there were data from 35 muscle samples, at the end of this study, there were only complete data from 28 patients (basal and final samples). * indicates statistically significant.

3.5. GH and CXCL12 (SDF-1): A Potential Collaboration for Collateral Growth

Another cytokine that plays an important role in arteriogenesis is SDF-1. This cytokine, produced mainly in platelets, can stimulate collateral growth in several ways. The role of SDF-1 was analyzed in a double animal model of ischemia with both types of processes, acute and gradual, and seems to have a less important function than expected since in the gradual model of ischemia in mice, a smaller increase in SDF-1 was found in both the thigh and calf compared to what occurs in the acute process [132]. However, in another interesting experimental study in mice, an important action of this molecule and its receptor, CXCR4, has been recently been described that could help to understand the real role of this cytokine in arteriogenesis [141]. SDF-1, released by activated platelets, recruits perivascular mast cells by interacting with CXCR-4, and mast cells are responsible for boosting the arteriogenic process by two main mechanisms: On the one hand, they recruit neutrophils, monocytes, and T cells in the vascular wall, and on the other hand, they directly release growth factors, mainly MCP-1 and VEGFA, that stimulate vascular remodeling. Therefore, SDF-1 could promote the inflammatory microenvironment necessary for collateral enlargement by recruiting perivascular mast cells that could play a key role that has never been clearly described. In addition, platelets facilitate the extravasation of neutrophils via GPIbα and uPA receptors, which in turn, activate mast cell degradation by releasing ROS. This is an important finding, and it represents another possible connection between shear stress (mechanical signal) and vascular growth (chemical signal) [141].

From this point of view, particularly striking is the relationship between SDF-1 and GH, since the receptor for SDF-1 (CXCR4) has been found in pituitary somatotrophs, where SDF-1 activates the expression of the GH gene and the production and secretion of GH from the anterior pituitary, regulating the normal physiological function of GH cells. In fact, when SDF-1β was administered to rats, both alone or with GHRH, the production of GH from the pituitary gland was increased by 2.5–3.5 times in a dose-dependent manner [143]. Interestingly, despite the different types of cells in the anterior pituitary gland, only somatotrophs express CXCR4. That means that SDF-1 and GH are closely related, at least at the pituitary level. The cellular mechanisms responsible for this stimulation have been studied in GH4C1 cells, showing two possible pathways: the Ca^{++}-independent stimulation of ERK1/2 activity and the Ca^{++}-dependent activation of Pyk2 and BK_{Ca} [144]. This positive relation is also supported by the finding that GH stimulates SDF-1, since high levels of the same can be seen in the thymus of GH-transgenic mice and in cultured primary thymic epithelial cells derived from these animals, as compared to age-matched wild-type counterparts. Additionally, thymocytes migration induced by SDF-1 is improved when these cells are exposed to GH [145]. Since both SDF-1 and GH are coordinated during embryological development for vasculogenesis and for immune system function [16,145], it is tempting to speculate that both may act together in situations such as ischemic injuries, mainly stimulating and leading the migration of macrophages, lymphocytes, and, probably, mast cells to the vascular wall during collateral enlargement.

The finding of Chillo et al. [141] about the possible role of mast cell on arteriogenesis by orchestrating leukocyte function has to be underlined again and could also support our finding of an increase of KDR/Flk-1 in human muscle samples. Mast cells activated by shear stress release VEGFA into the vascular wall that needs its receptor to achieve its action. In addition, as described before, KDR/Flk-1 is a critical factor for mechanotransduction because it induces the release of VWF by ECs. Therefore, GH must be a mediator in this context, enhancing ECs and mast cell activity.

3.6. GH and Mesenchymal Stem Cells (MSCs)

Another intriguing relationship of GH is that which the hormone has with MSCs. These cells migrate in the embryo to the newly formed vessels to release growth factors and stabilize the new vascular network, since they can differentiate into pericytes. However, these cells do not disappear in the postnatal period, and they can be identified in adults in many tissues, especially in the bone marrow but also in adipose tissue or in muscles near vascular structures. In adults, MSCs are also called resident stem cells and constitute a reserve to replace damaged cells because they are capable of differentiating into a wide variety of cellular types, which is why they have been advocated in tissue-regenerative therapies [146]. MSCs have also been utilized for limb ischemia in both animals and humans with a low level of benefit so far [147–150]. To improve their potential, some researchers have defended their combination with GH. First, as described, GHR have been found in these progenitor cells [151], facilitating differentiation and growth factor secretion from MSCs by GH. For example, it has been shown that MSCs that overexpress Akt improve their functions, increasing the power to repair damaged myocardium despite infrequent cellular fusion or differentiation [152]. However, MSCs, rather than stimulate growth factor secretion, facilitate the release of growth factors from surrounding tissues [149]. This insight confirms that paracrine mechanisms mediated by MSCs are authentic players in enhancing the survival of existing myocytes and that we could act on cytokines and growth factor secretion by stimulating the Akt pathway. GH might favor the stimulus of this signaling pathway in MSCs. In fact, knockout mice with a GH receptor (GHRKO) have shown how MSCs tend to differentiate into adipocytes, partially losing their potential, both in bone marrow and peripheral tissues. The Wnt/β-catenin signaling pathway seems to increase when GH is present, suggesting that it has a role in the modulation of MSCs' fate by GH [153]. This fact has also been confirmed in MSCs of human trabecular bones. Human bone marrow MSCs express GHR and respond to GH via JAK2/STAT5 intracellular signaling [154]. These findings support the idea that MSC activity might be modulated with independence of the origin of these cells and that GH can be a true stimulator for them. Thus, since MSCs are essential for vasculogenesis, they could also be crucial during adult arteriogenesis due to the similarity between both processes, and GH could be of help to increase the potential and modulate the action of MSCs or even to facilitate their differentiation in SMCs that favor collateral growth.

3.7. GH and Extracellular Matrix (ECM)

Collateral remodeling is the final step for arteriogenesis, and it occurs mainly in the media and adventitia layers. SMCs and fibroblasts play the main role in this phase, in which the external elastic lamina and the adventitia elastin are degraded by proteolytic enzymes such as metalloproteinases (MMP) and plasmin to make room for the growing vessel. FGF-2 or IGF-I, among others, trigger the maturation and proliferation of fibroblasts and SMCs [155]. Cell migration is key for both angiogenesis and arteriogenesis. However, migrating cells need of a scaffold to do so. For this, the extracellular matrix (ECM) plays a pivotal role, and GH can regulate it [156,157]. For instance, when the hormone is administered to cultured human SMCs, it produces a direct and dose-dependent increase of hyaluronic acid and chondroitin [157]. That is, the remodeling process takes place by the dynamic restructuring of the ECM with degradation and synthesis. GH, on the other hand, can act as a mitogenic factor, also favoring the release of growth factors and the migration of a major players in this process such as SMCs, fibroblasts, ECs, and the same macrophages in the vascular wall. In a study with cultured murine thymic endothelioma cells (tEnd.1), treatment with GH for 24 h induced an increase in the production of fibronectin and laminin from these ECs as compared to the control, and it also increased the expression of ECM receptors for fibronectin and laminin, as well as the migratory activity of the aforementioned cell line [156]. On the other hand, the activation of macrophages in the vascular wall facilitate MMP production, influencing ECM degradation. All these data confirm the ability of GH to influence ECM, playing an important role for vessel remodeling.

3.8. GH and NO-Independent Vascular Tone: the Role of Sympathetic System

Sympathetic innervation seems to be necessary for stabilizing vascular wall tone and cell phenotype, since in sympathectomized vessels, both SMCs and fibroblasts increase in numbers with collagen alterations (collagen III upregulation and collagen IV downregulation) [158]. This supports the hypothesis that the autonomic system participates in vascular homeostasis. In GHD patients, a marked increase in sympathetic activity has been found [159], but it tends to be reversed after GH replacement therapy [160], suggesting that the hormone may regulate central sympathetic activity, thus affecting vascular peripheral resistance. When sympathetic activity is increased, collaterals suffer an intimal thickening that diminishes SSF and collateral enlargement after ischemia [158]. In skeletal muscle arterioles from diabetic patients with neuropathy, an increased vasomotor tone has been described, while a higher α-adrenergic tone has been found in the iliac artery of diabetic animals [161,162]. Thereupon, proper innervation plays an important role in the development and remodeling of blood vessels, although the exact mechanism of impaired arteriogenesis, when altered, is still poorly understood.

That GH is related to the autonomous system has not only been described in GHD patients. In healthy humans, sympathetic activation and baroreflex resetting were found after GHRH administration in a microneurographic study of muscle sympathetic nerve activity as compared to a placebo group at rest, whereas blood pressure and heart rate were not altered [163]. Therefore, GH is related to sympathetic system during both the physiological and pathological situations of GH secretion. These findings could help to understand the connections of GH with the vascular system and the role of the hormone in arteriogenesis.

3.9. GH and Midkine (MDK) Relation should Be Investigated

Midkine (MK), a heparin-binding growth factor that seems to play an important role in arteriogenesis by mediating eNOS activity and increasing the bioavailability of VEGFA [164], has also been related with GH, as the expression of MK and its receptors have been detected in somatotrophs of both embryonic and adult rats, favoring the development of the pituitary gland and acting as a regulator of its function in adults [165]. MK seems to be secreted by follicle-stimulating cells in the pituitary gland, controlling GH production from GH cells in a paracrine way via protein tyrosine phosphatase receptor-type Z (Ptprz1) [166].

In MK-deficient mice, altered vascular remodeling has been seen due to the reduction in ECs proliferation [167]. This means that ECs proliferation plays a pivotal role in correcting vascular growth, and, as described before, GH is mainly involved in EC proliferation, participating, from this point of view, in this mitogenic and proliferative process.

Given that GH is a major regulator of eNOS expression and NO production in ECs for vasodilation that typically increases VEGF and KDR, and as a consequence of its participation in vascular homeostasis, it is tempting to speculate that both MK and GH might work together to maintain vascular homeostasis, as well as to activate vascular enlargement when an ischemic condition is present. MK could indirectly promote vasodilation by increasing the bioavailability of GH in ECs [168]. However, this hypothesis is not yet proved and needs confirmation.

3.10. GH and Klotho: the Perfect Combination?

Of interest is the special relationship between Klotho and GH. A comprehensive review of the relation between GH and Klotho has been previously described [16,169]. Here, the intention is just to highlight the importance of this relationship for arteriogenesis. As is known, Klotho is a type of transmembrane full-length protein mainly found in the kidneys which can act remotely by generating a circulating form (sKlotho) [170]. This form can work as a hormone that regulates the functions of cells that lack this protein, such as ECs and arterial SMCs [171]. It is known that sKlotho increases both GH production by the anterior pituitary [172] and the local production of the hormone by the endothelium. Additionally, sKlotho inhibits the negative feedback of IGF-I on GH secretion [173]. Both molecules are essential for vascular homeostasis, as well as when this process is altered. It is thought that the lack of Klotho production in chronic renal insufficiency is the reason for the aging and calcification of the vessel wall, even in collaterals, and, in consequence, it impairs atherosclerosis and arteriogenesis. In fact, mice overexpressing Klotho have a longer life expectancy due to the mentioned effect of Klotho and its anti-IGF-I action [174]. Thus, Klotho stimulates GH while blocking IGF-I, eliminating the deleterious effects of the latter. However, GH also exerts influences on Klotho levels, as patients with acromegaly show increased levels of Klotho, and they show a downregulation when the GH-produced pituitary adenoma is removed [169].

Klotho seems to be important in physiological states but also in pathological ones, since mice with Klotho deficiency show vascular hyperpermeability. This molecule seems to be necessary for the control of the action of VEGF on the vascular permeability. At the level of the endothelium, Klotho facilitates the association of both VEGFR2 and transient receptor potential canonical calcium channel 1 (TRPC-1) by promoting their cointernalization and regulating calcium entry to maintain homeostasis. Thus, KDR is needed by Klotho to accomplish its actions [175]. GH, as demonstrated before, increases KDR in the ischemic muscle of the leg and could collaborate with Klotho this way by facilitating this action.

Other important action of Klotho for arteriogenesis is that this factor also participates in the regulation of vascular tone, as it compensates for the vasoconstrictor action of some factors such as phosphates or FGF23 by increasing the production of NO [176], an action probably mediated by local GH. Interestingly, while Klotho favors vascular contraction in aortic ring samples from mice in *in vitro* studies by increasing ROS levels both in SMCs and ECs when is administered alone, the relaxation phenomenon predominates if SMCs are pretreated with FGF23 or phosphates, while ROS levels remain elevated. This is an effect that is mediated by an indirect NO production by Klotho from ECs stimulating both eNOS and iNOS [176]. In fact, when the endothelium is removed, this effect disappears.

The above data supports again that redox stress contributes to the regulation of vascular homeostasis, since eNOS is sensitive to ROS. It also supports the complex action that Klotho has depending of its environment, as happens with GH. The other important message is the main role of the ECs in the control of vascular tone and SMCs actions, and that Klotho and GH seem to collaborate in physiological and pathological conditions such as ischemia, although this aspect has to be confirmed.

4. Conclusions

Vascular homeostasis critically depends on the physiological response of endothelial cells to blood supply and the appropriate redox balance. The endothelium releases many factors to control vascular tone, the adhesion of circulating blood cells, the proliferation of smooth muscle cells, and inflammation.

Why should GH be considered a promising therapeutic agent for neovascularization? The GH/PRL/PL family regulates the physiological growth and regression of blood vessels in female reproductive organs, and this fact strongly support its vascular role in neovascularization. There is no doubt about the fact that the GH/IGF-I axis has to play an important role in neovascularization, both in physiological and pathological states, as evidence here presented has underlined. This axis suffers an important decline with aging, mainly affecting GH secretion. Considering that most patients with ischemic injuries are elderly, GH therapy could be considered of help in improving vascularization and mitigating symptoms.

However, information concerning the regulation of neovascularization by proangiogenic hormones such as GH is insufficient, since few physiological or pathological conditions have been deeply studied, with some exceptions. This fact could be explained by the use of different animal models of ischemia, types of tissue analyzed, disease status, hormone doses, or follow-up times. These effects also depend on the relative contribution of the local production of hormones or on the hormonal cleavage by proteases in cells or the clearance of these hormones by kidneys when they are exogenously administered. Surprisingly, data are also limited about endogenously produced antiangiogenic substances that might be overexpressed in chronic states such as ischemia and that could act with a harmful effect on GH actions.

The role of redox balance in arteriogenesis and how GH could aid in the mitigation of it were analyzed. We also proposed the possibility that GH and IGF-I could be parts of those mitogenic factors secreted by endothelial cells in response to shear stress forces. The large number of connections that both molecules have with cytokines, hormones, and cells involved in neovascularization reinforce their role in this process. Finally, in this review, it has been presented some molecular insights from the

GHAS trial in patients with critical limb ischemia that correlate perfectly with recent publications on arteriogenesis and that can help to understand the action of GH dealing with ischemia. Nevertheless, the molecular results of this initial clinical study still need to be confirmed in larger studies.

Author Contributions: Conceptualization, D.C., J.D., and P.D.; methodology, D.C. J.D. and C.V.A.; software, D.C.; validation, D.C. and J.D.; formal analysis, D.C. and J.D.; investigation, D.C., P.D. and C.V.A.; resources, D.C.; data curation, D.C., J.D. and C.V.A.; writing—original draft preparation, D.C. and J.D.; writing—review and editing, D.C. J.D. and C.V.A.; visualization, D.C. and J.C.; supervision, J.D.; project administration, D.C.; funding acquisition, D.C. All authors have read and agreed to the published version of the manuscript.

Funding: This review was funded by the Spanish Society of Angiology and Vascular Surgery (SEACV). Not this review, but the GHAS trial was funded by the Carlos III Health Institute and the European Regional Development Fund (ISCIII- FEDER), Madrid, Spain. Grant number PI 13-00790.

Acknowledgments: We thank Santiago Pérez Cachafeiro for providing an important stimulus to develop this review and the GHAS trial. Without his help and knowledge this article would not have been possible. We equally thank Sihara Pérez-Romero from the Center of Research in Molecular Medicine of the University of Santiago of Compostela (CIMUS), Spain, for her technical assistance in the molecular analysis in ischemic muscle samples from the GHAS study.

Conflicts of Interest: The authors declare no conflict of interest. The funders had no role in the design of the study; in the collection, analyses, or interpretation of data; in the writing of the manuscript, or in the decision to publish the results.

References

1. Devesa, J.; Almengló, C.; Devesa, P. Multiple Effects of Growth Hormone in the Body: Is It Really the Hormone for Growth? *Clin. Med. Insights Endocrinol. Diabetes* **2016**, *9*, 47–71. [CrossRef]
2. Pfeifer, M.; Verhovec, R.; Zizek, B.; Prezelj, J.; Poredoz, P.; Clayton, R.N. Growth Hormone (GH) Treatment Reverses Early Atherosclerotic Changes in GH-Deficient Adults. *J. Clin. Endocrinol. Metab.* **1999**, *84*, 453–457. [CrossRef] [PubMed]
3. Suzuki, K.; Yanagi, K.; Shimizu, M.; Wakamatsu, S.; Niitani, T.; Hosonuma, S.; Sagara, M.; Aso, Y. Effect of Growth Hormone Replacement Therapy on Plasma Diacron-Reactive Oxygen Metabolites and Endothelial Function in Japanese Patients: The GREAT Clinical Study. *Endocr. J.* **2017**, *65*, 101–111. [CrossRef] [PubMed]
4. Rosén, T.; Bengtsson, B.A. Premature Mortality Due to Cardiovascular Disease in Hypopituitarism. *Lancet (London, England)* **1990**, *336*, 285–288. [CrossRef]
5. Smith, J.C.; Evans, L.M.; Wilkinson, I.; Goodfellow, J.; Cockcroft, J.R.; Scanlon, M.F.; Davies, J.S. Effects of GH Replacement on Endothelial Function and Large-Artery Stiffness in GH-Deficient Adults: A Randomized, Double-Blind, Placebo-Controlled Study. *Clin. Endocrinol. (Oxf.)* **2002**, *56*, 493–501. [CrossRef] [PubMed]
6. Strazhesko, I.D.; Tkacheva, O.N.; Akasheva, D.U.; Dudinskaya, E.N.; Plokhova, E.V.; Pykhtina, V.S.; Kruglikova, A.S.; Brailova, N.V.; Sharashkina, N.V.; Kashtanova, D.A.; et al. Growth Hormone, Insulin-Like Growth Factor-1, Insulin Resistance, and Leukocyte Telomere Length as Determinants of Arterial Aging in Subjects Free of Cardiovascular Diseases. *Front. Genet.* **2017**, *8*, 198. [CrossRef] [PubMed]
7. Li, G.; Del Rincon, J.P.; Jahn, L.A.; Wu, Y.; Gaylinn, B.; Thorner, M.O.; Liu, Z. Growth Hormone Exerts Acute Vascular Effects Independent of Systemic or Muscle Insulin-like Growth Factor I. *J. Clin. Endocrinol. Metab.* **2008**, *93*, 1379–1385. [CrossRef] [PubMed]
8. Thum, T.; Tsikas, D.; Frölich, J.C.; Borlak, J. Growth Hormone Induces ENOS Expression and Nitric Oxide Release in a Cultured Human Endothelial Cell Line. *FEBS Lett.* **2003**, *555*, 567–571. [CrossRef]
9. Colao, A. The GH-IGF-I Axis and the Cardiovascular System: Clinical Implications. *Clin. Endocrinol.* **2008**, 347–358. [CrossRef]
10. Corbacho, A.M.; Martínez de la Escalera, G.; Clapp, C. Roles of Prolactin and Related Members of the Prolactin/Growth Hormone/Placental Lactogen Family in Angiogenesis. *J. Endocrinol.* **2002**, 219–238. [CrossRef]
11. Brunet-Dunand, S.E.; Vouyovitch, C.; Araneda, S.; Pandey, V.; Vidal, L.J.P.; Print, C.; Mertani, H.C.; Lobie, P.E.; Perry, J.K. Autocrine Human Growth Hormone Promotes Tumor Angiogenesis in Mammary Carcinoma. *Endocrinology* **2009**, *150*, 1341–1352. [CrossRef] [PubMed]
12. Verhelst, J.; Abs, R. Long-Term Growth Hormone Replacement Therapy in Hypopituitary Adults. *Drugs* **2002**, *62*, 2399–2412. [CrossRef] [PubMed]

13. Evans, L.M.; Davies, J.S.; Anderson, R.A.; Ellis, G.R.; Jackson, S.K.; Lewis, M.J.; Frenneaux, M.P.; Rees, A.; Scanlon, M.F. The Effect of GH Replacement Therapy on Endothelial Function and Oxidative Stress in Adult Growth Hormone Deficiency. *Eur. J. Endocrinol.* **2000**, *142*, 254–262. [CrossRef] [PubMed]
14. Napoli, R.; Guardasole, V.; Angelini, V.; D'Amico, F.; Zarra, E.; Matarazzo, M.; Sacca, L. Acute Effects of Growth Hormone on Vascular Function in Human Subjects. *J. Clin. Endocrinol. Metab.* **2003**, *88*, 2817–2820. [CrossRef]
15. Elhadd, T.A.; Abdu, T.A.; Oxtoby, J.; Kennedy, G.; McLaren, M.; Neary, R.; Belch, J.J.F.; Clayton, R.N. Biochemical and Biophysical Markers of Endothelial Dysfunction in Adults with Hypopituitarism and Severe GH Deficiency. *J. Clin. Endocrinol. Metab.* **2001**, *86*, 4223–4232. [CrossRef]
16. Caicedo, D.; Díaz, O.; Devesa, P.; Devesa, J. Growth Hormone (GH) and Cardiovascular System. *Int. J. Mol. Sci.* **2018**, *19*, 290. [CrossRef]
17. Palmeiro, C.R.; Anand, R.; Dardi, I.K.; Balasubramaniyam, N.; Schwarcz, M.D.; Weiss, I.A. Growth Hormone and the Cardiovascular System. *Cardiol. Rev.* **2012**, *20*, 197–207. [CrossRef]
18. Wahlberg, E. Angiogenesis and Arteriogenesis in Limb Ischemia. *J. Vasc. Surg.* **2003**, 198–203. [CrossRef]
19. Veldhuis, J.D.; Roemmich, J.N.; Richmond, E.J.; Bowers, C.Y. Somatotropic and Gonadotropic Axes Linkages in Infancy, Childhood, and the Puberty-Adult Transition. *Endocr. Rev.* **2006**, *27*, 101–140. [CrossRef]
20. Arce, V.M.; Devesa, J.; Fernández-Tresguerres, J.A. Hormona de Crecimiento. In *Fisiología Humana*; Fernández-Tresguerres, J.A., Ed.; Mcgraw-Hill Medical: Madrid, Spain, 2019; pp. 1–36.
21. Drake, C.J. Embryonic and Adult Vasculogenesis. *Birth Defects Res. Part C-Embryo Today Rev* **2003**, 73–82. [CrossRef]
22. Groothuis, P.G. Angiogenesis and Vascular Remodelling in Female Reproductive Organs. *Angiogenesis* **2005**, *8*, 87–88. [CrossRef] [PubMed]
23. Pugh, C.W.; Ratcliffe, P.J. Regulation of Angiogenesis by Hypoxia: Role of the HIF System. *Nat. Med.* **2003**, *9*, 677–684. [CrossRef] [PubMed]
24. Böger, R.H.; Skamira, C.; Bode-Böger, S.M.; Brabant, G.; Von Zur Mühlen, A.; Frölich, J.C. Nitric Oxide May Mediate the Hemodynamic Effects of Recombinant Growth Hormone in Patients with Acquired Growth Hormone Deficiency: A Double-Blind, Placebo-Controlled Study. *J. Clin. Investig.* **1996**, *98*, 2706–2713. [CrossRef] [PubMed]
25. Tsukahara, H.; Gordienko, D.V.; Tonshoff, B.; Gelato, M.C.; Goligorsky, M.S. Direct Demonstration of Insulin-Like Growth Factor-I-Induced Nitric Oxide Production by Endothelial Cells. *Kidney Int.* **1994**, *45*, 598–604. [CrossRef] [PubMed]
26. Bar, R.S.; Boes, M.; Dake, B.L.; Booth, B.A.; Henley, S.A.; Sandra, A. Insulin, Insulin-Like Growth Factors, and Vascular Endothelium. *Am. J. Med.* **1988**, *85*, 59–70. [CrossRef]
27. Wickman, A.; Jonsdottir, I.; Bergstrom, G.; Hedin, L. GH and IGF-I Regulate the Expression of Endothelial Nitric Oxide Synthase (ENOS) in Cardiovascular Tissues of Hypophysectomized Female Rats. *Eur. J. Endocrinol.* **2002**, *147*, 523–533. [CrossRef]
28. Warzecha, Z.; Dembiński, A.; Ceranowicz, P.; Konturek, S.J.; Tomaszewska, R.; Stachura, J.; Konturek, P.C. IGF-1 Stimulates Production of Interleukin-10 and Inhibits Development of Caerulein-Induced Pancreatitis. *J. Physiol. Pharmacol.* **2003**, *54*, 575–590.
29. Shimizu, Y.; Nagaya, N.; Teranishi, Y.; Imazu, M.; Yamamoto, H.; Shokawa, T.; Kangawa, K.; Kohno, N.; Yoshizumi, M. Ghrelin Improves Endothelial Dysfunction through Growth Hormone-Independent Mechanisms in Rats. *Biochem. Biophys. Res. Commun.* **2003**, *310*, 830–835. [CrossRef]
30. Waters, M.J. The Growth Hormone Receptor. *Growth Horm. IGF Res.* **2016**. [CrossRef]
31. Dehkhoda, F.; Lee, C.M.M.; Medina, J.; Brooks, A.J. The Growth Hormone Receptor: Mechanism of Receptor Activation, Cell Signaling, and Physiological Aspects. *Front. Endocrinol. (Lausanne)* **2018**, *9*, 35. [CrossRef]
32. Thum, T.; Bauersachs, J. Growth Hormone Regulates Vascular Function—What We Know from Bench and Bedside. *Eur. J. Clin. Pharmacol.* **2006**. [CrossRef]
33. Tanimura, S.; Takeda, K. ERK Signalling as a Regulator of Cell Motility. *J. Biochem.* **2017**, *162*, 145–154. [CrossRef] [PubMed]
34. Zhu, T.; Goh, E.L.K.; Lobie, P.E. Growth Hormone Stimulates the Tyrosine Phosphorylation and Association of P125 Focal Adhesion Kinase (FAK) with JAK2. *J. Biol. Chem.* **1998**, *273*, 10682–10689. [CrossRef] [PubMed]

35. Ryu, H.; Lee, J.-H.; Kim, K.S.; Jeong, S.-M.; Kim, P.-H.; Chung, H.-T. Regulation of Neutrophil Adhesion by Pituitary Growth Hormone Accompanies Tyrosine Phosphorylation of Jak2, P125 FAK, and Paxillin. *J. Immunol.* **2000**, *165*, 2116–2123. [CrossRef]
36. Milstien, S.; Katusic, Z. Oxidation of Tetrahydrobiopterin by Peroxynitrite: Implications for Vascular Endothelial Function. *Biochem. Biophys. Res. Commun.* **1999**, *263*, 681–684. [CrossRef] [PubMed]
37. Thum, T.; Borlak, J. Mechanistic Role of Cytochrome P450 Monooxygenases in Oxidized Low-Density Lipoprotein-Induced Vascular Injury: Therapy through LOX-1 Receptor Antagonism? *Circ. Res.* **2004**, *94*, 1–13. [CrossRef] [PubMed]
38. Nylander, E.; Grönbladh, A.; Zelleroth, S.; Diwakarla, S.; Nyberg, F.; Hallberg, M. Growth Hormone Is Protective against Acute Methadone-Induced Toxicity by Modulating the NMDA Receptor Complex. *Neuroscience* **2016**, *339*, 538–547. [CrossRef]
39. Nylander, E.; Zelleroth, S.; Nyberg, F.; Grönbladh, A.; Hallberg, M. The Protective and Restorative Effects of Growth Hormone and Insulin-Like Growth Factor-1 on Methadone-Induced Toxicity In Vitro. *Int. J. Mol. Sci.* **2018**, *19*, 3627. [CrossRef]
40. Erusalimsky, J.D. Vascular Endothelial Senescence: From Mechanisms to Pathophysiology. *J. Appl. Physiol.* **2009**, *106*, 326–332. [CrossRef]
41. Ungvari, Z.; Orosz, Z.; Labinskyy, N.; Rivera, A.; Xiangmin, Z.; Smith, K.; Csiszar, A. Increased Mitochondrial H2O2 Production Promotes Endothelial NF-KappaB Activation in Aged Rat Arteries. *Am. J. Physiol. Heart Circ. Physiol.* **2007**, *293*, H37–H47. [CrossRef]
42. Pierce, G.L.; Lesniewski, L.A.; Lawson, B.R.; Beske, S.D.; Seals, D.R. Nuclear Factor-KB Activation Contributes to Vascular Endothelial Dysfunction via Oxidative Stress in Overweight/Obese Middle-Aged and Older Humans. *Circulation* **2009**, *119*, 1284–1292. [CrossRef]
43. Ungvari, Z.; Gautam, T.; Koncz, P.; Henthorn, J.C.; Pinto, J.T.; Ballabh, P.; Yan, H.; Mitschelen, M.; Farley, J.; Sonntag, W.E.; et al. Vasoprotective Effects of Life Span-Extending Peripubertal GH Replacement in Lewis Dwarf Rats. *J. Gerontol.-Ser. A Biol. Sci. Med. Sci.* **2010**, *65A*, 1145–1156. [CrossRef]
44. Ungvari, Z.; Sosnowska, D.; Podlutsky, A.; Koncz, P.; Sonntag, W.E.; Csiszar, A. Free Radical Production, Antioxidant Capacity, and Oxidative Stress Response Signatures in Fibroblasts from Lewis Dwarf Rats: Effects of Life Span-Extending Peripubertal GH Treatment. *J. Gerontol. Ser. A Biol. Sci. Med. Sci.* **2011**, *66A*, 501–510. [CrossRef] [PubMed]
45. Perret-Vivancos, C.; Abbate, A.; Ardail, D.; Raccurt, M.; Usson, Y.; Lobie, P.; Morel, G. Growth Hormone Activity in Mitochondria Depends on GH Receptor Box 1 and Involves Caveolar Pathway Targeting. *Exp. Cell Res.* **2005**, *312*, 215–232. [CrossRef]
46. Ardail, D.; Debon, A.; Perret-Vivancos, C.; Biol-N'Garagba, M.-C.; Krantic, S.; Lobie, P.E.; Morel, G. Growth Hormone Internalization in Mitochondria Decreases Respiratory Chain Activity. *Neuroendocrinology* **2010**, *91*, 16–26. [CrossRef] [PubMed]
47. Csiszar, A.; Labinskyy, N.; Perez, V.; Recchia, F.A.; Podlutsky, A.; Mukhopadhyay, P.; Losonczy, G.; Pacher, P.; Austad, S.N.; Bartke, A.; et al. Endothelial Function and Vascular Oxidative Stress in Long-Lived GH/IGF-Deficient Ames Dwarf Mice. *AJP Hear. Circ. Physiol.* **2008**, *295*, H1882–H1894. [CrossRef]
48. Keane, J.; Tajouri, L.; Gray, B. Recombinant Human Growth Hormone and Insulin-Like Growth Factor-1 Do Not Affect Mitochondrial Derived Highly Reactive Oxygen Species Production in Peripheral Blood Mononuclear Cells under Conditions of Substrate Saturation In-Vitro. *Nutr. Metab. (Lond.)* **2016**, *13*, 45. [CrossRef]
49. Friedenstein, A.J.; Petrakova, K.V.; Kurolesova, A.I.; Frolova, G.P. Heterotopic of Bone Marrow. Analysis of Precursor Cells for Osteogenic and Hematopoietic Tissues. *Transplantation* **1968**, *6*, 230–247. [CrossRef]
50. da Silva Meirelles, L.; Fontes, A.M.; Covas, D.T.; Caplan, A.I. Mechanisms Involved in the Therapeutic Properties of Mesenchymal Stem Cells. *Cytokine Growth Factor Rev.* **2009**, *20*, 419–427. [CrossRef]
51. Kassis, I.; Zangi, L.; Rivkin, R.; Levdansky, L.; Samuel, S.; Marx, G.; Gorodetsky, R. Isolation of Mesenchymal Stem Cells from G-CSF-Mobilized Human Peripheral Blood Using Fibrin Microbeads. *Bone Marrow Transplant.* **2006**, *37*, 967–976. [CrossRef]
52. Zou, Z.; Zhang, Y.; Hao, L.; Wang, F.; Liu, D.; Su, Y.; Sun, H. More Insight into Mesenchymal Stem Cells and Their Effects inside the Body. *Expert Opin. Biol. Ther.* **2010**, *10*, 215–230. [CrossRef] [PubMed]
53. Lin, G.; Garcia, M.; Ning, H.; Banie, L.; Guo, Y.-L.; Lue, T.F.; Lin, C.-S. Defining Stem and Progenitor Cells within Adipose Tissue. *Stem Cells Dev.* **2008**, *17*, 1053–1063. [CrossRef] [PubMed]

54. Corselli, M.; Chen, C.-W.; Crisan, M.; Lazzari, L.; Péault, B. Perivascular Ancestors of Adult Multipotent Stem Cells. *Arterioscler. Thromb. Vasc. Biol.* **2010**, *30*, 1104–1109. [CrossRef] [PubMed]
55. Siow, R. Migration of Adventitial Myofibroblasts Following Vascular Balloon Injury: Insights from In Vivo Gene Transfer to Rat Carotid Arteries. *Cardiovasc. Res.* **2003**, *59*, 212–221. [CrossRef]
56. Li, G.; Chen, S.-J.; Oparil, S.; Chen, Y.-F.; Thompson, J.A. Direct In Vivo Evidence Demonstrating Neointimal Migration of Adventitial Fibroblasts After Balloon Injury of Rat Carotid Arteries. *Circulation* **2000**, *101*, 1362–1365. [CrossRef]
57. Faggin, E.; Puato, M.; Zardo, L.; Franch, R.; Millino, C.; Sarinella, F.; Pauletto, P.; Sartore, S.; Chiavegato, A. Smooth Muscle-Specific SM22 Protein Is Expressed in the Adventitial Cells of Balloon-Injured Rabbit Carotid Artery. *Arterioscler. Thromb. Vasc. Biol.* **1999**, *19*, 1393–1404. [CrossRef]
58. Haurani, M.; Pagano, P. Adventitial Fibroblast Reactive Oxygen Species as Autacrine and Paracrine Mediators of Remodeling: Bellwether for Vascular Disease? *Cardiovasc. Res.* **2007**, *75*, 679–689. [CrossRef]
59. Herrmann, J.; Samee, S.; Chade, A.; Porcel, M.R.; Lerman, L.O.; Lerman, A. Differential Effect of Experimental Hypertension and Hypercholesterolemia on Adventitial Remodeling. *Arterioscler. Thromb. Vasc. Biol.* **2005**, *25*, 447–453. [CrossRef]
60. Stenmark, K.R.; Davie, N.; Frid, M.; Gerasimovskaya, E.; Das, M. Role of the Adventitia in Pulmonary Vascular Remodeling. *Physiology* **2006**, *21*, 134–145. [CrossRef]
61. Jin, K.; Li, B.; Lou, L.; Xu, Y.; Ye, X.; Yao, K.; Ye, J.; Gao, C. In Vivo Vascularization of MSC-Loaded Porous Hydroxyapatite Constructs Coated with VEGF-Functionalized Collagen/Heparin Multilayers. *Sci. Rep.* **2016**, *6*, 19871. [CrossRef]
62. Khaki, M.; Salmanian, A.H.; Abtahi, H.; Ganji, A.; Mosayebi, G. Mesenchymal Stem Cells Differentiate to Endothelial Cells Using Recombinant Vascular Endothelial Growth Factor—A. *Rep. Biochem. Mol. Biol.* **2018**, *6*, 144–150. [PubMed]
63. Devesa, J.; Caicedo, D. The Role of Growth Hormone on Ovarian Functioning and Ovarian Angiogenesis. *Front. Endocrinol. (Lausanne)* **2019**, *10*, 450. [CrossRef] [PubMed]
64. Galvão, A.M.; Skarzynski, D.; Ferreira-Dias, G. Luteolysis and the Auto-, Paracrine Role of Cytokines from Tumor Necrosis Factor α and Transforming Growth Factor β Superfamilies. In *Vitamins and Hormones*; Academic Press: Cambridge, MA, USA, 2018; pp. 287–315. [CrossRef]
65. Xie, Q.; Cheng, Z.; Chen, X.; Lobe, C.G.; Liu, J. The Role of Notch Signalling in Ovarian Angiogenesis. *J. Ovarian Res.* **2017**, *10*, 13. [CrossRef]
66. Wójcik, M.; Krawczynska, A.; Antushevinch, H.; Przemyslaw, A. Post-Receptor Inhibitors of the GHR-JAK2-STAT Pathway in the Growth Hormone Signal Transduction. *Int. J. Mol. Sci.* **2018**, *19*, 1843. [CrossRef] [PubMed]
67. Schaper, W. Multiple Pathways Converge in the Development of a Collateral Circulation (Arteriogenesis). In *Arteriogenesis—Molecular Regulation, Pathophysiology and Therapeutics I*; Deindl, E., Schaper, W., Eds.; Shaker Verlag: Aachan, Germany, 2011; pp. 67–71.
68. Brooks, A.J.; Waters, M.J. The Growth Hormone Receptor: Mechanism of Activation and Clinical Implications. *Nat. Rev. Endocrinol.* **2010**, *6*, 515–525. [CrossRef]
69. Delafontaine, P.; Song, Y.H.; Li, Y. Expression, Regulation, and Function of IGF-1, IGF-1R, and IGF-1 Binding Proteins in Blood Vessels. *Arterioscler. Thromb. Vasc. Biol.* **2004**, 435–444. [CrossRef]
70. Lang, C.H.; Hong-Brown, L.; Frost, R.A. Cytokine Inhibition of JAK-STAT Signaling: A New Mechanism of Growth Hormone Resistance. *Pediatr. Nephrol.* **2005**, 306–312. [CrossRef]
71. Wickman, A.; Friberg, P.; Adams, M.A.; Matejka, G.L.; Brantsing, C.; Guron, G.; Isgaard, J. Induction of Growth Hormone Receptor and Insulin-Like Growth Factor-I MRNA in Aorta and Caval Vein during Hemodynamic Challenge. *Hypertension* **1997**, *29*, 123–130. [CrossRef]
72. Owens, G.K.; Reidy, M.A. Hyperplastic Growth Response of Vascular Smooth Muscle Cells Following Induction of Acute Hypertension in Rats by Aortic Coarctation. *Circ. Res.* **1985**, *57*, 695–705. [CrossRef]
73. Delafontaine, P.; Lou, H.; Alexander, R.W. Regulation of Insulin-Like Growth Factor I Messenger RNA Levels in Vascular Smooth Muscle Cells. *Hypertension* **1991**, *18*, 742–747. [CrossRef]
74. Hansson, H.-A.; Jennische, E.; Skottner, A. IGF-I Expression in Blood Vessels Varies with Vascular Load. *Acta Physiol. Scand.* **1987**, *129*, 165–169. [CrossRef] [PubMed]
75. Rowlinson, S.W.; Yoshizato, H.; Barclay, J.L.; Brooks, A.J.; Behncken, S.N.; Kerr, L.M.; Millard, K.; Palethorpe, K.; Nielsen, K.; Clyde-Smith, J.; et al. An Agonist-Induced Conformational Change in the Growth

Hormone Receptor Determines the Choice of Signalling Pathway. *Nat. Cell Biol.* **2008**, *10*, 740–747. [CrossRef] [PubMed]
76. Clapp, C.; Thebault, S.; Jeziorski, M.C.; Martínez De La Escalera, G. Peptide Hormone Regulation of Angiogenesis. *Physiol. Rev.* **2009**, *89*, 1177–1215. [CrossRef]
77. Brüel, A.; Oxlund, H. Growth Hormone Influences the Content and Composition of Collagen in the Aorta from Old Rats. *Mech. Ageing Dev.* **2002**, *123*, 627–635. [CrossRef]
78. Cittadini, A.; Strömer, H.; Katz, S.E.; Clark, R.; Moses, A.C.; Morgan, J.P.; Douglas, P.S. Differential Cardiac Effects of Growth Hormone and Insulin-Like Growth Factor-1 in the Rat. A Combined In Vivo and In Vitro Evaluation. *Circulation* **1996**, *93*, 800–809. [CrossRef]
79. Le Roith, D.; Scavo, L.; Butler, A. What Is the Role of Circulating IGF-I? *Trends Endocrinol. Metab.* **2001**, *12*, 48–52. [CrossRef]
80. Xu, X.Q.; Emerald, B.S.; Goh, E.L.K.; Kannan, N.; Miller, L.D.; Gluckman, P.D.; Liu, E.T.; Lobie, P.E. Gene Expression Profiling to Identify Oncogenic Determinants of Autocrine Human Growth Hormone in Human Mammary Carcinoma. *J. Biol. Chem.* **2005**, *280*, 23987–24003. [CrossRef]
81. Nakonechnaya, A.O.; Jefferson, H.S.; Chen, X.; Shewchuk, B.M. Differential Effects of Exogenous and Autocrine Growth Hormone on LNCaP Prostate Cancer Cell Proliferation and Survival. *J. Cell. Biochem.* **2013**, *114*, 1322–1335. [CrossRef]
82. Erman, A.; Wabitsch, M.; Goodyer, C.G. Human Growth Hormone Receptor (GHR) Expression in Obesity: II. Regulation of the Human GHR Gene by Obesity-Related Factors. *Int. J. Obes. (Lond.)* **2011**, *35*, 1520–1529. [CrossRef]
83. Schwartzbauer, G.; Menon, R.K. Regulation of Growth Hormone Receptor Gene Expression. *Mol. Genet. Metab.* **1998**, *63*, 243–253. [CrossRef]
84. Lobie, P.E.; Breipohl, W.; Aragón, J.G.; Waters, M.J. Cellular Localization of the Growth Hormone Receptor/Binding Protein in the Male and Female Reproductive Systems. *Endocrinology* **1990**, *126*, 2214–2221. [CrossRef] [PubMed]
85. Gonzalez, C.; Corbacho, A.M.; Eiserich, J.P.; Garcia, C.; Lopez-Barrera, F.; Morales-Tlalpan, V.; Barajas-Espinosa, A.; Diaz-Muñoz, M.; Rubio, R.; Lin, S.-H.; et al. 16K-Prolactin Inhibits Activation of Endothelial Nitric Oxide Synthase, Intracellular Calcium Mobilization, and Endothelium-Dependent Vasorelaxation. *Endocrinology* **2004**, *145*, 5714–5722. [CrossRef] [PubMed]
86. Govers, R.; Rabelink, T.J. Cellular Regulation of Endothelial Nitric Oxide Synthase. *Am. J. Physiol. Renal Physiol.* **2001**, *280*, F193–F206. [CrossRef] [PubMed]
87. Walford, G.; Loscalzo, J. Nitric Oxide in Vascular Biology. *J. Thromb. Haemost.* **2003**, 2112–2118. [CrossRef] [PubMed]
88. Böger, R.H. Nitric Oxide and the Mediation of the Hemodynamic Effects of Growth Hormone in Humans. *J. Endocrinol. Investig.* **1999**, *22* (Suppl. 5), 75–81.
89. Gonzalez, C.; Rosas-Hernandez, H.; Jurado-Manzano, B.; Ramirez-Lee, M.A.; Salazar-Garcia, S.; Martinez-Cuevas, P.P.; Velarde-Salcedo, A.J.; Morales-Loredo, H.; Espinosa-Tanguma, R.; Ali, S.F.; et al. The Prolactin Family Hormones Regulate Vascular Tone through NO and Prostacyclin Production in Isolated Rat Aortic Rings. *Acta Pharmacol. Sin.* **2015**, *36*, 572–586. [CrossRef]
90. Campión, J.; Maestro, B.; Calle, C.; Dávila, N.; Barceló, B. Receptor de La Hormona de Crecimiento Humano: Características Estructurales, Estudio de Su Expresión y Regulación Génica. *Endocrinol. Nutr.* **1999**, *46*, 235–240.
91. Caicedo, D.; Devesa, P.; Arce, V.M.; Requena, J.; Devesa, J. Chronic Limb-Threatening Ischemia Could Benefit from Growth Hormone Therapy for Wound Healing and Limb Salvage. *Ther. Adv. Cardiovasc. Dis.* **2017**, 1–20. [CrossRef]
92. Heil, M.; Schaper, W. Insights into Pathways of Arteriogenesis. *Curr. Pharm. Biotechnol.* **2007**, *8*, 35–42. [CrossRef] [PubMed]
93. Meazza, C.; Pagani, S.; Travaglino, P.; Bozzola, M. Effect of Growth Hormone (GH) on the Immune System. *Pediatr. Endocrinol. Rev.* **2004**, *1*, 490–495. [PubMed]
94. Fasshauer, M.; Klein, J.; Kralisch, S.; Klier, M.; Lossner, U.; Bluher, M.; Paschke, R. Monocyte Chemoattractant Protein 1 Expression Is Stimulated by Growth Hormone and Interleukin-6 in 3T3-L1 Adipocytes. *Biochem. Biophys. Res. Commun.* **2004**, *317*, 598–604. [CrossRef] [PubMed]

95. Van der Laan, A.; Piek, J.; Van Royen, N. Collateral Artery Growth in Man, from Assesment to Stimulation. In *Arteriogenesis—Molecular Regulation, Pathophysiology and Therapeutics I*; Deindl, E., Schaper, W., Eds.; Shaker Verlag: Aachen, Germany, 2011; pp. 167–175.
96. Shireman, P.K.; Contreras-Shannon, V.; Reyes-Reyna, S.M.; Robinson, S.C.; McManus, L.M. MCP-1 Parallels Inflammatory and Regenerative Responses in Ischemic Muscle. *J. Surg. Res.* **2006**, *134*, 145–157. [CrossRef] [PubMed]
97. Hansen, T.K.; Fisker, S.; Dall, R.; Ledet, T.; Jørgensen, J.O.L.; Rasmussen, L.M. Growth Hormone Increases Vascular Cell Adhesion Molecule 1 Expression: In Vivo and In Vitro Evidence. *J. Clin. Endocrinol. Metab.* **2004**, *89*, 909–916. [CrossRef] [PubMed]
98. Sun, W.; Yu, W.-Y.; Yu, D.-J.; Zhao, T.-L.; Wu, L.-J.; Han, W.-Y. The Effects of Recombinant Human Growth Hormone (RHGH) on Survival of Slender Narrow Pedicle Flap and Expressions of Vascular Endothelial Growth Factor (VEGF) and Classification Determinant 34 (CD34). *Eur. Rev. Med. Pharmacol. Sci.* **2018**, *22*, 771–777. [CrossRef]
99. Nielsen, J.S.; McNagny, K.M. Novel Functions of the CD34 Family. *J. Cell Sci.* **2008**, *121*, 3683–3692. [CrossRef] [PubMed]
100. van der Klaauw, A.A.; Pereira, A.M.; Rabelink, T.J.; Corssmit, E.P.M.; Zonneveld, A.-J.; Pijl, H.; de Boer, H.C.; Smit, J.W.A.; Romijn, J.A.; de Koning, E.J.P. Recombinant Human GH Replacement Increases CD34+ Cells and Improves Endothelial Function in Adults with GH Deficiency. *Eur. J. Endocrinol.* **2008**, *159*, 105–111. [CrossRef]
101. Kiess, W.; Butenandt, O. Specific Growth Hormone Receptors on Human Peripheral Mononuclear Cells: Reexpression, Identification, and Characterization. *J. Clin. Endocrinol. Metab.* **1985**, *60*, 740–746. [CrossRef]
102. Bresson, J.L.; Jeay, S.; Gagnerault, M.C.; Kayser, C.; Beressi, N.; Wu, Z.; Kinet, S.; Dardenne, M.; Postel-Vinay, M.C. Growth Hormone (GH) and Prolactin Receptors in Human Peripheral Blood Mononuclear Cells: Relation with Age and GH-Binding Protein. *Endocrinology* **1999**, *140*, 3203–3209. [CrossRef]
103. Hattori, N. Expression, Regulation and Biological Actions of Growth Hormone (GH) and Ghrelin in the Immune System. *Growth Horm. IGF Res.* **2009**, *19*, 187–197. [CrossRef]
104. Stuart, C.; Meehan, R.; Neale, L.; Cintron, N.; Furlanetto, R. Insulin-Like Growth Factor-I Binds Selectively to Human Peripheral Blood Monocytes and B-Lymphocytes*. *J. Clin. Endocrinol. Metab.* **1991**, *72*, 1117–1122. [CrossRef]
105. Arkins, S.; Rebeiz, N.; Biragyn, A.; Reese, D.L.; Kelley, K.W. Murine Macrophages Express Abundant Insulin-Like Growth Factor-I Class I Ea and Eb Transcripts. *Endocrinology* **1993**, *133*, 2334–2343. [CrossRef] [PubMed]
106. Lehoux, S.; Castier, Y.; Tedgui, A. Molecular Mechanisms of the Vascular Responses to Haemodynamic Forces. *J. Intern. Med.* **2006**, *259*, 381–392. [CrossRef]
107. Yang, H. Effect of Aging on Angiogenesis and Arteriogenesis. *Curr. Cardiol. Rev.* **2007**, *3*, 65–74. [CrossRef]
108. Hellingman, A.; Seghers, L.; Quax, P.; Van Weel, V. Bone Marrow Derived Cells in Artriogenesis: A Crucial Role for Leukocytes. In *Arteriogenesis—Molecular Regulation, Pathophysiology and Therapeutics I*; Deindl, E., Scahper, W., Eds.; Shaker Verlag: Aachen, Germany, 2011; pp. 145–150.
109. Wiedermann, C.J.; Reinisch, N.; Kähler, C.; Geisen, F.; Zilian, U.; Herold, M.; Braunsteiner, H. In Vivo Activation of Circulating Monocytes by Exogenous Growth Hormone in Man. *Brain Behav. Immun.* **1992**, *6*, 387–393. [CrossRef]
110. Zhu, T.; Goh, E.L.K.; LeRoith, D.; Lobie, P.E. Growth Hormone Stimulates the Formation of a Multiprotein Signaling Complex Involving P130(Cas) and CrkII: Resultant Activation of c-Jun N-Terminal Kinase/Stress-Activated Protein Kinase (JNK/SAPK). *J. Biol. Chem.* **1998**, *273*, 33864–33875. [CrossRef] [PubMed]
111. Tanaka, S.; Ouchi, T.; Hanafusa, H. Downstream of Crk Adaptor Signaling Pathway: Activation of Jun Kinase by v-Crk through the Guanine Nucleotide Exchange Protein C3G. *Proc. Natl. Acad. Sci. USA* **1997**, *94*, 2356–2361. [CrossRef]
112. Wiktor-Jedrzejczak, W.; Urbanowska, E.; Aukerman, S.L.; Pollard, J.W.; Stanley, E.R.; Ralph, P.; Ansari, A.A.; Sell, K.W.; Szperl, M. Correction by CSF-1 of Defects in the Osteopetrotic Op/Op Mouse Suggests Local, Developmental, and Humoral Requirements for This Growth Factor. *Exp. Hematol.* **1991**, *19*, 1049–1054.
113. Baxter, J.; Blalock, J.; Weigent, D. Characterization of Immunoreactive Insulin-Like Growth Factor-I from Leukocytes and Its Regulation by Growth Hormone*. *Endocrinology* **1991**, *129*, 1727–1734. [CrossRef]

114. Gow, D.J.; Sester, D.P.; Hume, D.A. CSF-1, IGF-1, and the Control of Postnatal Growth and Development. *J. Leukoc. Biol.* **2010**, *88*, 475–481. [CrossRef]
115. Hume, D.A.; Halpin, D.; Charlton, H.; Gordon, S. The Mononuclear Phagocyte System of the Mouse Defined by Immunohistochemical Localization of Antigen F4/80: Macrophages of Endocrine Organs. *Proc. Natl. Acad. Sci. USA* **1984**, *81*, 4174–4177. [CrossRef]
116. Park, B.; Hoffman, A.; Yang, Y.; Yan, J.; Tie, G.; Bagshahi, H.; Nowicki, P.T.; Messina, L.M. Endothelial Nitric Oxide Synthase Affects Both Early and Late Collateral Arterial Adaptation and Blood Flow Recovery after Induction of Hind Limb Ischemia in Mice. *J. Vasc. Surg.* **2010**, *51*, 165–173. [CrossRef] [PubMed]
117. González, D.; Tamay, F.; Álvarez, S.; Mendieta, J. Current Advances in the Biochemical and Physiological Aspects of the Treatment of Type 2 Diabetes Mellitus with Thiazolidinediones. *PPAR Res.* **2016**, *2016*, 14–17. [CrossRef]
118. Prior, B.M.; Lloyd, P.G.; Ren, J.; Li, H.; Yang, H.T.; Laughlin, M.H.; Terjung, R.L. Time Course of Changes in Collateral Blood Flow and Isolated Vessel Size and Gene Expression after Femoral Artery Occlusion in Rats. *Am. J. Physiol. Circ. Physiol.* **2004**, *287*, H2434–H2447. [CrossRef] [PubMed]
119. Mees, B.; Wagner, S.; Ninci, E.; Tribulova, S.; Martin, S.; Van Haperen, R.; Kostin, S.; Heil, M.; De Crom, R.; Schaper, W. Endothelial Nitric Oxide Synthase Activity Is Essential for Vasodilation during Blood Flow Recovery but Not for Arteriogenesis. *Arterioscler. Thromb. Vasc. Biol.* **2007**, *27*, 1926–1933. [CrossRef]
120. Unthank, J.; Haas, T.L.; Miller, S. Impact of Shear Level and Cardiovascular Risk Factors on Bioavailable Nitric Oxide and Outward Vascular Remodeling in Mesenteric Arteries. In *Arteriogenesis-Molecular Regulation, Pathophysiology, and Therapeutics I*; Shaker Verlag Publishing: Aachen, Germany, 2011; No. May 2014; pp. 89–119.
121. Stasch, J.P.; Schmidt, P.M.; Nedvetsky, P.I.; Nedvetskaya, T.Y.; Arun Kumar, H.S.; Meurer, S.; Deile, M.; Taye, A.; Knorr, A.; Lapp, H.; et al. Targeting the Heme-Oxidized Nitric Oxide Receptor for Selective Vasodilatation of Diseased Blood Vessels. *J. Clin. Investig.* **2006**, *116*, 2552–2561. [CrossRef]
122. Gladwin, M.T. Deconstructing Endothelial Dysfunction: Soluble Guanylyl Cyclase Oxidation and the NO Resistance Syndrome. *J. Clin. Investig.* **2006**, *116*, 2330–2332. [CrossRef]
123. Bauersachs, J.; Bouloumié, A.; Mülsch, A.; Wiemer, G.; Fleming, I.; Busse, R. Vasodilator Dysfunction in Aged Spontaneously Hypertensive Rats: Changes in NO Synthase III and Soluble Guanylyl Cyclase Expression, and in Superoxide Anion Production. *Cardiovasc. Res.* **1998**, *37*, 772–779. [CrossRef]
124. Bir, S.C.; Kolluru, G.K.; Fang, K.; Kevil, C.G. Redox Balance Dynamically Regulates Vascular Growth and Remodeling. In *Seminars in Cell and Developmental Biology*; Elsevier Ltd.: Amsterdam, The Netherlands, 2012; pp. 745–757. [CrossRef]
125. Gardner, A.W.; Parker, D.E.; Montgomery, P.S.; Sosnowska, D.; Casanegra, A.I.; Esponda, O.L.; Ungvari, Z.; Csiszar, A.; Sonntag, W.E. Impaired Vascular Endothelial Growth Factor A and Inflammation in Patients with Peripheral Artery Disease. *Angiology* **2014**, *65*, 683–690. [CrossRef]
126. Maekawa, Y.; Ishikawa, K.; Yasuda, O.; Oguro, R.; Hanasaki, H.; Kida, I.; Takemura, Y.; Ohishi, M.; Katsuya, T.; Rakugi, H. Klotho Suppresses TNF-Alpha-Induced Expression of Adhesion Molecules in the Endothelium and Attenuates NF-KappaB Activation. *Endocrine* **2009**, *35*, 341–346. [CrossRef]
127. Yi, C.; Cao, Y.; Mao, S.H.; Liu, H.; Ji, L.L.; Xu, S.Y.; Zhang, M.; Huang, Y. Recombinant Human Growth Hormone Improves Survival and Protects against Acute Lung Injury in Murine Staphylococcus Aureus Sepsis. *Inflamm. Res.* **2009**, *58*, 855–862. [CrossRef]
128. Adamopoulos, S. Effects of Growth Hormone on Circulating Cytokine Network, and Left Ventricular Contractile Performance and Geometry in Patients with Idiopathic Dilated Cardiomyopathy. *Eur. Heart J.* **2003**, *24*, 2186–2196. [CrossRef]
129. Masternak, M.M.; Bartke, A. Growth Hormone, Inflammation and Aging. *Pathobiol. Aging Age-Relat. Dis.* **2012**, *2*, 17293. [CrossRef]
130. Rentrop, K.P.; Feit, F.; Sherman, W.; Thornton, J.C. Serial Angiographic Assessment of Coronary Artery Obstruction and Collateral Flow in Acute Myocardial Infarction. Report from the Second Mount Sinai-New York University Reperfusion Trial. *Circulation* **1989**, *80*, 1166–1175. [CrossRef]
131. Piek, J.J.; van Liebergen, R.A.; Koch, K.T.; Peters, R.J.G.; David, G.K. Clinical, Angiographic and Hemodynamic Predictors of Recruitable Collateral Flow Assessed During Balloon Angioplasty Coronary Occlusion. *J. Am. Coll. Cardiol.* **1997**, *29*, 275–282. [CrossRef]

132. Yang, Y.; Tang, G.; Yan, J.; Park, B.; Hoffman, A.; Tie, G.; Messina, L.M. Cellular and Molecular Mechanism Regulating Blood Flow Recovery in Acute versus Gradual Femoral Artery Occlusion Are Distinct in the Mouse. *J. Vasc. Surg.* **2009**, *48*, 1546–1558. [CrossRef] [PubMed]
133. Rabinovsky, E.D.; Draghia-Akli, R. Insulin-Like Growth Factor I Plasmid Therapy Promotes In Vivo Angiogenesis. *Mol. Ther.* **2004**, *9*, 46–55. [CrossRef]
134. Kusano, K.; Tsutsumi, Y.; Dean, J.; Gavin, M.; Ma, H.; Silver, M.; Thorne, T.; Zhu, Y.; Losordo, D.W.; Aikawa, R. Long-Term Stable Expression of Human Growth Hormone by RAAV Promotes Myocardial Protection Post-Myocardial Infarction. *J. Mol. Cell. Cardiol.* **2007**, *42*, 390–399. [CrossRef] [PubMed]
135. Dobruckia, L.W.; Tsutsumib, Y.; Kalinowskia, L.; Deanb, J.; Gavinb, M.; Senb, S.; Mendizabald, M.; Sinusasa, A.J.; Aikawab, R. Analysis of Angiogenesis Induced by Local IGF-1 Expression after Myocardial Infarction Using MicroSPECT-CT Imaging. *J. Mol. Cell. Cardiol.* **2009**, *6*, 247–253. [CrossRef]
136. Pelisek, J.; Shimizu, M.; Nikol, S. Differential Developmental Origin of Arteries: Impact on Angiogenesis and Arteriogenesis. *Med. Chem. Rev.-Online* **2004**, *1*, 317–326. [CrossRef]
137. Palmer-Kazen, U.; Wariaro, D.; Luo, F.; Wahlberg, E. Vascular Endothelial Cell Growth Factor and Fibroblast Growth Factor 2 Expression in Patients with Critical Limb Ischemia. *J. Vasc. Surg.* **2004**, *39*, 621–628. [CrossRef]
138. Rissanen, T.T.; Vajanto, I.; Hiltunen, M.O.; Rutanen, J.; Kettunen, M.I.; Niemi, M.; Leppänen, P.; Turunen, M.P.; Markkanen, J.E.; Arve, K.; et al. Expression of Vascular Endothelial Growth Factor and Vascular Endothelial Growth Factor Receptor-2 (KDR/Flk-1) in Ischemic Skeletal Muscle and Its Regeneration. *Am. J. Pathol.* **2002**, *160*, 1393–1403. [CrossRef]
139. Klinnikova, M.G.; Bakarev, M.A.; Nikityuk, D.B.; Lushnikova, E.L. Immunohistochemical Study of the Expression of Vascular Endothelial Growth Factor Receptor-2 (KDR/Flk-1) during Myocardial Infarction. *Bull. Exp. Biol. Med.* **2017**, *163*, 500–505. [CrossRef] [PubMed]
140. Lasch, M.; Kleinert, E.C.; Meister, S.; Kumaraswami, K.; Buchheim, J.-I.; Grantzow, T.; Lautz, T.; Salpisti, S.; Fischer, S.; Troidl, K.; et al. Extracellular RNA Released Due to Shear Stress Controls Natural Bypass Growth by Mediating Mechanotransduction in Mice. *Blood* **2019**, *134*, 1469–1479. [CrossRef] [PubMed]
141. Chillo, O.; Kleinert, E.C.; Lautz, T.; Lasch, M.; Pagel, J.I.; Heun, Y.; Troidl, K.; Fischer, S.; Caballero-Martinez, A.; Mauer, A.; et al. Perivascular Mast Cells Govern Shear Stress-Induced Arteriogenesis by Orchestrating Leukocyte Function. *Cell Rep.* **2016**, *16*, 2197–2207. [CrossRef] [PubMed]
142. Di Lorenzo, A.; Lin, M.I.; Murata, T.; Landskroner-Eiger, S.; Schleicher, M.; Kothiya, M.; Iwakiri, Y.; Yu, J.; Huang, P.L.; Sessa, W.C. ENOS-Derived Nitric Oxide Regulates Endothelial Barrier Function through VE-Cadherin and Rho GTPases. *J. Cell Sci.* **2013**, *126* (Pt 24), 5541–5552. [CrossRef]
143. Lee, Y.; Kim, J.M.; Lee, E.J. Functional Expression of CXCR4 in Somatotrophs: CXCL12 Activates GH Gene, GH Production and Secretion, and Cellular Proliferation. *J. Endocrinol.* **2008**, *199*, 191–199. [CrossRef]
144. Barbieri, F.; Bajetto, A.; Porcile, C.; Pattarozzi, A.; Schettini, G.; Florio, T. Role of Stromal Cell-Derived Factor 1 (SDF1/CXCL12) in Regulating Anterior Pituitary Function. *J. Mol. Endocrinol.* **2007**, *38*, 383–389. [CrossRef]
145. Smaniotto, S.; Martins-Neto, A.A.; Dardenne, M.; Savino, W. Growth Hormone Is a Modulator of Lymphocyte Migration. *Neuroimmunomodulation* **2011**, *18*, 309–313. [CrossRef] [PubMed]
146. Bolamperti, S.; Guidobono, F.; Rubinacci, A.; Villa, I. The Role of Growth Hormone in Mesenchymal Stem Cell Commitment. *Int. J. Mol. Sci.* **2019**, *20*, 5264. [CrossRef]
147. Zhang, B.; Adesanya, T.M.A.; Zhang, L.; Xie, N.; Chen, Z.; Fu, M.; Zhang, J.; Zhang, J.; Tan, T.; Kilic, A.; et al. Delivery of Placenta-Derived Mesenchymal Stem Cells Ameliorates Ischemia Induced Limb Injury by Immunomodulation. *Cell. Physiol. Biochem.* **2014**, *34*, 1998–2006. [CrossRef]
148. Katare, R.; Riu, F.; Rowlinson, J.; Lewis, A.; Holden, R.; Meloni, M.; Reni, C.; Wallrapp, C.; Emanueli, C.; Madeddu, P. Perivascular Delivery of Encapsulated Mesenchymal Stem Cells Improves Postischemic Angiogenesis Via Paracrine Activation of VEGF-A. *Arterioscler. Thromb. Vasc. Biol.* **2013**, *33*, 1872–1880. [CrossRef] [PubMed]
149. Laurila, J.P.; Laatikainen, L.; Castellone, M.D.; Trivedi, P.; Heikkila, J.; Hinkkanen, A.; Hematti, P.; Laukkanen, M.O. Human Embryonic Stem Cell-Derived Mesenchymal Stromal Cell Transplantation in a Rat Hind Limb Injury Model. *Cytotherapy* **2009**, *11*, 726–737. [CrossRef] [PubMed]
150. Giordano, A.; Galderisi, U.; Marino, I.R. From the Laboratory Bench to the Patient's Bedside: An Update on Clinical Trials with Mesenchymal Stem Cells. *J. Cell. Physiol.* **2007**, *211*, 27–35. [CrossRef] [PubMed]

151. Werther, G.A.; Haynes, K.; Waters, M.J. Growth Hormone (GH) Receptors Are Expressed on Human Fetal Mesenchymal Tissues—Identification of Messenger Ribonucleic Acid and GH-Binding Protein. *J. Clin. Endocrinol. Metab.* **1993**, *76*, 1638–1646. [CrossRef] [PubMed]
152. Noiseux, N.; Gnecchi, M.; Lopez-Ilasaca, M.; Zhang, L.; Solomon, S.D.; Deb, A.; Dzau, V.J.; Pratt, R.E. Mesenchymal Stem Cells Overexpressing Akt Dramatically Repair Infarcted Myocardium and Improve Cardiac Function despite Infrequent Cellular Fusion or Differentiation. *Mol. Ther.* **2006**, *14*, 840–850. [CrossRef] [PubMed]
153. Olarescu, N.C.; Berryman, D.E.; Householder, L.A.; Lubbers, E.R.; List, E.O.; Benencia, F.; Kopchick, J.J.; Bollerslev, J. GH Action Influences Adipogenesis of Mouse Adipose Tissue-Derived Mesenchymal Stem Cells. *J. Endocrinol.* **2015**, *226*, 13–23. [CrossRef]
154. Bolamperti, S.; Signo, M.; Spinello, A.; Moro, G.; Fraschini, G.; Guidobono, F.; Rubinacci, A.; Villa, I. GH Prevents Adipogenic Differentiation of Mesenchymal Stromal Stem Cells Derived from Human Trabecular Bone via Canonical Wnt Signaling. *Bone* **2018**, *112*, 136–144. [CrossRef] [PubMed]
155. Scholz, D.; Ito, W.; Fleming, I.; Deindl, E.; Sauer, A.; Wiesnet, M.; Busse, R.; Schaper, J.; Schaper, W. Ultrastructure and Molecular Histology of Rabbit Hind-Limb Collateral Artery Growth (Arteriogenesis). *Virchows Arch.* **2000**, *436*, 257–270. [CrossRef]
156. Messias de Lima, C.F.; Dos Santos Reis, M.D.; da Silva Ramos, F.W.; Ayres-Martins, S.; Smaniotto, S. Growth Hormone Modulates In Vitro Endothelial Cell Migration and Formation of Capillary-Like Structures. *Cell Biol. Int.* **2017**, *41*, 577–584. [CrossRef]
157. Erikstrup, C.; Pedersen, L.M.; Heickendorff, L.; Ledet, T.; Rasmussen, L.M. Production of Hyaluronan and Chondroitin Sulphate Proteoglycans from Human Arterial Smooth Muscle—The Effect of Glucose, Insulin, IGF-I or Growth Hormone. *Eur. J. Endocrinol.* **2001**, *145*, 193–198. [CrossRef]
158. Cen, Y.; Liu, J.; Qin, Y.; Liu, R.; Wang, H.; Zhou, Y.; Wang, S.; Hu, Z. Denervation in Femoral Artery-Ligated Hindlimbs Diminishes Ischemic Recovery Primarily via Impaired Arteriogenesis. *PLoS ONE* **2016**, *11*, e0154941. [CrossRef] [PubMed]
159. Sverrisdottir, Y.B.; Elam, M.; Herlitz, H.; Bengtsson, B.A.; Johannsson, G. Intense Sympathetic Nerve Activity in Adults with Hypopituitarism and Untreated Growth Hormone Deficiency. *J. Clin. Endocrinol. Metab.* **1998**, *83*, 1881–1885. [CrossRef]
160. Sverrisdóttir, Y.B.; Elam, M.; Caidahl, K.; Söderling, A.-S.; Herlitz, H.; Johannsson, G. The Effect of Growth Hormone (GH) Replacement Therapy on Sympathetic Nerve Hyperactivity in Hypopituitary Adults: A Double-Blind, Placebo-Controlled, Crossover, Short-Term Trial Followed by Long-Term Open GH Replacement in Hypopituitary Adults. *J. Hypertens.* **2003**, *21*, 1905–1914. [CrossRef]
161. Martínez-Nieves, B.; Dunbar, J.C. Vascular Dilatatory Responses to Sodium Nitroprusside (SNP) and Alpha-Adrenergic Antagonism in Female and Male Normal and Diabetic Rats. *Proc. Soc. Exp. Biol. Med.* **1999**, *222*, 90–98. [CrossRef] [PubMed]
162. Ruiter, M.S.; van Golde, J.M.; Schaper, N.C.; Stehouwer, C.D.; Huijberts, M.S. Diabetes Impairs Arteriogenesis in the Peripheral Circulation: Review of Molecular Mechanisms. *Clin. Sci. (Lond.)* **2010**, *119*, 225–238. [CrossRef] [PubMed]
163. Meusel, M.; Herrmann, M.; Machleidt, F.; Franzen, K.F.; Krapalis, A.F.; Sayk, F. GHRH-Mediated GH Release Is Associated with Sympathoactivation and Baroreflex Resetting: A Microneurographic Study in Healthy Humans. *Am. J. Physiol. Regul. Integr. Comp. Physiol.* **2019**, *317*, R15–R24. [CrossRef]
164. Lautz, T.; Lasch, M.; Borgolte, J.; Troidl, K.; Pagel, J.-I.; Caballero-Martinez, A.; Kleinert, E.C.; Walzog, B.; Deindl, E. Midkine Controls Arteriogenesis by Regulating the Bioavailability of Vascular Endothelial Growth Factor A and the Expression of Nitric Oxide Synthase 1 and 3. *EBioMedicine* **2018**, *27*, 237–246. [CrossRef]
165. Fujiwara, K.; Maliza, R.; Tofrizal, A.; Batchuluun, K.; Ramadhani, D.; Tsukada, T.; Azuma, M.; Horiguchi, K.; Kikuchi, M.; Yashiro, T. In Situ Hybridization Analysis of the Temporospatial Expression of the Midkine/Pleiotrophin Family in Rat Embryonic Pituitary Gland. *Cell Tissue Res.* **2014**, *357*, 337–344. [CrossRef]
166. Fujiwara, K.; Horiguchi, K.; Maliza, R.; Tofrizal, A.; Batchuluun, K.; Ramadhani, D.; Syaidah, R.; Tsukada, T.; Azuma, M.; Kikuchi, M.; et al. Expression of the Heparin-Binding Growth Factor Midkine and Its Receptor, Ptprz1, in Adult Rat Pituitary. *Cell Tissue Res.* **2015**, *359*, 909–914. [CrossRef]
167. Mulvany, M. Vascular Remodelling of Resistance Vessels: Can We Define This? *Cardiovasc. Res.* **1999**, *41*, 9–13. [CrossRef]

168. Weckbach, L.; Preissner, K.; Deindl, E. The Role of Midkine in Arteriogenesis, Involving Mechanosensing, Endothelial Cell Proliferation, and Vasodilation. *Int. J. Mol. Sci.* **2018**, *19*, 2559. [CrossRef] [PubMed]
169. Schmid, C.; Neidert, M.C.; Tschopp, O.; Sze, L.; Bernays, R.L. Growth Hormone and Klotho. *J. Endocrinol.* **2013**, *219*, R37–R57. [CrossRef] [PubMed]
170. Kuro-o, M.; Matsumura, Y.; Aizawa, H.; Kawaguchi, H.; Suga, T.; Utsugi, T.; Ohyama, Y.; Kurabayashi, M.; Kaname, T.; Kume, E.; et al. Mutation of the Mouse Klotho Gene Leads to a Syndrome Resembling Ageing. *Nature* **1997**, *390*, 45–51. [CrossRef] [PubMed]
171. Xu, Y.; Sun, Z. Molecular Basis of Klotho: From Gene to Function in Aging. *Endocr. Rev.* **2015**. [CrossRef] [PubMed]
172. Rubinek, T.; Modan-Moses, D. Klotho and the Growth Hormone/Insulin-Like Growth Factor 1 Axis: Novel Insights into Complex Interactions. In *Vitamins and Hormones*; Academic Press: Cambridge, MA, USA, 2016; Volume 101, pp. 85–118. [CrossRef]
173. Chung, C.-P.; Chang, Y.-C.; Ding, Y.; Lim, K.; Liu, Q.; Zhu, L.; Zhang, W.; Lu, T.-S.; Molostvov, G.; Zehnder, D.; et al. α-Klotho Expression Determines Nitric Oxide Synthesis in Response to FGF-23 in Human Aortic Endothelial Cells. *PLoS ONE* **2017**, *12*, e0176817. [CrossRef] [PubMed]
174. Kurosu, H. Suppression of Aging in Mice by the Hormone Klotho. *Science* **2005**, *309*, 1829–1833. [CrossRef]
175. Kusaba, T.; Okigaki, M.; Matui, A.; Murakami, M.; Ishikawa, K.; Kimura, T.; Sonomura, K.; Adachi, Y.; Shibuya, M.; Shirayama, T.; et al. Klotho Is Associated with VEGF Receptor-2 and the Transient Receptor Potential Canonical-1 Ca2+ Channel to Maintain Endothelial Integrity. *Proc. Natl. Acad. Sci. USA* **2010**, *107*, 19308–19313. [CrossRef]
176. Six, I.; Okazaki, H.; Gross, P.; Cagnard, J.; Boudot, C.; Maizel, J.; Drueke, T.B.; Massy, Z.A. Direct, Acute Effects of Klotho and FGF23 on Vascular Smooth Muscle and Endothelium. *PLoS ONE* **2014**, *9*. [CrossRef]

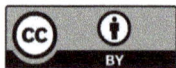

© 2020 by the authors. Licensee MDPI, Basel, Switzerland. This article is an open access article distributed under the terms and conditions of the Creative Commons Attribution (CC BY) license (http://creativecommons.org/licenses/by/4.0/).

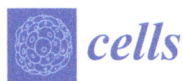

Review

Exercise-Induced Vascular Adaptations under Artificially Versus Pathologically Reduced Blood Flow: A Focus Review with Special Emphasis on Arteriogenesis

Johanna Vogel [1], Daniel Niederer [1], Georg Jung [2] and Kerstin Troidl [2,3,*]

1. Department of Sports Medicine and Exercise Physiology, Goethe University Frankfurt/Main, Ginnheimer Landstr. 39, 60487 Frankfurt, Germany; johvogel@em.uni-frankfurt.de (J.V.); niederer@sport.uni-frankfurt.de (D.N.)
2. Department of Vascular and Endovascular Surgery, University Hospital Frankfurt, Theodor-Stern-Kai 7, 60590 Frankfurt, Germany; Georg.Jung@kgu.de
3. Department of Pharmacology, Max-Planck-Institute for Heart and Lung Research, Ludwigstrasse 43, 61231 Bad Nauheim, Germany
* Correspondence: Kerstin.Troidl@mpi-bn.mpg.de

Received: 20 December 2019; Accepted: 30 January 2020; Published: 31 January 2020

Abstract: Background: The vascular effects of training under blood flow restriction (BFR) in healthy persons can serve as a model for the exercise mechanism in lower extremity arterial disease (LEAD) patients. Both mechanisms are, inter alia, characterized by lower blood flow in the lower limbs. We aimed to describe and compare the underlying mechanism of exercise-induced effects of disease- and external application-BFR methods. Methods: We completed a narrative focus review after systematic literature research. We included only studies on healthy participants or those with LEAD. Both male and female adults were considered eligible. The target intervention was exercise with a reduced blood flow due to disease or external application. Results: We identified 416 publications. After the application of inclusion and exclusion criteria, 39 manuscripts were included in the vascular adaption part. Major mechanisms involving exercise-mediated benefits in treating LEAD included: inflammatory processes suppression, proinflammatory immune cells, improvement of endothelial function, remodeling of skeletal muscle, and additional vascularization (arteriogenesis). Mechanisms resulting from external BFR application included: increased release of anabolic growth factors, stimulated muscle protein synthesis, higher concentrations of heat shock proteins and nitric oxide synthase, lower levels in myostatin, and stimulation of S6K1. Conclusions: A main difference between the two comparators is the venous blood return, which is restricted in BFR but not in LEAD. Major similarities include the overall ischemic situation, the changes in microRNA (miRNA) expression, and the increased production of NOS with their associated arteriogenesis after training with BFR.

Keywords: lower extremity arterial disease; peripheral arterial disease; blood flow restriction; activity-based benefits; training effects; effect mechanism

1. Introduction

Of all deaths caused by major non-communicable diseases (coronary disease, type 2 diabetes, breast, and colon cancer), a considerable share of up to 10 percent results from physical inactivity [1]. That results in 5.3 million out of 57 million deaths worldwide per year [1]. Approximately one-third of the global population does not fulfil the minimum requirements for physical activity to maintain health [2,3]. However, retrospective studies have suggested that regular physical activity is associated with a lower risk of cardiovascular mortality and morbidity [4,5]. Prospective studies provide direct evidence that adopting a physically active lifestyle delays all-cause mortality, extends longevity [6], and reduces risk for cardiovascular mortality by 42 to 44 percent [7,8]. Several vascular diseases such as arteriosclerosis, thrombosis, embolic diseases, accidental vascular damages, or dissections are known risk factors for LEAD [9]. Beyond that, smoking, diabetes, dyslipidemia, hypertension, and, in particular, physical inactivity are major risk factors for LEAD [10,11]. Exercising and physical activity are, thus, of great relevance in the context of LEAD.

Peripheral arterial disease is characterized by limited blood flow through the arteries supplying the (usually lower) extremities. Peripheral arterial disease commonly refers to stenosis or occlusion of the peripheral arteries. The global prevalence was estimated to be 202 million [11]. Approximately 30 percent of these individuals suffer from intermittent claudication and subsequent impairment of mobility [12]. Major assessable impacts include impaired performance in lower extremity performance tests and, due to its effect on everyday activities, a significant impairment of health-related quality of life [13,14]. The walking performance of these patients is 50 percent or less lower [15]. In addition, a lower peak oxygen uptake is approximately 50 percent lower in patients with intermittent claudication as compared with the normal population [15]. There is clear evidence that supervised exercise therapies aimed at improving lower extremity performance, including supervised exercise programs, home-based walking interventions, and resistance training, improve lower limb symptoms and quality of life among LEAD patients [13,14,16]. The training is effective if it takes place at least two times per week over a period of three months [17]. A single training session should be approximately 45 min to achieve cardiovascular adjustments [13]. A well-established screening tool for individuals with LEAD, even when it is still in a mild asymptomatic state, is the measurement of ankle-brachial index (ABI). In order to diagnose most individuals with LEAD, regular measurements of the ankle-brachial index (ABI) in the whole population starting at an age of about 40 years seem to be useful [18].

The clinical manifestation and the clinical course of LEAD are heterogenous. Symptoms of varying severity occur depending on the degree of stenosis and insufficiency of blood (i.e., oxygen) supply to the distal tissues [19]. At a low grade of stenosis, LEAD usually remains clinically asymptomatic and individuals do not have any adverse effects in their everyday activities. As the disease progresses, LEAD is characterized by leg pain, induced during exercise or when walking (intermittent claudication) [20]. At a higher grade of LEAD, the patients suffer from resting pain in the affected leg, and in end stage from ulceration and gangrene of the foot (critical limb ischemia) [20]. Peripheral arterial disease is a major cause of decreased mobility, functional capacity, quality of life, and increases the risks of amputation or death [21,22]. This risk is triggered by the prevalence of atherosclerotic manifestations in the coronary and cerebral circulation [22,23]. That leads to a high cardiovascular mortality risk [24]. Therefore, the early identification and treatment of LEAD patients is one of the key elements in LEAD therapy. According to international guidelines, any patient suffering from LEAD should receive the best medical treatment (BMT), whereas in Fontaine stage I or IIA/B (Rutherford 1–3), conservative treatment by BMT and exercise training is recommended [10,25]. In higher stages of LEAD, surgical or interventional treatment could be indicated.

Skeletal muscle is constantly adapting to its environment [26]. It responds to stress by stimulating muscle development, and it responds to disuse with atrophy [27]. Traditional training methods use loads greater than 70 percent of one repetition maximum (1RM) to stimulate muscle hypertrophy [26,28]. This is not be safe for all patients and healthy people who are unable to tolerate high-load resistance due to stress, for example, placed on the joints and soft tissues. Therefore, there is adapted low-load resistance training that can also stimulate the anabolic pathway. This training method with lower loads, additionally, uses a blood flow restriction (BFR) to receive a similar stimulus than high-load training. The BFR is, thereby, artificially induced, usually by applying a blood pressure cuff. The cuff is attached at the origin of the target extremity (arms or legs). Low-load resistance training alone has not been shown to promote muscle development, but when combined with BFR, positive effects have been demonstrated to occur. A meta-analysis investigating 20 studies showed that low-load BFR training was more effective at increased muscle strength as compared with low-load training alone [29]. In healthy populations, training under reduced blood flow aims to reach low-loaded training effects comparable to those under high-loaded conditions. To achieve systematic effects during BFR, a resistance load lower than that in classic (resistance/strength) training without using BFR is used. An intensity of 20 percent of the one repetition maximum (the weight which can be moved once over the total range of motion, 1RM) and a reduced training time of about four to eight weeks have been demonstrated to have systematic effects on muscle hypertrophy and muscular strength [30]. More specifically, BFR training with a reduced load can lead to the same results as resistance training with significantly higher loads (at 65% 1RM) and longer intervention time. In particular, increases in muscle thickness and strength gains are comparable between these two strategies [31,32]. A wide variety of suggested, known, and potential mechanisms of how BFR during exercise leads to training benefits is given.

Both BFR and exercising with LEAD seems to elicit physical benefits over exercising effects solely and combined with the reduced blood flow. This makes BFR a promising model for studying exercise effects in LEAD patients without putting the vulnerable target population at an undue risk of (for example) adverse events. There is a multitude of known, potential, and suggested mechanisms of exercising during BFR or with LEAD, and therefore designing a study to prove one or more similarities or differences is of importance in order to collect and present all known mechanisms. This could lead, in a second step, to the selection of outcomes for experimental confirmatory studies.

Against this background, it is important (1) to identify the exercise-induced effects under both blood flow reduced conditions (disease vs. external application) and (2) to compare the underlying mechanism to point out differences and similarities. With this review on systematic reviews and original data publications, we aim to describe the current evidence of vascular adaption due to training under blood flow restriction.

2. Materials and Methods

This review adopts a narrative (focus) comparative design. A priori systematic literature research was performed to find and select suitable evidence. We followed up-to-date guidelines for systematic literature research.

2.1. Search Strategy

In July 2019, systematic literature research was performed. For that purpose, the peer review-based bibliographic database MEDLINE (PubMed) was used. Two investigators (JV, KT) independently searched for relevant primary and secondary analyses using the following predefined Boolean search syntax, especially adaptable to PubMed): ("peripheral arterial disease" [All Fields] OR "intermittent claudication" [All Fields] OR "blood flow restriction" [All Fields] OR "reduced blood flow" [All Fields]) AND ("effects" [All Fields] OR "exercise response" [All Fields] OR "mechanism" [All Fields] OR "vascular adaption" [All Fields]) AND ("training" [All Fields]). An initial exploratory electronic database search was conducted by the two reviewers to define the final search terms. Both reviewers independently conducted the main research afterwards. The herewith identified studies were screened for eligibility using (1) titles and (2) abstracts. The remaining full texts were assessed to ascertain whether they are fulfilling the inclusion and not fulfilling the exclusion criteria. The search was restricted to peer-review publications authored in English or German (publication date: 01.01.2010 to 02.07.2019). The references of all manuscripts included were screened for further sources with potential relevance for the review.

2.2. Participants' Inclusion Criteria

Both male and female adults (>18 years of age) were considered eligible. Participants had to be healthy or LEAD patients. On participant level, no further inclusion criteria were applied.

2.3. Study Inclusion Criteria

Primary and secondary data studies (RCTs, CTs, systematic reviews or meta-analyses, cohort and case-control studies) were considered eligible if they adopted an (exercise, training, physical activity, and movement) intervention that consisted of exercises without additional specific treatment. Position papers, consensus papers, letters to the editor, and editorials were excluded. Primary aim (of the studies to be included) had to be training with reduced blood flow due to disease or external superficial (non-invasive) application.

2.4. Study Selection

All studies initially found were individually screened for relevance. Final inclusion (or exclusion) into the review followed a standardized procedure: for each of the messages found in the literature, the publication with the highest level of evidence (Oxford Centre for Evidence-Based Medicine, Levels of Evidence) and the highest relevance was selected and included. The description of the results and findings were, thus, preferably selected from systematic reviews, randomized controlled trials, controlled trials, and cohort and case-control studies. The order followed a decrease in the evidence levels, starting from Level 1 (meta-analyses and systematic reviews on RCTs) downwards to Level 5 (narrative reviews and consensus papers). The relevance rating was conducted based on the special focus on vascular adaption and arteriogenesis. All types of controls were included; and no restrictions were undertaken for outcomes.

3. Results and Discussion

3.1. Study Selection

We identified 416 manuscripts. After inclusion and exclusion criteria application and study selection (evidence slope), $n = 39$ manuscripts were included in the vascular adaption part.

3.2. Evidence on LEAD and Exercise

As the major effect, exercise improves walking in patients with LEAD. More specifically, the walking distance until pain occurs and the maximum walking distance can be improved with exercise therapy. Beyond the general exercise effects, a variety of involved mechanisms for the effect of exercise on walking ability have been proposed in studies investigating exercise in populations exposed to LEAD risk factors such as suppression of inflammation, as shown by a decrease in circulating chemokines (interleukin (IL)-8 and monocyte chemoattractant protein-1) after endurance training [33]. A decrease in number of proinflammatory immune cells (leucocytes, monocytes, and neutrophils) has been observed in overweight participants [34,35].

Furthermore, an improvement in the endothelial function in hypertensive patients [36] was attributed to an improved endothelium-dependent vasorelaxation. The latter was triggered through an increase in the release of nitric oxide. A remodeling of the involved skeletal muscles during strength training in LEAD patients [37,38] affects not only muscle histology but also their metabolism. The remodeling characteristics in skeletal muscle are as follows: change in capillary density, alterations in the ratio of type I to type II muscle fibers, arteriogenesis, and increases in mitochondrial activity [37,39].

3.2.1. Neovascularization

Beyond that, physical training has the potential to promote neovascularization in hypoxic and ischemic tissues, such as in the myocardium or peripheral limbs [40,41]. Two forms of neovascularization can be distinguished, angiogenesis and arteriogenesis. Angiogenesis is driven by hypoxia and is usually characterized by the sprouting of newly formed capillaries [42]. Arteriogenesis is defined as the growth of functional collateral arteries from pre-existing arterio-arteriolar anastomoses [43]. The latter, arteriogenesis, can be induced by exercise, in humans [44–46], rats [46], and in mice [25,47]. A fluid shear stress-associated transient receptor potential cation channel, subfamily V, member 4 (trpv4) [48], turned out to be upregulated transiently after endurance training [46].

3.2.2. Fluid Shear Stress

The driving force of arteriogenesis is the altered fluid shear stress (FSS) in preformed collateral arteries. It is triggered by increased blood flow [49]. Although this FSS can be impacted by exercise training, the initiation of vascular remodeling and diameter growth [50] remains incomplete. The FSS, as well as the induction of related molecules, returned to baseline values already 6 h post exercise. A more frequent exercise to chronically increase FSS was proposed to be required for sufficient arteriogenesis to compensate for a peripheral occlusion [46].

Several mechano-sensors and transducers that convey the FSS message during collateral remodeling have been proposed. These include ion channels [51], the glycocalyx layer of endothelial cells (ECs) [52], and nitric oxide (NO) [53]. Recently, microRNAs (miRNAs) have also been proposed as potential factors to control the response of vascular cells to hemodynamic stress [54]. In addition, miRNAs can be secreted, and thereby can contribute to intercellular communication [55]. Hence, miRNAs have also been linked to FSS-induced arteriogenesis [56].

In addition, structural and functional adaptations of the vasculature can also be induced by exercise training in humans. These changes have been shown in young endurance athletes who presented larger diameters of the main conduit arteries of their trained limbs as compared with matched legs of untrained controls [44–46,57].

3.3. Evidence of BFR Exercise Effects

Although not finally delineated, some identical, some comparable, and some completely different vascular mechanisms for the effects of blood flow restriction exercises are known. The mechanisms of BFR exercise are based on the combination of two primary factors, metabolic and mechanical stress. These two factors act synergistically to signal a number of secondary mechanisms such as tissue hypoxia, metabolite formation, and cellular swelling, which, afterwards, stimulate autocrine and paracrine signaling pathways, ultimately leading to protein synthesis, type II muscle fiber recruitment, local and systemic anabolic hormone synthesis, and stimulation of myogenic stem cells [28].

3.3.1. Hypoxia

As a major effect, exercises under BFR reduce oxygen concentration, leading to hypoxia and, consequently, increase the number of metabolic products [58]. Mostly named as such are blood lactate and muscle cell lactate [58]. The blood lactate concentrations are significantly increased following low-intensity resistance training under ischemic conditions, such as BFR as compared with a performed exercise protocol under normal conditions [59]. Thereby, a pressure gradient is built which favors the flow of blood into the muscle fibers in the intracellular space [28]. The result is an increased cell volume which leads to altered cell structure and ultimately drives anabolic signal pathways. This cellular swelling supports the increased protein synthesis in many different cell types including muscle fibers [28,60]. Cell swelling can indicate muscle growth through the proliferation and fusion of satellite cells [61].

Tissue hypoxia can also trigger an increase in localized and systemic hormone synthesis. These effectors are likely to lead to an increased release of anabolic growth factors [58]. In training with BFR, the growth hormone levels are up to 290 times greater as compared with a matched control group that trained without vascular occlusion [59]. Consequently, training under BFR leads to skeletal muscle remodeling in connection with anabolic growth factors expression. Resistance training under BFR seems to stimulate 1.8 times greater muscle recruitment than volume-matched non-BFR strength trainings [59]. As a consequence thereof, muscle protein synthesis could be stimulated [62].

3.3.2. Vascular Adaption

The application of BFR also influences the vascular system supply by promoting post-exercise blood flow, oxygenation, and arteriogenesis. Here, an increase of angiogenetic and arteriogenetic factors after BFR trainings, such as vascular endothelial growth factor and hypoxia inducible factor 1 alpha [63], are commonly described. Additionally, an increase in protein biosynthesis, higher concentrations of heat shock proteins (HSP), and the enzyme nitric oxide synthase (NOS) are present in blood serum after BFR training [64]. Nitric oxide (NO) is an important cellular signaling molecule which is produced in high levels in muscle by neuronal NOS. The production of NO is connected with the mammalian target of rapamycin (mTOR) activation and, subsequently, with protein synthesis [65]. In practice, the role of NO in vasodilatation under ischemic conditions is increased as compared with normoxic conditions, which results in an upregulation of endothelial NOS (eNOS) [66]. BFR training evokes similar mechanisms of vascular adaption and promotes arteriogenesis, such as increased fluid shear stress as a consequence of a slowly progressing vascular stenosis does. One known process following arteriogenesis is "pruning", which means that the number of collateral arteries decreases after a certain level of arteriogenesis is reached and fluid shear stress decreases by self-limitation due to a diminishing pressure gradient. Similar phenomena occur after successful revascularization; collateral arteries shrink or disappear as the main blood flow is directed through the vascular reconstruction, e.g., a bypass. In this situation, the effect of BFR on vascular adaption remains unclear. With respect to the risk of mechanical damage to the reconstruction or its occlusion caused by reduced blood flow during the compression period, BFR is considered to be a potential therapeutic option in chronic PAD patients under conservative treatment. Furthermore, after revascularization, the potential benefit of BFR regarding vascular adaption is questionable.

3.3.3. Myostatin

All these pathways are additional potential exercise under-BFR mechanisms and are mostly accompanied by lower myostatin levels [64]. Previous research has shown that the expression of myostatin is reduced in response to BFR training and is associated with increased muscle mass and strength after eight weeks of resistance training with the BFR application [67]. As myostatin harms protein synthesis, lower levels thereof can lead to larger training effects. Furthermore, ribosomal protein S6 kinase beta-1 (S6K1) is stimulated under BFR after a single low-intensity strength training of the lower extremities (20% of 1RM, duration approximately four to five minutes) [62]. The S6K1 is involved in the regulation of mRNA translation and, again, may be an important contributor to muscular protein biosynthesis [62].

The mechanisms of how BFR leads to positive training effects are, conclusively, found in metabolic stress, ischemic hypoxia, and an increased expression of vascular endothelial growth factors [68], elicited by the training, BFR, or a combination of both. The increased fluid shear stress caused by ischemia and reperfusion between the repetitions and sets during the training intervention with BFR could be a stimulator for arteriogenesis [69,70]. The hemodynamic stimuli amplified by BFR lead to an increased release of endothelial NO synthase, among other responses [71]. Additionally, recent studies have shown that a single bout of strength training under BFR leads to changes in the miRNA expression profile [72]. So far, the parameters in animal and human studies to determine the mechanisms have only been identified by invasive measures such as muscle biopsies and whole blood samples. The exact mechanism of low-load training under BFR has not yet been finally clarified.

3.3.4. BFR and LEAD

Summarizing the findings, both exercising with LEAD and BFR share, inter alia, reduced blood flow, altered miRNA expression, and changes in the hemodynamic stimuli (e.g., fluid shear stress) as the main mechanisms of the adaptions to training. One of the main differences is the return of blood through the veins. When the blood flow is reduced via an external application (in BFR), the pressure on the veins increases, as well. That leads to a reduced backflow of the (venous) blood. At the same time, the transport of metabolic products is elicited by the applied reduced blood flow. This mechanism does not occur in LEAD. Furthermore, in LEAD, mitochondrial activity is increased. Under BFR (in training), myostatin levels decrease, whereas S6K1, heat shock proteins, surrounding tissue pressure, fast-twitch muscle fibers involvement, and venous blood flow increase. Both mechanisms (exercising with LEAD or under BFR application) have in common that blood and mucous cell lactate, nitric oxide synthase, miRNA, fluid shear stress, and VEGF concentrations are increased; hypoxia/ischemia is induced and the arterial blood flow is decreased. These micro and macro level adaptations lead to neovascularization (LEAD), a decrease of inflammatory processes, and expression of proinflammatory immune cells. Furthermore, the endothelial function is increased, the involved skeletal muscles are remodeled, and alterations in capillary density and in the ratio of type I to type II muscle fibers occur.

Despite considerable differences, there are, thus, many mechanisms that the two conditions have in common. Especially, the ischemic situation, the changes in miRNA expression, and the increased production of NOS, with their associated arteriogenesis after training with blood flow reduction, attract attention when comparing the underlying adaptation mechanisms to reduced blood flow applied via BFR or pathophysiologically via LEAD. An overview of the similarities and differences in the mechanisms of exercise in LEAD and under BFR is provided in Figure 1. At the bottom level, the differences and commonalities are displayed as Venn diagrams. These exercise (plus BFR or LEAD)-induced mechanisms lead to (upper level of the figure) several effects on different biophysiological levels. These are, again, displayed as Venn diagrams, to show commonalities and differences between the exercise effects of the training with LEAD or under BFR. Despite broad knowledge on several factors, many of the mechanisms are only suggested by anecdotical evidence and not yet proven by high quality studies.

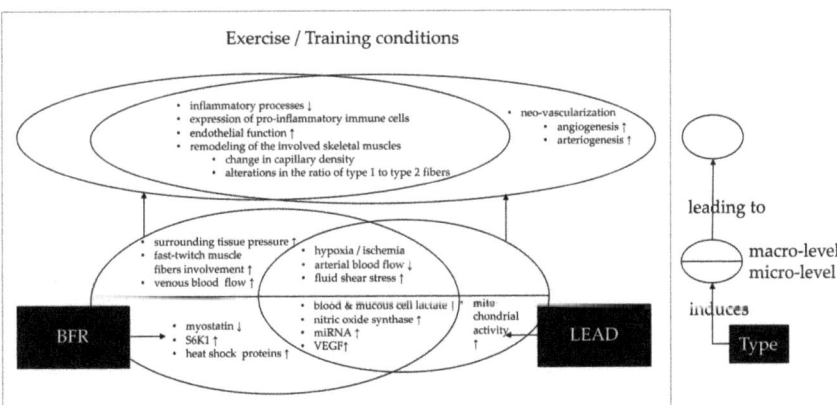

Figure 1. Mechanisms and pathways of how exercise leads to training success in peripheral arterial disease (lower extremity arterial disease (LEAD), right side) and under blood flow restriction (blood flow restriction (BFR) left side).

4. Conclusions

This review addresses a new field of LEAD therapy. Thus, at first glance, therapeutic use of blood flow restriction and peripheral artery disease and LEAD are of a contradictory nature, but both induce physiological vessel growth by hemodynamic forces and hemodynamic adaptions. We want to emphasize overlaps in effects on vessel physiology and function and the need for new clinical trials that would focus on the effects of BFR in cardiovascular patients.

There is a lack of evidence regarding studies focused on BFR with resistance exercise, particular in seniors [73]. Promising results are presented by Shimizu et al. They showed that BFR training improved endothelial function and blood circulation in active elderly people [74].

A long-term effect of structured exercise training is a decrease in blood flow-associated hypoxia, which is also mediated by effects of fluid shear. Similar physiological changes occur as a consequence. Additionally, BFR could serve as a model for how exercise leads to adaptations in LEAD, and further beneficial effects of BFR could also work when implemented in exercise training for LEAD patients.

However, many mechanisms are not yet proven by high quality evidence. As further considerable differences between the mechanism of the two comparators in this review exist; a final statement (or even recommendation) regarding whether BFR can act as a model for the mechanism of how exercise affects LEAD cannot be given. Considering the differences and (of course) contraindications for exercising, BFR can, nevertheless, be used as a model for certain outcomes of LEAD exercise intervention effects modeling or, from a practical point of view, sample size calculation. As future clinical applications of BFR training in LEAD patients should be evaluated, the most beneficial effect is expected in patients with stable lower grade LEAD. Patients with previous vascular interventions (stent or bypass surgery) might not be suitable for BFR due to the risk of occlusion of the vascular reconstruction by external mechanical forces. By simulating hypoxic metabolism in BFR intervals, the physiological activation of autogenious pro-arteriogenetic changes could be triggered. Due to the reduction in mechanical forces during BFR and low-load training, the method could be suitable in particular for patients with limited physical resilience. A known problem, when mobility is yet limited by LEAD to lower than 100 m, is that effective exercise is difficult to conduct. Regarding this problem, BFR training could be useful for the preconditioning of a structured exercise program for patients with advanced Fontaine IIb LEAD.

Funding: This research received no external funding

Acknowledgments: The Goethe Research Academy for Early Career Researchers (GRADE) provided editorial assistance during preparation of this manuscript.

Conflicts of Interest: The authors declare no conflict of interest.

References

1. Lee, I.-M.; Shiroma, E.J.; Lobelo, F.; Puska, P.; Blair, S.N.; Katzmarzyk, P.T. Effect of physical inactivity on major non-communicable diseases worldwide: An analysis of burden of disease and life expectancy. *Lancet* **2012**, *380*, 219–229. [CrossRef]
2. Guthold, R.; Stevens, G.A.; Riley, L.M.; Bull, F.C. Worldwide trends in insufficient physical activity from 2001 to 2016: A pooled analysis of 358 population-based surveys with 1.9 million participants. *Lancet Glob. Health* **2018**, *6*, e1077–e1086. [CrossRef]
3. Hallal, P.C.; Andersen, L.B.; Bull, F.C.; Guthold, R.; Haskell, W.; Ekelund, U. Global physical activity levels: Surveillance progress, pitfalls, and prospects. *Lancet* **2012**, *380*, 247–257. [CrossRef]
4. Manson, J.E.; Hu, F.B.; Rich-Edwards, J.W.; Colditz, G.A.; Stampfer, M.J.; Willett, W.C.; Speizer, F.E.; Hennekens, C.H. A prospective study of walking as compared with vigorous exercise in the prevention of coronary heart disease in women. *N. Engl. J. Med.* **1999**, *341*, 650–658. [CrossRef] [PubMed]
5. Paffenbarger, R.S.; Hyde, R.T.; Wing, A.L.; Hsieh, C.C. Physical activity, all-cause mortality, and longevity of college alumni. *N. Engl. J. Med.* **1986**, *314*, 605–613. [CrossRef] [PubMed]
6. Paffenbarger, R.S.; Kampert, J.B.; Lee, I.M.; Hyde, R.T.; Leung, R.W.; Wing, A.L. Changes in physical activity and other lifeway patterns influencing longevity. *Med. Sci. Sports Exerc.* **1994**, *26*, 857–865. [CrossRef] [PubMed]
7. Blair, S.N.; Kohl, H.W.; Barlow, C.E.; Paffenbarger, R.S.; Gibbons, L.W.; Macera, C.A. Changes in physical fitness and all-cause mortality. A prospective study of healthy and unhealthy men. *JAMA* **1995**, *273*, 1093–1098. [CrossRef]
8. Lee, D.-c.; Sui, X.; Artero, E.G.; Lee, I.-M.; Church, T.S.; McAuley, P.A.; Stanford, F.C.; Kohl, H.W.; Blair, S.N. Long-term effects of changes in cardiorespiratory fitness and body mass index on all-cause

and cardiovascular disease mortality in men: The Aerobics Center Longitudinal Study. *Circulation* **2011**, *124*, 2483–2490. [CrossRef]
9. Duvall, W.L.; Vorchheimer, D.A. Multi-bed vascular disease and atherothrombosis: Scope of the problem. *J. Thromb. Thrombolysis* **2004**, *17*, 51–61. [CrossRef]
10. Tendera, M.; Aboyans, V.; Bartelink, M.-L.; Baumgartner, I.; Clément, D.; Collet, J.-P.; Cremonesi, A.; de Carlo, M.; Erbel, R.; Fowkes, F.G.R.; et al. ESC Guidelines on the diagnosis and treatment of peripheral artery diseases: Document covering atherosclerotic disease of extracranial carotid and vertebral, mesenteric, renal, upper and lower extremity arteries: The Task Force on the Diagnosis and Treatment of Peripheral Artery Diseases of the European Society of Cardiology (ESC). *Eur. Heart J.* **2011**, *32*, 2851–2906. [CrossRef]
11. Fowkes, F.G.R.; Rudan, D.; Rudan, I.; Aboyans, V.; Denenberg, J.O.; McDermott, M.M.; Norman, P.E.; Sampson, U.K.A.; Williams, L.J.; Mensah, G.A.; et al. Comparison of global estimates of prevalence and risk factors for peripheral artery disease in 2000 and 2010: A systematic review and analysis. *Lancet* **2013**, *382*, 1329–1340. [CrossRef]
12. Vodnala, D.; Rajagopalan, S.; Brook, R.D. Medical management of the patient with intermittent claudication. *Cardiol. Clin.* **2011**, *29*, 363–379. [CrossRef] [PubMed]
13. Guidon, M.; McGee, H. Exercise-based interventions and health-related quality of life in intermittent claudication: A 20-year (1989–2008) review. *Eur. J. Cardiovasc. Prev. Rehabil.* **2010**, *17*, 140–154. [CrossRef] [PubMed]
14. McDermott, M.M.; Liu, K.; Guralnik, J.M.; Criqui, M.H.; Spring, B.; Tian, L.; Domanchuk, K.; Ferrucci, L.; Lloyd-Jones, D.; Kibbe, M.; et al. Home-based walking exercise intervention in peripheral artery disease: A randomized clinical trial. *JAMA* **2013**, *310*, 57–65. [CrossRef]
15. Barker, G.A.; Green, S.; Green, A.A.; Walker, P.J. Walking performance, oxygen uptake kinetics and resting muscle pyruvate dehydrogenase complex activity in peripheral arterial disease. *Clin. Sci.* **2004**, *106*, 241–249. [CrossRef]
16. Morris, D.R.; Rodriguez, A.J.; Moxon, J.V.; Cunningham, M.A.; McDermott, M.M.; Myers, J.; Leeper, N.J.; Jones, R.E.; Golledge, J. Association of lower extremity performance with cardiovascular and all-cause mortality in patients with peripheral artery disease: A systematic review and meta-analysis. *J. Am. Heart Assoc.* **2014**, *3*. [CrossRef]
17. Leng, G.C.; Fowler, B.; Ernst, E. Exercise for intermittent claudication. *Cochrane Database Syst. Rev.* **2000**, CD000990. [CrossRef]
18. Kieback, A.G.; Espinola-Klein, C.; Lamina, C.; Moebus, S.; Tiller, D.; Lorbeer, R.; Schulz, A.; Meisinger, C.; Medenwald, D.; Erbel, R.; et al. One simple claudication question as first step in Peripheral Arterial Disease (PAD) screening: A meta-analysis of the association with reduced Ankle Brachial Index (ABI) in 27,945 subjects. *PLoS ONE* **2019**, *14*, e0224608. [CrossRef]
19. McDermott, M.M.; Greenland, P.; Liu, K.; Guralnik, J.M.; Criqui, M.H.; Dolan, N.C.; Chan, C.; Celic, L.; Pearce, W.H.; Schneider, J.R.; et al. Leg symptoms in peripheral arterial disease: Associated clinical characteristics and functional impairment. *JAMA* **2001**, *286*, 1599–1606. [CrossRef]
20. Hardman, R.L.; Jazaeri, O.; Yi, J.; Smith, M.; Gupta, R. Overview of classification systems in peripheral artery disease. *Semin. Intervent. Radiol.* **2014**, *31*, 378–388. [CrossRef]
21. Ouma, G.O.; Zafrir, B.; Mohler, E.R.; Flugelman, M.Y. Therapeutic angiogenesis in critical limb ischemia. *Angiology* **2013**, *64*, 466–480. [CrossRef] [PubMed]
22. Hirsch, A.T.; Haskal, Z.J.; Hertzer, N.R.; Bakal, C.W.; Creager, M.A.; Halperin, J.L.; Hiratzka, L.F.; Murphy, W.R.C.; Olin, J.W.; Puschett, J.B.; et al. ACC/AHA 2005 guidelines for the management of patients with peripheral arterial disease (lower extremity, renal, mesenteric, and abdominal aortic): Executive summary a collaborative report from the American Association for Vascular Surgery/Society for Vascular Surgery, Society for Cardiovascular Angiography and Interventions, Society for Vascular Medicine and Biology, Society of Interventional Radiology, and the ACC/AHA Task Force on Practice Guidelines (Writing Committee to Develop Guidelines for the Management of Patients With Peripheral Arterial Disease) endorsed by the American Association of Cardiovascular and Pulmonary Rehabilitation; National Heart, Lung, and Blood Institute; Society for Vascular Nursing; TransAtlantic Inter-Society Consensus; and Vascular Disease Foundation. *J. Am. Coll. Cardiol.* **2006**, *47*, 1239–1312. [CrossRef] [PubMed]

23. Bhatt, D.L.; Steg, P.G.; Ohman, E.M.; Hirsch, A.T.; Ikeda, Y.; Mas, J.-L.; Goto, S.; Liau, C.-S.; Richard, A.J.; Röther, J.; et al. International prevalence, recognition, and treatment of cardiovascular risk factors in outpatients with atherothrombosis. *JAMA* **2006**, *295*, 180–189. [CrossRef] [PubMed]
24. Norgren, L.; Hiatt, W.R.; Dormandy, J.A.; Nehler, M.R.; Harris, K.A.; Fowkes, F.G.R.; Rutherford, R.B. Inter-society consensus for the management of peripheral arterial disease. *Int. Angiol.* **2007**, *26*, 81–157.
25. Anderson, J.L.; Halperin, J.L.; Albert, N.M.; Bozkurt, B.; Brindis, R.G.; Curtis, L.H.; DeMets, D.; Guyton, R.A.; Hochman, J.S.; Kovacs, R.J.; et al. Management of patients with peripheral artery disease (compilation of 2005 and 2011 ACCF/AHA guideline recommendations): A report of the American College of Cardiology Foundation/American Heart Association Task Force on Practice Guidelines. *Circulation* **2013**, *127*, 1425–1443. [CrossRef]
26. Scott, B.R.; Loenneke, J.P.; Slattery, K.M.; Dascombe, B.J. Blood flow restricted exercise for athletes: A review of available evidence. *J. Sci. Med. Sport* **2016**, *19*, 360–367. [CrossRef]
27. Takarada, Y.; Takazawa, H.; Ishii, N. Applications of vascular occlusion diminish disuse atrophy of knee extensor muscles. *Med. Sci. Sports Exerc.* **2000**, *32*, 2035–2039. [CrossRef]
28. Pearson, S.J.; Hussain, S.R. A review on the mechanisms of blood-flow restriction resistance training-induced muscle hypertrophy. *Sports Med.* **2015**, *45*, 187–200. [CrossRef]
29. Hughes, L.; Paton, B.; Rosenblatt, B.; Gissane, C.; Patterson, S.D. Blood flow restriction training in clinical musculoskeletal rehabilitation: A systematic review and meta-analysis. *Br. J. Sports Med.* **2017**, *51*, 1003–1011. [CrossRef]
30. Loenneke, J.P.; Abe, T.; Wilson, J.M.; Thiebaud, R.S.; Fahs, C.A.; Rossow, L.M.; Bemben, M.G. Blood flow restriction: An evidence based progressive model (Review). *Acta Physiol. Hung.* **2012**, *99*, 235–250. [CrossRef]
31. Bagley, J.R.; Rosengarten, J.J.; Galpin, A.J. Is Blood Flow Restriction Training Beneficial for Athletes? *Strength Cond. J.* **2015**, *37*, 48–53. [CrossRef]
32. Loenneke, J.P.; Pujol, T.J. The Use of Occlusion Training to Produce Muscle Hypertrophy. *Strength Cond. J.* **2009**, *31*, 77–84. [CrossRef]
33. Niessner, A.; Richter, B.; Penka, M.; Steiner, S.; Strasser, B.; Ziegler, S.; Heeb-Elze, E.; Zorn, G.; Leitner-Heinschink, A.; Niessner, C.; et al. Endurance training reduces circulating inflammatory markers in persons at risk of coronary events: Impact on plaque stabilization? *Atherosclerosis* **2006**, *186*, 160–165. [CrossRef]
34. Michishita, R.; Shono, N.; Inoue, T.; Tsuruta, T.; Node, K. Effect of exercise therapy on monocyte and neutrophil counts in overweight women. *Am. J. Med. Sci.* **2010**, *339*, 152–156. [CrossRef]
35. Timmerman, K.L.; Flynn, M.G.; Coen, P.M.; Markofski, M.M.; Pence, B.D. Exercise training-induced lowering of inflammatory (CD14+CD16+) monocytes: A role in the anti-inflammatory influence of exercise? *J. Leukoc. Biol.* **2008**, *84*, 1271–1278. [CrossRef]
36. Higashi, Y.; Sasaki, S.; Kurisu, S.; Yoshimizu, A.; Sasaki, N.; Matsuura, H.; Kajiyama, G.; Oshima, T. Regular aerobic exercise augments endothelium-dependent vascular relaxation in normotensive as well as hypertensive subjects: Role of endothelium-derived nitric oxide. *Circulation* **1999**, *100*, 1194–1202. [CrossRef]
37. Hiatt, W.R.; Regensteiner, J.G.; Wolfel, E.E.; Carry, M.R.; Brass, E.P. Effect of exercise training on skeletal muscle histology and metabolism in peripheral arterial disease. *J. Appl. Physiol.* **1996**, *81*, 780–788. [CrossRef]
38. Regensteiner, J.G.; Steiner, J.F.; Hiatt, W.R. Exercise training improves functional status in patients with peripheral arterial disease. *J. Vasc. Surg.* **1996**, *23*, 104–115. [CrossRef]
39. Clyne, C.A.; Mears, H.; Weller, R.O.; O'Donnell, T.F. Calf muscle adaptation to peripheral vascular disease. *Cardiovasc. Res.* **1985**, *19*, 507–512. [CrossRef] [PubMed]
40. Guerreiro, L.F.; Rocha, A.M.; Martins, C.N.; Ribeiro, J.P.; Wally, C.; Strieder, D.L.; Carissimi, C.G.; Oliveira, M.G.; Pereira, A.A.; Biondi, H.S.; et al. Oxidative status of the myocardium in response to different intensities of physical training. *Physiol. Res.* **2016**, *65*, 737–749. [PubMed]
41. Menêses, A.L.; Ritti-Dias, R.M.; Parmenter, B.; Golledge, J.; Askew, C.D. Combined Lower Limb Revascularisation and Supervised Exercise Training for Patients with Peripheral Arterial Disease: A Systematic Review of Randomised Controlled Trials. *Sports Med.* **2017**, *47*, 987–1002. [CrossRef] [PubMed]
42. Risau, W. Mechanisms of angiogenesis. *Nature* **1997**, *386*, 671–674. [CrossRef] [PubMed]
43. Schaper, W. On arteriogenesis—A reply. *Basic Res. Cardiol.* **2003**, *98*, 183–184. [CrossRef] [PubMed]

44. Dopheide, J.F.; Rubrech, J.; Trumpp, A.; Geissler, P.; Zeller, G.C.; Schnorbus, B.; Schmidt, F.; Gori, T.; Münzel, T.; Espinola-Klein, C. Supervised exercise training in peripheral arterial disease increases vascular shear stress and profunda femoral artery diameter. *Eur. J. Prev. Cardiol.* **2017**, *24*, 178–191. [CrossRef] [PubMed]
45. Nash, M.S.; Montalvo, B.M.; Applegate, B. Lower extremity blood flow and responses to occlusion ischemia differ in exercise-trained and sedentary tetraplegic persons. *Arch. Phys. Med. Rehabil.* **1996**, *77*, 1260–1265. [CrossRef]
46. Sayed, A.; Schierling, W.; Troidl, K.; Rüding, I.; Nelson, K.; Apfelbeck, H.; Benli, I.; Schaper, W.; Schmitz-Rixen, T. Exercise linked to transient increase in expression and activity of cation channels in newly formed hind-limb collaterals. *Eur. J. Vasc. Endovasc. Surg.* **2010**, *40*, 81–87. [CrossRef]
47. Bresler, A.; Vogel, J.; Niederer, D.; Gray, D.; Schmitz-Rixen, T.; Troidl, K. Development of an Exercise Training Protocol to Investigate Arteriogenesis in a Murine Model of Peripheral Artery Disease. *Int. J. Mol. Sci.* **2019**, *20*. [CrossRef]
48. Troidl, C.; Troidl, K.; Schierling, W.; Cai, W.-J.; Nef, H.; Möllmann, H.; Kostin, S.; Schimanski, S.; Hammer, L.; Elsässer, A.; et al. Trpv4 induces collateral vessel growth during regeneration of the arterial circulation. *J. Cell. Mol. Med.* **2009**, *13*, 2613–2621. [CrossRef]
49. Heil, M.; Eitenmüller, I.; Schmitz-Rixen, T.; Schaper, W. Arteriogenesis versus angiogenesis: Similarities and differences. *J. Cell. Mol. Med.* **2006**, *10*, 45–55. [CrossRef]
50. Ben Driss, A.; Benessiano, J.; Poitevin, P.; Levy, B.I.; Michel, J.B. Arterial expansive remodeling induced by high flow rates. *Am. J. Physiol.* **1997**, *272*, H851–H858. [CrossRef]
51. Gerhold, K.A.; Schwartz, M.A. Ion Channels in Endothelial Responses to Fluid Shear Stress. *Physiol. (Bethesda)* **2016**, *31*, 359–369. [CrossRef] [PubMed]
52. Shi, Z.-D.; Tarbell, J.M. Fluid flow mechanotransduction in vascular smooth muscle cells and fibroblasts. *Ann. Biomed. Eng.* **2011**, *39*, 1608–1619. [CrossRef] [PubMed]
53. Tronc, F.; Mallat, Z.; Lehoux, S.; Wassef, M.; Esposito, B.; Tedgui, A. Role of matrix metalloproteinases in blood flow-induced arterial enlargement: Interaction with NO. *Arterioscler. Thromb. Vasc. Biol.* **2000**, *20*, E120–E126. [CrossRef] [PubMed]
54. Neth, P.; Nazari-Jahantigh, M.; Schober, A.; Weber, C. MicroRNAs in flow-dependent vascular remodelling. *Cardiovasc. Res.* **2013**, *99*, 294–303. [CrossRef] [PubMed]
55. Hergenreider, E.; Heydt, S.; Tréguer, K.; Boettger, T.; Horrevoets, A.J.G.; Zeiher, A.M.; Scheffer, M.P.; Frangakis, A.S.; Yin, X.; Mayr, M.; et al. Atheroprotective communication between endothelial cells and smooth muscle cells through miRNAs. *Nat. Cell Biol.* **2012**, *14*, 249–256. [CrossRef] [PubMed]
56. Wang, G.-K.; Zhu, J.-Q.; Zhang, J.-T.; Li, Q.; Li, Y.; He, J.; Qin, Y.-W.; Jing, Q. Circulating microRNA: A novel potential biomarker for early diagnosis of acute myocardial infarction in humans. *Eur. Heart J.* **2010**, *31*, 659–666. [CrossRef]
57. Huonker, M.; Halle, M.; Keul, J. Structural and functional adaptations of the cardiovascular system by training. *Int. J. Sports Med.* **1996**, *17* Suppl 3, S164–S172. [CrossRef] [PubMed]
58. Reeves, G.V.; Kraemer, R.R.; Hollander, D.B.; Clavier, J.; Thomas, C.; Francois, M.; Castracane, V.D. Comparison of hormone responses following light resistance exercise with partial vascular occlusion and moderately difficult resistance exercise without occlusion. *J. Appl. Physiol.* **2006**, *101*, 1616–1622. [CrossRef]
59. Takarada, Y.; Nakamura, Y.; Aruga, S.; Onda, T.; Miyazaki, S.; Ishii, N. Rapid increase in plasma growth hormone after low-intensity resistance exercise with vascular occlusion. *J. Appl. Physiol.* **2000**, *88*, 61–65. [CrossRef]
60. Scott, B.R.; Slattery, K.M.; Sculley, D.V.; Dascombe, B.J. Hypoxia and resistance exercise: A comparison of localized and systemic methods. *Sports Med.* **2014**, *44*, 1037–1054. [CrossRef]
61. Dangott, B.; Schultz, E.; Mozdziak, P.E. Dietary creatine monohydrate supplementation increases satellite cell mitotic activity during compensatory hypertrophy. *Int. J. Sports Med.* **2000**, *21*, 13–16. [CrossRef] [PubMed]
62. Fujita, S.; Abe, T.; Drummond, M.J.; Cadenas, J.G.; Dreyer, H.C.; Sato, Y.; Volpi, E.; Rasmussen, B.B. Blood flow restriction during low-intensity resistance exercise increases S6K1 phosphorylation and muscle protein synthesis. *J. Appl. Physiol.* **2007**, *103*, 903–910. [CrossRef] [PubMed]
63. Pope, Z.K.; Willardson, J.M.; Schoenfeld, B.J. Exercise and blood flow restriction. *J. Strength Cond. Res.* **2013**, *27*, 2914–2926. [CrossRef] [PubMed]

64. Loenneke, J.P.; Wilson, G.J.; Wilson, J.M. A mechanistic approach to blood flow occlusion. *Int. J. Sports Med.* **2010**, *31*, 1–4. [CrossRef]
65. Ito, N.; Ruegg, U.T.; Kudo, A.; Miyagoe-Suzuki, Y.; Takeda, S. Activation of calcium signaling through Trpv1 by nNOS and peroxynitrite as a key trigger of skeletal muscle hypertrophy. *Nat. Med.* **2013**, *19*, 101–106. [CrossRef]
66. Casey, D.P.; Madery, B.D.; Curry, T.B.; Eisenach, J.H.; Wilkins, B.W.; Joyner, M.J. Nitric oxide contributes to the augmented vasodilatation during hypoxic exercise. *J. Physiol. (Lond.)* **2010**, *588*, 373–385. [CrossRef]
67. Laurentino, G.C.; Ugrinowitsch, C.; Roschel, H.; Aoki, M.S.; Soares, A.G.; Neves, M.; Aihara, A.Y.; Fernandes, A.d.R.C.; Tricoli, V. Strength training with blood flow restriction diminishes myostatin gene expression. *Med. Sci. Sports Exerc.* **2012**, *44*, 406–412. [CrossRef]
68. Takano, H.; Morita, T.; Iida, H.; Asada, K.-i.; Kato, M.; Uno, K.; Hirose, K.; Matsumoto, A.; Takenaka, K.; Hirata, Y.; et al. Hemodynamic and hormonal responses to a short-term low-intensity resistance exercise with the reduction of muscle blood flow. *Eur. J. Appl. Physiol.* **2005**, *95*, 65–73. [CrossRef]
69. Amani-Shalamzari, S.; Rajabi, S.; Rajabi, H.; Gahreman, D.E.; Paton, C.; Bayati, M.; Rosemann, T.; Nikolaidis, P.T.; Knechtle, B. Effects of Blood Flow Restriction and Exercise Intensity on Aerobic, Anaerobic, and Muscle Strength Adaptations in Physically Active Collegiate Women. *Front. Physiol.* **2019**, *10*, 810. [CrossRef]
70. Hudlicka, O.; Brown, M.D. Adaptation of skeletal muscle microvasculature to increased or decreased blood flow: Role of shear stress, nitric oxide and vascular endothelial growth factor. *J. Vasc. Res.* **2009**, *46*, 504–512. [CrossRef]
71. Green, D.J.; Hopman, M.T.E.; Padilla, J.; Laughlin, M.H.; Thijssen, D.H.J. Vascular Adaptation to Exercise in Humans: Role of Hemodynamic Stimuli. *Physiol. Rev.* **2017**, *97*, 495–528. [CrossRef] [PubMed]
72. Vogel, J.; Niederer, D.; Engeroff, T.; Vogt, L.; Troidl, C.; Schmitz-Rixen, T.; Banzer, W.; Troidl, K. Effects on the Profile of Circulating miRNAs after Single Bouts of Resistance Training with and without Blood Flow Restriction-A Three-Arm, Randomized Crossover Trial. *Int. J. Mol. Sci.* **2019**, *20*. [CrossRef] [PubMed]
73. Amorim, S.; Degens, H.; Passos Gaspar, A.; de Matos, L.D.N.J. The Effects of Resistance Exercise With Blood Flow Restriction on Flow-Mediated Dilation and Arterial Stiffness in Elderly People With Low Gait Speed: Protocol for a Randomized Controlled Trial. *Jmir Res. Protoc.* **2019**, *8*, e14691. [CrossRef] [PubMed]
74. Shimizu, R.; Hotta, K.; Yamamoto, S.; Matsumoto, T.; Kamiya, K.; Kato, M.; Hamazaki, N.; Kamekawa, D.; Akiyama, A.; Kamada, Y.; et al. Low-intensity resistance training with blood flow restriction improves vascular endothelial function and peripheral blood circulation in healthy elderly people. *Eur. J. Appl. Physiol.* **2016**, *116*, 749–757. [CrossRef] [PubMed]

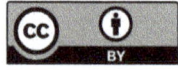

© 2020 by the authors. Licensee MDPI, Basel, Switzerland. This article is an open access article distributed under the terms and conditions of the Creative Commons Attribution (CC BY) license (http://creativecommons.org/licenses/by/4.0/).

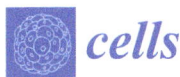

Review

Arteriogenesis of the Spinal Cord—The Network Challenge

Florian Simon [1,*], Markus Udo Wagenhäuser [1], Albert Busch [2], Hubert Schelzig [1] and Alexander Gombert [3]

1. Department of Vascular and Endovascular Surgery, Heinrich-Heine-University of Düsseldorf, 40225 Düsseldorf, Germany; markus.wagenhaeuser@med.uni-duesseldorf.de (M.U.W.); hubert.schelzig@med.uni-duesseldorf.de (H.S.)
2. Department of Vascular and Endovascular Surgery, Klinikum rechts der Isar, Technical University of Munich, 81675 Munich, Germany; albert.busch@mri.tum.de
3. Department of Vascular Surgery, University Hospital RWTH Aachen, 52074 Aachen, Germany; agombert@ukaachen.de
* Correspondence: florian.simon@med.uni-duesseldorf.de

Received: 12 December 2019; Accepted: 21 February 2020; Published: 22 February 2020

Abstract: Spinal cord ischemia (SCI) is a clinical complication following aortic repair that significantly impairs the quality and expectancy of life. Despite some strategies, like cerebrospinal fluid drainage, the occurrence of neurological symptoms, such as paraplegia and paraparesis, remains unpredictable. Beside the major blood supply through conduit arteries, a huge collateral network protects the central nervous system from ischemia—the paraspinous and the intraspinal compartment. The intraspinal arcades maintain perfusion pressure following a sudden inflow interruption, whereas the paraspinal system first needs to undergo arteriogenesis to ensure sufficient blood supply after an acute ischemic insult. The so-called steal phenomenon can even worsen the postoperative situation by causing the hypoperfusion of the spine when, shortly after thoracoabdominal aortic aneurysm (TAAA) surgery, muscles connected with the network divert blood and cause additional stress. Vessels are a conglomeration of different cell types involved in adapting to stress, like endothelial cells, smooth muscle cells, and pericytes. This adaption to stress is subdivided in three phases—initiation, growth, and the maturation phase. In fields of endovascular aortic aneurysm repair, pre-operative selective segmental artery occlusion may enable the development of a sufficient collateral network by stimulating collateral vessel growth, which, again, may prevent spinal cord ischemia. Among others, the major signaling pathways include the phosphoinositide 3 kinase (PI3K) pathway/the antiapoptotic kinase (AKT) pathway/the endothelial nitric oxide synthase (eNOS) pathway, the Erk1, the delta-like ligand (Dll), the jagged (Jag)/NOTCH pathway, and the midkine regulatory cytokine signaling pathways.

Keywords: spinal cord ischemia; arteriogenesis; paraplegia; aortic disease; TAAA; collateral network; paraspinous compartment; NO; VEGF; NOTCH

1. Introduction

Spinal cord ischemia (SCI) is a major clinical complication of aortic repair. A complex aortic aneurysm, such as thoracoabdominal aortic aneurysm (TAAA), is a rare and potentially lethal condition. Even in experienced centers, both open and endovascular repair of, specially, type II TAAA is associated with severe complications and in-hospital mortality, evidently provoked by the replacement of the entire descending thoracic and abdominal aorta, often associated with iliac artery repair. Improved surgical techniques and protective measures have improved outcomes preoperatively and during follow up [1,2].

Back in the 1980s, about one third of the patients that underwent thoracic or thoracoabdominal aortic surgery suffered from neurological disabilities afterwards. Even with the introduction of endovascular approaches into the clinical routine, SCI remains a devastating complication that is associated with the extent of aortic replacement and/or stent graft coverage. Thoracic endovascular aortic repair (TEVAR) has undergone a tremendous evolution in past decades. In the case of a complicated aortic type B dissection, according to the Stanford classification, which is defined as a malperfusion of sprouting aortic branches resulting in, e.g., paraplegia, endovascular aortic repair seems to be favorable today, as it seems to be related to a decreased mortality rate and a reduced complication rate when compared with open aortic repair [3–7]. The incidence of SCI ranges from 1.2% to 8% following TEVAR and is of utmost interest since neurological dysfunctions significantly impair the quality of life, and even reduce life expectancy in the long-term [8]. The incidence of SCI following open surgical procedures for thoracic aortic aneurysm is as high as 2%–19%, which exceeds the rates seen after TEVAR. There is a clear preference for TEVAR in all major industrial countries, because of the reduced rates of paraplegia [9,10]. However, even pararenal endovascular aortic repair holds the risk of spinal cord ischemia, especially when the hypogastric artery becomes occluded during the procedure [11,12]. More specifically, there are numerous risk factors that influence the patient outcome, such as, e.g., the extended length of covered aortic segments, the placement of stent grafts between TH9-Th12, the occlusion of the left subclavian artery, perioperative hypotension, and long total procedure time [8]. Considering these risk factors, there are strategies which have proven to be capable to reduce the incidence of SCI. These strategies include cerebrospinal fluid drainage (CSFD), local spinal cord cooling, re-implantation of segmental arteries during open surgical procedures, and prevention of hypotensive episodes during and after surgery. Although all these measures follow a comprehensive physiological theory, the current literature reveals only limited clinical success [7,13–15]. The beneficial application of somatosensoric (SSEP) and motoric-evoked potentials (MEP) during TAAA surgery has been described before [16]. A reduction in MEP amplitude to less than 50% of the baseline is considered an indication of ischemic spinal cord dysfunction. If the signals remain normal, intercostal arteries can be reattached if the aortic wall allowed a safe anastomosis during open TAAA repair. In case of a decrease, patent intercostal or lumbar arteries are revascularized. Even when applying somatosensoric and motoric-evoked potentials during surgery to identify relevant segmental arteries to maintain a sufficient blood supply to the spinal cord, paraplegia is not preventable for all cases and the application of these potentials is not clearly recommended according to the current guidelines of the European Society for Vascular Surgery (ESVS) [7,17].

As a perspective, the application of biomarkers, which can be measured in patients' blood and cerebrospinal fluid (CSF), could be a further option to detect spinal cord ischemia postoperatively. These could be a possibility to monitor the spinal cord function pre-, intra-, and postoperatively. Based on the experience in the fields of traumatology, several biomarkers have been assessed which could be associated with acute spinal cord trauma [18]. Elevated levels of lactate in the CSF as well as elevated levels of neurone-specific enolase (NSE), glial fibrillary acidic protein (GFAP), and S100B in CSF and serum have been assessed as promising biomarkers to monitor acute spinal cord damage due to ischemia [19–21]. In fields of complex aortic surgery, only a few studies evaluated the applicability of biomarkers to detect spinal cord ischemia. Regarding S-100β in the CSF, ambiguous results could be observed in the existent studies, as levels of S-100β were not significantly higher in some studies for patients who suffered from SCI compared to the control group [22]. NSE, a dominant enolase-isoenzyme found in neuronal and neuroendocrine tissues, is a 78 kD gamma-homodimer. The biological half-life of NSE in body fluids is approximately 24 h. NSE levels in CSF were measured in the study of Lases et al. and have been compared with standard MEP monitoring. The authors found a poor correlation between CSF levels of NSE and postoperative paraplegia, although patients suffering from SCI had greater levels of NSE than the 90th percentile of patients with no adverse neurological outcomes. GFAP, an intermediate filament protein expressed by many cell types of the central nervous system, was first described in 1971 [23]. GFAp, which it was first named, isolated and characterized by Eng et al. in 1969, is estimated to maintain astrocyte mechanical strength [24]. In their study, Anderson et al. reported GFAP measurements in 11 patients that underwent complex open TAAA repair [25]. Only a rather weak correlation of biomarker levels and clinically relevant endpoints, such as SCI, could be observed; only one patient suffered from SCI. In this case, a significant elevation of biomarker levels could be assessed. This finding is typical for studies focusing on biomarkers and SCI in fields of aortic surgery. No study leading to clear results which would support a recommendation for the routine application of biomarkers has been conducted so far.

As described above, there is a wide range of established factors which may predict a patient's risk for spinal cord ischemia. However, we are unable to predict which patient will develop postoperative problems. One possible reason for this issue is the rather unknown arteriogenesis of the spinal cord blood supply, because the loss of a single segmental artery probably causes maturation of the paraspinal collaterals, which might be a fostering condition for patients undergoing therapy of an aortic disease [26,27]. The sweeping relevance of these complications and the lack of treatment options make it worth studying every possibility to increase the positive outcome of a patient's quality of life. Therefore, this review aims to illuminate arteriogenesis in general, with the focus on the special needs of the spinal cord blood supply.

2. Blood Supply of the Spinal Cord

Most of what is known today about the arterial supply to the spinal cord goes back to some studies from the last century [28–31].

When entering the medulla, various branches are sprouting from the vertebral arteries that merge to form the anterior spinal artery (ASA). The ASA courses midline on the ventral sulcus of the spinal cord and merge with approximately 10–12 segmental arteries, which arise from various branches of the aorta. These segmental arteries are known as medullary arteries. Furthermore, paired posterior spinal arteries (PSAs) arise from the vertebral arteries or the posterior inferior cerebellar artery adjacent to the medulla oblongata and course on the surface of the spinal cord medial to the posterior root entry zone. The ASA gives rise to numerous sulcal branches that supply the anterior two thirds of the spinal cord. The PSAs supply much of the dorsal horn and the dorsal columns. A tightly organized network of vessels, known as the vasocorona, connects these two sources of supply and sends branches into the white matter around the margin of the spinal cord [32].

So far, this is the doctrine of the blood supply of the spinal cord, but there is emerging evidence of a huge collateral network protecting the central nervous system from ischemia [33]. However, the structure and functionality of this network might be very different than initially thought. For instance, there is a network in close relation to the spinal cord—the paraspinous and the intraspinal compartment. The paraspinous vessels are small, nonconducting arterioles, whereas the intraspinal system consists of circle- or pentagon-shaped small conducting arteries. These arteries connect adjacent segments [34,35]. It is noteworthy that the anatomical structure of the vessel system of paraspinous and intraspinal arteries accounts for their disproportionate impact in restoring the blood flow in cases of an acute interruption of the segmental inflow. In more detail, the intraspinal arcades are essential to maintain blood pressure immediately after blood inflow interruption. Without these arcades, the blood flow would almost drop to zero and the perfusion pressure would not recover, which, in turn, does not allow reactive hyperemia, resulting in a severe ischemia of the spinal cord with following paraplegia [36]. On the other hand, the paraspinal system of immature nonconducting arterioles needs to undergo arteriogenesis to ensure ongoing blood flow after the acute ischemic insult [36]. The emergency system of epidural arcades of the intraspinal system remains functional if the anterior radiculomedullary arteries (ARMAs) are sufficiently established to ensure blood flow to the anterior spinal artery (ASA). All these vessels are closely related to each other and are connected via longitudinal anastomoses. In case of suddenly losing parts of the segmental inflow, there is a repetitive ring-shaped arterial pattern on the dorsal surface of the vertebral bodies, which, until recently, remained unnoticed. These arterial vessels might be part of a stopgap to ensure blood supply to the spinal cord [34].

The collateral network does not consist only of the blood vessels directly surrounding the spinal cord, but also includes segmental arteries, the subclavian and/or iliac arteries, the aforementioned vessels of the central nervous system, the vessels of the paraspinous muscles, and the vessels of other paravertebral tissues [33,34,37]. The entirety of this vessel system merges with the internal thoracic, epigastric, intercostal, and lumbar arteries to form a network that can be filled even from distant inputs. The reason for this is so that the network ensures a redistribution of the blood volume as long as the blood pressure as driving force is high enough [34]. The varying roles of such major vessels are of specific interest in modern (endo)vascular surgery, where the ambition is to preserve as many vessels connected to the lumbar feed as possible. However, this dogma is challenged by specific surgical approaches needing specific coverage of such vessels.

As well as blood pressure being one of the most important forces to keep up the perfusion of the spinal cord, the radius of the arteries is also of special importance. In particular, in the vessels suffering from chronic ischemia caused by increasing stenosis of the feeding arteries, the arterial radius is a powerful driver of pressure drop across the stenosis. This significance is described when considering Poiseuille's law. Here, Poiseuille stated that the fourth power of the radius of an artery is reciprocally associated with the pressure, as shown below:

Poiseuille's law "Pressure drop across stenosis = (blood flow × 8Lη)/πr4", where L is the length of stenosis, η is viscosity, and r is the radius of the artery [38].

This may underline the flexibility of the blood vessel system, resulting in the ability to re-distribute significant blood volumes through longitudinal artery anastomoses. In fact, there should not be too much fear of losing one segmental artery or of the artery of Adamkiewicz, because these vessels may be appropriately compensated by the spinal cord network [13,39–41]. In contrast, the paravertebral muscles not only ensure blood supply to the spinal cord but can also endanger the central nerves by so-called steal phenomena. During a steal phenomenon, blood is redistributed by alternate routes or reversed flow, causing hypoperfusion in the vessel bed from which blood is withdrawn. That said, the steal phenomena can cause considerable hypoperfusion of the spine when muscles that are connected with the network bypass blood. This may happen during body movements and may be of particular importance during the first 24–72 h after TAAA surgery [17,42,43]. In this regard, the delayed rewarming and shivering of patients might cause steal phenomena. However, not only the musculature can endanger the blood supply of the spinal cord via a steal phenomenon. Additionally, or especially, the intestinal aortic passages can lead to a critical undersupply of blood to the spinal cord during endovascular TAAA surgery. It was observed that patients undergoing such an intervention showed a collapse of the motor evoked potentials (MEP) during the procedure and necessary but temporary balloon occlusion of the aorta. The reason for this is the reduced pressure in the aneurysm sac during vessel cannulation, which, due to the temporary pressure gradient, withdraws blood retrogradely from the spinal cord blood network [44] (Figure 1). Last but not least, the venous system can also contribute to reduced arterial perfusion via an elevated venous pressure and/or the expansion of the venous system [17]. For these reasons, therapists have established measures during and after surgery, such as, e.g., intraoperative hypothermia and the use of relaxants during the first postoperative hours to reduce the metabolic demands of the paraspinal muscles [45,46].

Although little is known about arteriogenesis in the vessel network of the spinal cord, it seems very likely that findings from other locations in the body are transferable, since the arteries of the spinal cord and collateral arteries of the extremities both originate from skeletal muscle arterioles. This means, in particular, that findings that mostly concerned arteries of the lower extremities should also be true for other arteries of same origin but different anatomical position [47,48]. That being said, it is the paraspinal collaterals that most likely undergo arteriogenesis during chronic thoracic or thoraco-abdominal aortic diseases. In particular, the typical corkscrew formation, which is well known from collaterals in peripheral arterial occlusive disease, can also be observed for TAAA [26,49]. Patients with extensive aortic disease often form large arteriogenic collaterals in the paraspinous region, which connect adjacent segmental arteries in the case of isolated segmental occlusion [35].

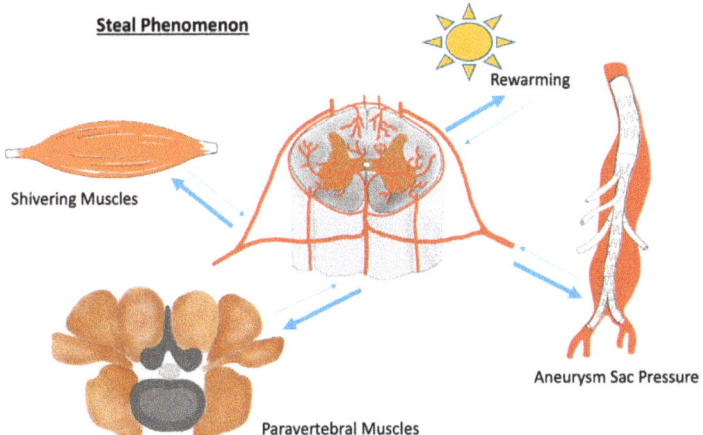

Figure 1. During a steal phenomenon blood becomes redistributed endangering spinal cord blood supply by hypoperfusion.

3. Stress-Related Changes in Blood Vessels

Due to the highly adaptive nature of the vascular system connecting all organs and systems in the body, it is a landmark for the progression and prevention of diseases. Vessels are a conglomeration of different cell types and consist of more than just endothelial cells (ECs). Each of them is involved in adapting to stress, ultimately resulting in vessel formation during arteriogenesis, like smooth muscle cells and pericytes [50,51]. Pericytes, for example, encompass endothelial cells and contribute to vessel integrity [52]. To this end, arteriogenesis is defined as dilation and remodeling of pre-existing small arteries or capillaries into vessels that can foster more blood volume [53,54]. This kind of vessel adaptation follows flow volume alterations and can also be observed in the paraspinal network. Here, the immature collaterals dilatate and increase in length to meet the elevated demand of blood volume of the spinal cord. Moreover, the pre-existing unstructured arterioles react with parallel realignment [55]. Again, these arteriogenic adaptions are somewhat comparable to observations in other tissues [35].

The phenotype of the vasculature of each organ is not a given, inflexible, or even unadaptable situation after embryogenic maturation. It is more a vivid system that might change depending on, e.g., metabolic needs, oxygen availability, oxygen radicals, and shear stress [56–60]. Under pathological conditions, like chronic ischemia, the identifying markers of the vessel walls change, indicating the convertibility of this biological system [61]. More specifically, enhanced shear stress might result in arteriogenesis, which establishes a biological bypass to circumvent the slowly growing stenosis of a vessel [62–64]. During this adaption, the collateral vessels dilatate to compensate for the reduced blood flow through a stenosis in a vessel [65]. As far as we know, a vessel's adaption can be described as follows:

During initiation, the local endothelium gets activated by the enhanced shear stress, resulting in the recruitment of local and bone marrow inflammatory cells [66,67]. These cells release several chemokines, e.g., tumor necrosis factor (TNF) and vascular endothelial growth factor (VEGF). VEGF is an important factor for vessel formation during angiogenesis. However, the expression level decreases during the late embryonic phases. This observation is given particular interest, since the mature central nervous system only expresses very low levels of VEGF to prevent blood–brain barrier leakage. In contrast, fenestrated capillaries release high VEGF levels. Such vessels may be found in the kidneys. Inflammatory cells are recruited and bind to the surface of the endothelial cells through various adhesion molecules, such as selectins, intercellular adhesion molecule 1 (iCAM1), and vascular adhesion molecule 1 (vCAM1). Following transmigration, it is the neutrophil cells that degrade the extracellular matrix to create space for expanding vessels. The recruitment of circulating monocytes paves the way for the next step of arteriogenesis [63,68–74].

During the growth phase, macrophages recruit other bone marrow-derived cells, vascular smooth muscle cells, and endothelial cells. Several chemokines, like TNF, VEGF, fibroblast growth factor (FGF), platelet derived growth factor (PDGF), granulocyte macrophage-colony stimulating factor (GM-CSF), monocyte chemoattractant protein-1 (MCP-1), and transforming growth factor are released, amongst others, by macrophages and the smooth muscle cells coordinate these actions [75]. matrix metallopeptidases 2 (MMP-2) and 9 (MMP-9) contribute to the remodeling of the basement membrane. Following a reversible shift along a continuum from a quiescent, contractile phenotype to a synthetic phenotype, vascular smooth muscle cells (VSMC) start to migrate and proliferate. The sequence of extracellular matrix (ECM) degradation and altered differentiation towards the synthesis and proliferation in the cells of the vessel wall contribute to the "new" vessels with their typical tortuous elongation and increased overall cross-section. Comprehensively, all these adaptive alterations ultimately decrease the local resistance of the vasculature, aiming to restore blood flow, as described by Poiseuille's law [38,63,66,74,76–80].

During the last phase, the so-called maturation, all processes characterizing arteriogenesis return to normal levels. That said, the shear stress decreases because the blood flow is distributed through the collateral network, causing pressure, flow, and stress reduction to the vessels. Likewise, the endothelium function normalizes, and the inflammatory activity gets downregulated. Furthermore, cell proliferation declines and the phenotypic shift of the vascular smooth muscle cells revokes. During maturation, the fate of the newly formed collaterals is different. While the collaterals at high flow rates stabilize, smaller collaterals at low flow rates regress [63,74,81,82]. To get an idea of the dimensions in which arteriogenesis may alter collateralization, experimental data in pigs were applied. Five days after the occlusion of all segmental arteries, vessels from different anatomical structures grew significantly. In more detail, the epidural arcades expanded from 150 to 249 µm. Likewise, an increase in diameter was observed for the ASA, ranging from 90 to 137 µm [55].

After considering all the aforementioned aspects, one should not miss one of the most significant determinates of tissue survival and cell death. This factor is the timespan. Due to its significance, there might be a huge difference in outcome depending on how the timespan within the alterations is established and how many pre-existing collaterals already exist. In fact, different tissues take different times to adapt. In animals, there is evidence that arteriogenesis in ischemic tissue is fast in the nervous system, where it takes only three days to reach the maximum of collateral remodeling, while it takes up to seven days in hearts, or even up to four weeks in skeletal muscles. This observation can be translated to what is seen in patients and correlated to their outcome. Here, the more pre-existing collaterals with the appropriate capability of remodeling, the better the clinical outcome [62,67,74,83–86]. Experimental findings also support this paradigm. In these settings, recent experimental data suggest that the blood supply to the spinal cord is mainly dependent on a well-established feeding vessel network and on its subsequent improvements via arteriogenesis [87,88]. Of note, there is data suggesting that these beneficial adaptions could be mimicked prior to surgery in the form of pre-conditioning the blood supply to the spinal cord. Preconditioning, in this context, means that segmental arteries become occluded by, e.g., coil embolization, to stimulate collateral network growth. Anatomical and physiological knowledge of the spinal cord circulation could improve open and endovascular TAAA repair by enabling or promoting a staged procedure that could improve spinal cord protection. Furthermore, preconditioning of the spinal cord before open or endovascular TAAA repair could result in the reduced vulnerability of the spinal cord during the first postoperative days. Animal studies, conducted in 2015 by the same research group, underline the beneficial application of the pre-operative embolization of intercostal and lumbar arteries before TEVAR; pigs with pre-interventional coil-embolization before TEVAR suffered significantly less frequently from SCI than the control group [89,90]. Moreover, there is clinical evidence that pre-conditioning enhances arteriogenesis, improving the blood supply to the central nervous system. That being said, such pre-conditioning has the potential to reduce the risk of paraplegia or paraparesis after TEVAR and might, therefore, be integrated into the clinical routine [91,92].

In the central nervous system (CNS), the barrier between the bloodstream and the underlying tissue is built up of special ECs that are less thick compared to the ECs of skeletal muscle. In addition, the blood–brain barrier (BBB) controls the passage of selected substances, such as ions, etc., into the brain. Hence, the ECs of the central nervous system (CNS) are continuous and non-fenestrated, with only a few exceptions [93]. For these reasons, the adaptions in this vascular bed are of particular interest, since they differ from other locations. In the case of an ischemic insult or chronic worsening ischemia caused by a severe narrowing of the feeding arteries of the spinal cord, the disruption of the BBB is unfavorable since its consequences, such as spinal edema or superinfections, are severe. Arteriogenesis serves as biological bypass for such stenoses and effectively maintains the blood–brain barrier since it is "only" an expansion of pre-existing collaterals.

4. Signaling Pathways

There are some important signaling pathways that contribute to arteriogenesis. For instance, the activation of the phosphoinositide 3 kinase (PI3K)/antiapoptotic kinase (AKT)/endothelial nitric oxide synthase (eNOS) pathway plays a major role in the remodeling of the collaterals. The PI3K/AKT pathway has an impact on many processes, like metabolism, apoptosis, cell survival in general, and cell proliferation. The most important effects during arteriogenesis are cell proliferation, cell growth, and reduction in apoptosis. PI3K is an intracellular signal transducer that activates the downstream target AKT that is able to phosphorylate eNOS. The activated eNOS is responsible for an increase of NO expression, which ameliorates cell survival, among other things. NO is a landmark effector and its production causes vasodilatation that enhances the blood flow, which, in turn, stabilizes vessel remodeling effects. The pathway also maintains interactions between ECs and other cell types of the surrounding tissue, such as VSMC and pericytes. Both cell types are significantly involved in the promotion and maintenance of ateriogenesis and its stabilization. In this regard, there are different sources of NO. The endothelial nitric oxide synthase (eNOS), neuronal nitric oxide synthase (nNOS), and the inducible nitric oxide synthase (iNOS) contribute to arteriogenesis and can replace each other's production to meet the demand of the required NO levels [94–101].

The extent of arteriogenesis is directly linked to the activation of the extracellular signal-regulated kinase 1 and 2 (ERK1/2) pathway. The two isoforms have different roles, but work hand-in-hand in arteriogenesis. VEGF is an important signal molecule for the activation of the endothelial ERK1/2, pathway resulting in increased arteriogenesis or, rather, the absence of VEGF causes a reduction in arteriogenesis. As mentioned above, inflammatory cells are necessary for arteriogenesis, especially as these cells are a major source of VEGF in absence of tissue ischemia. ERK1 is a key holder of macrophage infiltration. When ERK1 is absent, it creates a massive macrophage infiltration with excessive VEGF expression. This oversupply does not result in improved functional vessels—quite the opposite. The seemingly improved arteriogenesis is built up of only poorly functional vessels that do not increase blood flow sufficiently. In contrast to the effects of ERK1, the loss of the endothelial ERK2 pathway does not affect arteriogensis at first sight, but does end in reduced blood flow recovery. The reason for the diminished function of arteriogenesis is the positive stimulation of endothelial cell proliferation and eNOS expression that fails in the absence of ERK2. In particular, the missing NO production results in vasoconstriction with the aforementioned reduced blood flow [102–106].

Another important pathway is the delta-like ligand (Dll) and jagged (Jag)/NOTCH pathway that is responsible for perivascular macrophage maturation and the inflammatory response, resulting in the remodeling of the newly formed collaterals. NOTCH is a family of transmembrane proteins that get cleaved following ligand binding. After such cleavage, the intracellular domain is translocated into the nucleus. NOTCH signaling is also of particular significance in the close interaction between ECs and VSMCs. Here, cytokines, such as VEGF and FGF, enhance the expression of Dll, which, in turn, elevates EPHB-2/4 plasma levels by NOTCH signaling. The aforementioned process is essential for the precise coordination of vessel remodeling during arteriogenesis [54,74,107–114]. VEGF signaling improves EC survival, because the above-mentioned phosphoinositide 3 kinases (PI3Ks) and antiapoptotic kinases (AKTs) are increased by VEGF. Additionally, the elevation of NO levels, caused by vascular endothelial growth factor receptor 2/neuropilin 1 (VEGFR-2/NRP-1), influence lumen expansion, vascular remodeling, and maturation/stabilization [115]. Moreover, VEGF also stimulates other receptors, such as the erythropoietin-producing hepatocellular (Eph) receptor. This tyrosin kinase is categorized into two subtypes—Eph-A and Eph-B. Those two receptors are bound to ephrin-A and ephrin-B. Ephrin-B, for example, internalizes via endocytosis VEGFR-2 and prevents PDGF endocytosis. Thus, it contributes to VSMC maturation, which plays a key role in stabilizing the arterial wall. These ligands and receptors are not only found on vessels where they serve as identification marker, but are also found in the nervous system [116–121]. Tumor growth factor ß (TGF-ß) cytokine is also involved in arteriogenesis. Interestingly, the expression of this cytokine is stimulated in hypoxic conditions through HIF-1α and oxidative stress. TGF-ß up-regulates collagen and produces and promotes vascular remodeling, although it is not the primary effector in arteriogenesis [122]. Macrophages are inflammatory cells and also contribute to the remodeling of the vessel wall. During arteriogenesis, macrophages increase the number of VSMCs within the arterial wall, which stabilizes the newly formed vessel [74,123,124].

A midkine (MK) is a regulatory cytokine during embryonic vessel angiogenesis, and its dysfunctional signaling causes malignant diseases. Meanwhile, rising evidence has linked this cytokine to arteriogenesis via, e.g., elevated VEGF-A levels [94,125–127]. The positively charged molecule binds to the endothelium, where several receptors/receptor complexes interact with MK and mediate its downstream signaling. Due to its high significance for key processes, it is worth mentioning that the endothelium itself might be a relevant source of MK [128,129]. Interestingly, MK interferes with the above-mentioned NOTCH receptor, suggesting significant potential for altering the inflammatory response via iCAM1. This is further supported by animal experiments, since MK-deficient mice revealed reduced leucocyte infiltration, which has a severe impact on arteriogenesis [130–133].

5. Conclusions

The feeding vessel network to the spinal cord is well known. Since SCI is a persisting clinical problem after open and endovascular aortic procedures, the scientific community has focused, once again, on the paraspinous and the intraspinal compartment. The aortic intervention-related steal phenomena can cause the hypoperfusion of the spine since large-volume muscles connected with the network and body movements can shift significant blood volumes shortly after TAAA surgery, which may be of importance during the first 24–72 h postoperatively. Even delayed rewarming and shivering might enhance the steal phenomena which contribute to SCI. Pre-conditioning with selective segmental artery occlusion reduces the blood supply to the CNS artificially, enhancing arteriogenesis. Both, arteries of the spinal cord as well as of the extremities are of skeletal muscle arterioles origin with transferable mechanisms according to arteriogenesis, involving signaling pathways like PI3K/AKT/eNOS, Erk1, the delta-like ligand, jagged (Jag)/NOTCH pathway, and the Midkine regulatory cytokine signaling. In the future, both arteriogenesis enhanced by the preconditioning of the blood supply of the central nervous system via selective segmental artery occlusion and the validation of biomarkers, e.g., NSE, GFAP, and S100B, might become additional cornerstones in the treatment of elective thoracic aortic repair, leading to a reduced risk of paraplegia or paraparesis.

Funding: This research received no external funding.

Conflicts of Interest: The authors declare no conflict of interest.

References

1. Coselli, J.S.; LeMaire, S.A.; Preventza, O.; de la Cruz, K.I.; Cooley, D.A.; Price, M.D. Outcomes of 3309 thoracoabdominal aortic aneurysm repairs. *J. Thorac. Cardiovasc. Surg.* **2016**, *151*, 1323–1337. [CrossRef] [PubMed]
2. Crawford, E.S. Thoraco-abdominal and abdominal aortic aneurysms involving renal, superior mesenteric, celiac arteries. *Ann. Surg.* **1974**, *179*, 763–772. [CrossRef] [PubMed]
3. Svensson, L.G.; Crawford, E.S. Aortic dissection and aortic aneurysm surgery: Clinical observations, experimental investigations, and statistical analyses. Part III. *Curr. Probl. Surg.* **1993**, *30*, 1–163. [CrossRef]
4. Greenberg, R.K.; Lu, Q.; Roselli, E.E.; Svensson, L.G.; Moon, M.C.; Hernandez, A.V. Contemporary analysis of descending thoracic and thoracoabdominal aneurysm repair: A comparison of endovascular and open techniques. *Circulation* **2008**, *118*, 808–817. [CrossRef] [PubMed]
5. Fattori, R.; Cao, P.; De Rango, P.; Czerny, M.; Evangelista, A.; Nienaber, C.; Rousseau, H.; Schepens, M. Interdisciplinary expert consensus document on management of type B aortic dissection. *J. Am. Coll. Cardiol.* **2013**, *61*, 1661–1678. [CrossRef] [PubMed]
6. Luebke, T.; Brunkwall, J. Outcome of patients with open and endovascular repair in acute complicated type B aortic dissection: A systematic review and meta-analysis of case series and comparative studies. *J. Cardiovasc. Surg. (Torino)* **2010**, *51*, 613–632.
7. Riambau, V.; Böckler, D.; Brunkwall, J. Editor's Choice - Management of Descending Thoracic Aorta Diseases: Clinical Practice Guidelines of the European Society for Vascular Surgery (ESVS). *Eur. J. Vasc. Endovasc. Surg.* **2017**, *53*, 4–52. [CrossRef]
8. Wortmann, M.; Böckler, D.; Geisbüsch, P. Perioperative cerebrospinal fluid drainage for the prevention of spinal ischemia after endovascular aortic repair. *Gefasschirurgie* **2017**, *22*, 35–40. [CrossRef]
9. Lettinga-van de Poll, T.; Schurink, G.W.; De Haan, M.W.; Verbruggen, J.P.; Jacobs, M.J. Endovascular treatment of traumatic rupture of the thoracic aorta. *Br. J. Surg.* **2007**, *94*, 525–533. [CrossRef]
10. Cheng, D.; Martin, J.; Shennib, H. Endovascular aortic repair versus open surgical repair for descending thoracic aortic disease a systematic review and meta-analysis of comparative studies. *J. Am. Coll. Cardiol.* **2010**, *55*, 986–1001. [CrossRef]
11. Hiramoto, J.S.; Fernandez, C.; Gasper, W.; Vartanian, S.; Reilly, L.; Chuter, T. Lower extremity weakness is associated with elevated blood and cerebrospinal fluid glucose levels following multibranched endovascular aortic aneurysm repair. *J. Vasc. Surg.* **2017**, *65*, 311–317. [CrossRef] [PubMed]
12. Peppelenbosch, N.; Cuypers, P.W.; Vahl, A.C.; Vermassen, F.; Buth, J. Emergency endovascular treatment for ruptured abdominal aortic aneurysm and the risk of spinal cord ischemia. *J. Vasc. Surg.* **2005**, *42*, 608–614. [CrossRef]
13. Acher, C.W.; Wynn, M.M.; Mell, M.W.; Tefera, G.; Hoch, J.R. A quantitative assessment of the impact of intercostal artery reimplantation on paralysis risk in thoracoabdominal aortic aneurysm repair. *Ann. Surg.* **2008**, *248*, 529–540. [CrossRef] [PubMed]
14. Acher, C. It is not just assisted circulation, hypothermic arrest, or clamp and sew. *J. Thorac. Cardiovasc. Surg.* **2010**, *140*, 136–146. [CrossRef] [PubMed]
15. Erbel, R.; Aboyans, V.; Boileau, C. ESC Committee for Practice Guidelines. 2014 ESC Guidelines on the diagnosis and treatment of aortic diseases: Document covering acute and chronic aortic diseases of the thoracic and abdominal aorta of the adult. The Task Force for the Diagnosis and Treatment of Aortic Diseases of the European Society of Cardiology (ESC). *Eur. Heart J.* **2014**, *35*, 2873–2926. [PubMed]
16. Jacobs, M.J.; Meylaerts, S.A.; de Haan, P.; de Mol, B.A.; Kalkman, C.J. Strategies to prevent neurologic deficit based on motor-evoked potentials in type I and II thoracoabdominal aortic aneurysm repair. *J. Vasc. Surg.* **1999**, *29*, 48–57. [CrossRef]
17. Etz, C.D.; Luehr, M.; Kari, F.A.; Bodian, C.A.; Smego, D.; Plestis, K.A. Paraplegia after extensive thoracic and thoracoabdominal aortic aneurysm repair: Does critical spinal cord ischemia occur postoperatively? *J. Thorac. Cardiovasc. Surg.* **2008**, *135*, 324–330. [CrossRef] [PubMed]
18. Pouw, M.H.; Hosman, A.J.; van Middendorp, J.J.; Verbeek, M.M.; Vos, P.E.; van de Meent, H. Biomarkers in spinal cord injury. *Spinal. Cord.* **2009**, *47*, 519–525. [CrossRef]

19. Winnerkvist, A.; Anderson, R.E.; Hansson, L.O.; Rosengren, L.; Estrera, A.E.; Huynh, T.T. Multilevel somatosensory evoked potentials and cerebrospinal proteins: Indicators of spinal cord injury in thoracoabdominal aortic aneurysm surgery. *Eur J. Cardiothorac. Surg.* **2007**, *31*, 637–642. [CrossRef]
20. Khaladj, N.; Teebken, O.E.; Hagl, C.; Wilhelmi, M.H.; Tschan, C.; Weissenborn, K. The role of cerebrospinal fluid S100 and lactate to predict clinically evident spinal cord ischaemia in thoraco-abdominal aortic surgery. *Eur. J. Vasc. Endovasc. Surg.* **2008**, *36*, 11–19. [CrossRef]
21. Lases, E.C.; Schepens, M.A.; Haas, F.J.; Aarts, L.P.; ter Beek, H.T.; van Dongen, E.P. Clinical prospective study of biochemical markers and evoked potentials for identifying adverse neurological outcome after thoracic and thoracoabdominal aortic aneurysm surgery. *Br. J. Anaesth.* **2005**, *95*, 651–661. [CrossRef] [PubMed]
22. Harky, A.; Fok, M.; Fraser, H.; Howard, C.; Rimmer, L.; Bashir, M. Could Cerebrospinal Fluid Biomarkers Offer Better Predictive Value for Spinal Cord Ischaemia Than Current Neuromonitoring Techniques During Thoracoabdominal Aortic Aneurysm Repair - A Systematic Review. *Braz. J. Cardiovasc. Surg.* **2019**, *34*, 464–471. [CrossRef]
23. Fuchs, E.; Weber, K. Intermediate filaments: Structure, dynamics, function, and disease. *Annu. Rev. Biochem.* **1994**, *63*, 345–382. [CrossRef] [PubMed]
24. Eng, L.F.; Ghirnikar, R.S.; Lee, Y.L. Glial fibrillary acidic protein: GFAP-thirty-one years (1969-2000). *Neurochem. Res.* **2000**, *25*, 1439–1451. [CrossRef] [PubMed]
25. Anderson, R.E.; Winnerkvist, A.; Hansson, L.O.; Nilsson, O.; Rosengren, L.; Settergren, G. Biochemical markers of cerebrospinal ischemia after repair of aneurysms of the descending and thoracoabdominal aorta. *J. Cardiothorac. Vasc. Anesth.* **2003**, *17*, 598–603. [CrossRef]
26. Backes, W.H.; Nijenhuis, R.J.; Mess, W.H. Magnetic resonance angiography of collateral blood supply to spinal cord in thoracic and thoracoabdominal aortic aneurysm patients. *J. Vasc. Surg.* **2008**, *48*, 261–271. [CrossRef] [PubMed]
27. Nijenhuis, R.J.; Backes, W.H. Optimal preopera- tive imaging of spinal cord blood supply. *AJNR Am. J. Neuroradiol.* **2009**, *30*, 38–39. [CrossRef]
28. Lazorthes, G.; Poulhes, J.; Bastide, G.; Roulleau, J.; Chancholle, A.R. Research on the arterial vascularization of the medulla; applications to medullary pathology. *Bull. Acad. Natl. Med.* **1957**, *141*, 464–477.
29. Lazorthes, G.; Poulhes, J.; Bastide, G.; Roulleau, J.; Chancholle, A.R. Arterial vascularization of the spine; anatomic research and applications in pathology of the spinal cord and aorta. *Neurochirurgie* **1958**, *4*, 3–19.
30. Lazorthes, G.; Gouaze, A.; Zadeh, J.O.; Santini, J.J.; Lazorthes, Y.; Burdin, P. Arterial vascularization of the spinal cord. *J. Neurosurg.* **1971**, *35*, 253–262. [CrossRef]
31. Adamkiewicz, A. *Die Blutgefäße des menschlichen Rückenmarks. II. Teil. Die Gefäße der Rückenmarksoberfläche*; Sitz der Akad Wiss: Berlin, Germany, 1882; pp. 101–130.
32. Purves, D.; Augustine, G.J.; Fitzpatrick, D. *Neuroscience*, 2nd ed.; Sinauer Associates: Oxford, MS, USA, 2001; pp. 145–165.
33. Griepp, R.B.; Griepp, E.B. Spinal cord perfusion and protection during descending thoracic and thoracoabdominal aortic surgery: The collateral network concept. *Ann. Thorac. Surg.* **2007**, *83*, 865–869. [CrossRef] [PubMed]
34. Etz, C.D.; Kari, F.A.; Mueller, C.S. The collateral network concept: A reassessment of the anatomy of spinal cord perfusion. *J. Thorac. Cardiovasc. Surg.* **2011**, *141*, 1020–1028. [CrossRef] [PubMed]
35. Meffert, P.; Bischoff, M.S.; Brenner, R.; Siepe, M.; Beyersdorf, F.; Kari, F.A. Significance and function of different spinal collateral compartments following thoracic aortic surgery: Immediate versus long-term flow compensation. *Eur. J. Cardio-Thorac. Surg.* **2014**, *45*, 799–804. [CrossRef] [PubMed]
36. Kari, F.A.; Wittmann, K.; Saravi, B.; Puttfarcken, L.; Krause, S.; Förster, K.; Maier, S.; Göbel, U.; Beyersdorf, F. Immediate Spinal Cord Collateral Blood Flow During Thoracic Aortic Procedures: The Role of Epidural Arcades. *Semin. Thorac. Cardiovasc. Surg.* **2016**, *28*, 378–387. [CrossRef]
37. Strauch, J.T.; Spielvogel, D.; Lauten, A.; Zhang, N.; Shiang, H.; Weisz, D. Importance of extrasegmental vessels for spinal cord blood supply in a chronic porcine model. *Eur J. Cardiothorac. Surg.* **2003**, *24*, 817–824. [CrossRef]
38. Hiatt, W.R. *Pathophysiology of Peripheral Artery Disease, Intermittent Claudication, and Critical Limb Ischemia*, 2nd ed.; Elsevier: Amsterdam, The Netherlands, 2012; pp. 223–230.
39. Safi, H.J.; Miller, C.C.; Carr, C.; Iliopoulos, D.C.; Dorsay, D.A.; Baldwin, J.C. Importance of intercostal artery reattachment during thoracoabdominal aortic aneurysm repair. *J. Vasc. Surg.* **1998**, *27*, 58–66. [CrossRef]

40. Coselli, J.S.; LeMaire, S.A.; de Figueiredo, L.P.; Kirby, R.P. Paraplegia after thoracoabdominal aortic aneurysm repair: Is dissection a risk factor? *Ann. Thorac. Surg.* **1997**, *63*, 28–36. [CrossRef]
41. Williams, G.M.; Roseborough, G.S.; Webb, T.H.; Perler, B.A.; Krosnick, T. Preoperative selective intercostal angiography in patients undergoing thoracoabdominal aneurysm repair. *J. Vasc. Surg.* **2004**, *39*, 314–321. [CrossRef]
42. Etz, C.D.; Homann, T.M.; Plestis, K.A.; Zhang, N.; Luehr, M.; Weisz, D.J. Spinal cord perfusion after extensive segmental artery sacrifice: Can paraplegia be prevented? *Eur. J. Cardiothorac. Surg.* **2007**, *31*, 643–648. [CrossRef]
43. Etz, C.D.; Di Luozzo, G.; Zoli, S.; Lazala, R.; Plestis, K.A.; Bodian, C.A. Direct spinal cord perfusion pressure monitoring in extensive distal aortic aneurysm repair. *Ann. Thorac. Surg.* **2009**, *87*, 1764–1774. [CrossRef] [PubMed]
44. Schurink, G.W.; De Haan, M.W.; Peppelenbosch, A.G. Spinal cord function monitoring during endovascular treatment of thoracoabdominal aneurysms: Implications for staged procedures. *J. Cardiovasc. Surg. (Torino)* **2013**, *54*, 117–124.
45. Bischoff, M.S.; Di Luozzo, G.; Griepp, E.B.; Griepp, R.B. Spinal cord preservation in thoracoabdominal aneurysm repair. *Perspect. Vasc. Surg. Endovasc.* **2011**, *23*, 214–222. [CrossRef] [PubMed]
46. De Haan, P.; Kalkman, C.J.; Jacobs, M.J. Pharmacologic neuroprotection in experimental spinal cord ischemia: A systematic review. *J. Neurosurg. Anesth.* **2001**, *13*, 3–12. [CrossRef]
47. Heil, M.; Schaper, W. Influence of mechanical, cellular, and molecular factors on collateral artery growth (arteriogenesis). *Circ. Res.* **2004**, *95*, 449–458. [CrossRef]
48. Heil, M.; Schaper, W. Pathophysiology of collateral development. *Coron. Artery Dis.* **2004**, *15*, 373–378. [CrossRef]
49. Nijenhuis, R.J.; Jacobs, M.J.; Schurink, G.W. Magnetic resonance angiography and neuro-monitoring to assess spinal cord blood supply in thoracic and thoracoabdominal aortic aneurysm surgery. *J. Vasc. Surg.* **2007**, *45*, 71–77. [CrossRef]
50. Potente, M.; Makinen, T. Vascular heterogeneity and specialization in development and disease. *Nat. Rev. Mol. Cell Biol.* **2017**, *18*, 477–494. [CrossRef]
51. Kashiwagi, S.; Izumi, Y.; Gohongi, T. NO mediates mural cell recruitment and vessel morphogenesis in murine melanomas and tissue-engineered blood vessels. *J. Clin. Investig.* **2005**, *115*, 1816–1827. [CrossRef]
52. Dar, A.; Domev, H.; Ben-Yosef, O. Multipotent vasculogenic pericytes from human pluripotent stem cells promote recovery of murine ischemic limb. *Circulation* **2011**, *125*, 87–99. [CrossRef]
53. Grundmann, S.; Piek, J.J.; Pasterkamp, G.; Hoefer, I.E. Arteriogenesis: Basic mechanisms and therapeutic stimulation. *Eur. J. Clin. Investig.* **2007**, *37*, 755–766. [CrossRef] [PubMed]
54. Helisch, A.; Schaper, W. Arteriogenesis: The development and growth of collateral arteries. *Microcirculation* **2003**, *10*, 83–97. [CrossRef] [PubMed]
55. Etz, C.D.; Kari, F.A.; Mueller, C.S.; Brenner, R.M.; Lin, H.M.; Griepp, R.B. The collateral network concept: Remodeling of the arterial collateral network after experimental segmental artery sacrifice. *J. Thorac. Cardiovasc. Surg.* **2011**, *141*, 1029–1036. [CrossRef] [PubMed]
56. Aird, W.C. Endothelial cell heterogeneity. *Cold Spring Harb. Perspect. Med.* **2012**, *2*, 1. [CrossRef] [PubMed]
57. Buschmann, I.; Pries, A.; Styp-Rekowska, B. Pulsatile shear and Gja5 modulate arterial identity and remodeling events during flow-driven arteriogenesis. *Development* **2010**, *137*, 2187–2196. [CrossRef] [PubMed]
58. Kawano, H.; Motoyama, T.; Hirai, N.; Kugiyama, K.; Yasue, H.; Ogawa, H. Endothelial dysfunction in hypercholesterolemia is improved by L-arginine admnistration: Possible role of oxidative stress. *Atherosclerosis* **2002**, *161*, 375–380. [CrossRef]
59. Lloyd, P.G.; Yang, H.T.; Terjung, R.L. Arteriogenesis and angiogenesis in rat ischemic hindlimb: Role of nitric oxide. *Am. J. Physiol. Heart Circ. Physiol.* **2001**, *281*, 2528–2538. [CrossRef]
60. Van Dijk, C.G.M.; Nieuweboer, F.E.; Pei, J.Y. The complex mural cell: Pericyte function in health and disease. *Int. J. Cardiol.* **2015**, *190*, 75–89. [CrossRef]
61. Hashimoto, T.; Tsuneki, M.; Foster, T.R.; Santana, J.M.; Bai, H.; Wang, M. Membrane-mediated regulation of vascular identity. *Birth Defects Res. Part C Embryo Today* **2016**, *108*, 65–84. [CrossRef]
62. Zhang, H.; Faber, J.E. De-novo collateral formation following acute myocardial infarction: Dependence on CCR2+ bone marrow cells. *J. Mol. Cell. Cardiol.* **2015**, *87*, 4–16. [CrossRef]

63. Scholz, D.; Ito, W.; Fleming, I. Ultrastructure and molecular histology of rabbit hind-limb collateral artery growth (arteriogenesis). *Virchows Archiv.* **2000**, *436*, 257–270. [CrossRef] [PubMed]
64. Pipp, F.; Boehm, S.; Cai, W.J.; Adili, F.; Ziegler, B.; Karanovic, G.; Ritter, R.; Balzer, J.; Scheler, C.; Schaper, W. Elevated fluid shear stress enhances postocclusive collateral artery growth and gene expression in the pig hind limb. *Arter. Thromb. Vasc. Biol.* **2004**, *24*, 1664–1668. [CrossRef] [PubMed]
65. Hakimzadeh, N.; Verberne, H.J.; Siebes, M.; Piek, J.J. The future of collateral artery research. *Curr. Cardiol. Rev.* **2014**, *10*, 73–86. [CrossRef] [PubMed]
66. Carmeliet, P. Mechanisms of angiogenesis and arteriogenesis. *Nat. Med.* **2000**, *6*, 389. [CrossRef] [PubMed]
67. Deindl, E.; Schaper, W. The art of arteriogenesis. *Cell Biochem. Biophys.* **2005**, *43*, 1–15. [CrossRef]
68. Jazwa, A.; Florczyk, U.; Grochot-Przeczek, A.; Krist, B.; Loboda, A.; Jozkowicz, A.; Dulak, J. Limb ischemia and vessel regeneration: Is there a role for VEGF? *Vasc. Pharmacol.* **2016**, *86*, 18–30. [CrossRef] [PubMed]
69. Lee, C.W.; Stabile, E.; Kinnaird, T. Temporal patterns of gene expression after acute hindlimb ischemia in mice. *JACC* **2004**, *43*, 474–482. [CrossRef]
70. Behm, C.Z.; Kaufmann, B.A.; Carr, C. Molecular imaging of endothelial vascular cell adhesion molecule-1 expression and inflammatory cell recruitment during vasculogenesis and ischemia-mediated arteriogenesis. *Circulation* **2008**, *117*, 2902–2911. [CrossRef]
71. Risau, W. Development and differentiation of endothelium. *Kidney Int.* **1998**, *54*, 3–6. [CrossRef]
72. Schaper, W.; Flameng, W.; Winkler, B. Quantification of collateral resistance in acute and chronic experimental coronary occlusion in the dog. *Circ. Res.* **1976**, *39*, 371–377. [CrossRef]
73. Hoefer, I.E.; van Royen, N.; Rectenwald, J.E. Arteriogenesis proceeds via ICAM-1/Mac-1-mediated mechanisms. *Circ. Res.* **2004**, *94*, 1179–1185. [CrossRef] [PubMed]
74. Castro, P.R.; Barbosa, A.S.; Pereira, J.M. Cellular and Molecular Heterogeneity Associated with Vessel Formation Processes. *Biomed. Res. Int.* **2018**, 6740408. [CrossRef] [PubMed]
75. Van Royen, N. Stimulation of arteriogenesis; a new concept for the treatment of arterial occlusive disease. *Cardiovasc. Res.* **2001**, *49*, 543–553. [CrossRef]
76. Arras, M.; Ito, W.D.; Scholz, D.; Winkler, B.; Schaper, J.; Schaper, W. Monocyte activation in angiogenesis and collateral growth in the rabbit hindlimb. *J. Clin. Investig.* **1998**, *101*, 40–50. [CrossRef] [PubMed]
77. Cai, W.J.; Kocsis, E.; Wu, X. Remodeling of the vascular tunica media is essential for development of collateral vessels in the canine heart. *Mol. Cell. Biochem.* **2004**, *264*, 201–210. [CrossRef]
78. Chillo, O.; Kleinert, E.C.; Lautz, T.; Lasch, M.; Pagel, J.I.; Heun, Y.; Troidl, K.; Fischer, S.; Caballero-Martinez, A.; Mauer, A. Perivascular Mast Cells Govern Shear Stress-Induced Arteriogenesis by Orchestrating Leukocyte Function. *Cell Rep.* **2016**, *16*, 2197–2207. [CrossRef]
79. Dodd, T.; Jadhav, R.; Wiggins, L. MMPs 2 and 9 are essential for coronary collateral growth and are prominently regulated by p38 MAPK. *J. Mol. Cell. Cardiol.* **2011**, *51*, 1015–1025. [CrossRef]
80. Cai, W.J.; Koltai, S.; Kocsis, E. Remodeling of the adventitia during coronary arteriogenesis. *Am. J. Physiol. Heart Circ. Physiol.* **2003**, *284*, 31–40. [CrossRef]
81. Wolf, C.; Cai, W.J.; Vosschulte, R. Vascular remodeling and altered protein expression during growth of coronary collateral arteries. *J. Mol. Cell. Cardiol.* **1998**, *30*, 2291–2305. [CrossRef]
82. Hoefer, I.E.; van Royen, N.; Buschmann, I.R.; Piek, J.J.; Schaper, W. Time course of arteriogenesis following femoral artery occlusion in the rabbit. *Cardiovasc. Res.* **2001**, *49*, 609–617. [CrossRef]
83. Seiler, C.; Stoller, M.; Pitt, B.; Meier, P. The human coronary collateral circulation: Development and clinical importance. *Eur. Heart J.* **2013**, *34*, 2674–2682. [CrossRef]
84. Zhang, H.; Prabhakar, P.; Sealock, R.; Faber, J.E. Wide genetic variation in the native pial collateral circulation is a major determinant of variation in severity of stroke. *J. Cereb. Blood Flow Metab.* **2010**, *30*, 923–934. [CrossRef]
85. Heil, M.; Eitenmüller, I.; Schmitz-Rixen, T.; Schaper, W. Arteriogenesis versus angiogenesis: Similarities and differences. *J. Cell. Mol. Med.* **2006**, *10*, 45–55. [CrossRef]
86. Chalothorn, D.; Clayton, J.A.; Zhang, H.; Pomp, D.; Faber, J.E. Collateral density, remodeling, and VEGF-A expression differ widely between mouse strains. *Physiol. Genomics.* **2007**, *30*, 179–191. [CrossRef]
87. Bischoff, M.S.; Scheumann, J.; Brenner, R.M.; Ladage, D.; Bodian, C.A.; Kleinman, G. Staged approach prevents spinal cord injury in hybrid surgical endovascular thoracoabdominal aortic aneurysm repair: An experimental model. *Ann. Thorac. Surg.* **2011**, *92*, 138–146. [CrossRef]

88. Zoli, S.; Etz, C.D.; Roder, F.; Brenner, R.M.; Bodian, C.A.; Kleinman, G. Experimental two-stage simulated repair of extensive thoracoabdominal aneurysms reduces paraplegia risk. *Ann. Thorac. Surg.* **2010**, *90*, 722–729. [CrossRef]
89. Geisbusch, S.; Stefanovic, A.; Koruth, J.S.; Lin, H.M.; Morgello, S.; Weisz, D.J. Endovascular coil embolization of segmental arteries prevents paraplegia after subsequent thoracoabdominal aneurysm repair: An experimental model. *J. Thorac. Cardiovasc. Surg.* **2014**, *147*, 220–226. [CrossRef]
90. Griepp, E.B.; Di Luozzo, G.; Schray, D.; Stefanovic, A.; Geisbüsch, S.; Griepp, R.B. The anatomy of the spinal cord collateral circulation. *Ann. Cardiothorac. Surg.* **2012**, *1*, 350–357.
91. Etz, C.D.; Zoli, S.; Mueller, C.S.; Bodian, C.A.; Di Luozzo, G.; Lazala, R. Staged repair significantly reduces paraplegia rate after extensive thoracoabdominal aortic aneurysm repair. *J. Thorac. Cardiovasc. Surg.* **2010**, *139*, 1464–1472. [CrossRef]
92. Etz, C.D.; Debus, E.S.; Mohr, F.W.; Kölbel, T. First-in-man endovascular preconditioning of the paraspinal collateral network by segmental artery coil embolization to prevent ischemic spinal cord injury. *J. Thorac. Cardiovasc. Surg.* **2015**, *149*, 1074–1079. [CrossRef]
93. Ufnal, M.; Skrzypecki, J. Blood borne hormones in a crosstalk between peripheral and brain mechanisms regulating blood pressure, the role of circumventricular organs. *Neuropeptides* **2014**, *48*, 65–73. [CrossRef] [PubMed]
94. Lautz, T.; Lasch, M.; Borgolte, J.; Troidl, K.; Pagel, J.I.; Caballero-Martinez, A.; Kleinert, E.C.; Walzog, B.; Deindl, E. Midkine Controls Arteriogenesis by Regulating the Bioavailability of Vascular Endothelial Growth Factor A and the Expression of Nitric Oxide Synthase 1 and 3. *EBioMedicine* **2018**, *27*, 237–246. [CrossRef] [PubMed]
95. Pagel, J.I.; Borgolte, J.; Hoefer, I.; Fernandez, B.; Schaper, W.; Deindl, E. Involvement of neuronal NO synthase in collateral artery growth. *Indian J. Biochem. Biophys.* **2011**, *48*, 270–274.
96. Troidl, K.; Tribulova, S.; Cai, W.J.; Ruding, I.; Apfelbeck, H.; Schierling, W.; Troidl, C.; Schmitz-Rixen, T.; Schaper, W. Effects of endogenous nitric oxide and of DETA NONOate in arteriogenesis. *J. Cardiovasc. Pharm.* **2010**, *55*, 153–160. [CrossRef]
97. Son, H.; Hawkins, R.D.; Martin, K.; Kiebler, M.; Huang, P.L.; Fishman, M.C.; Kandel, E.R. Long-term potentiation is reduced in mice that are doubly mutant in endothelial and neuronal nitric oxide synthase. *Cell* **1996**, *87*, 1015–1023. [CrossRef]
98. Datta, S.R.; Dudek, H.; Tao, X.; Masters, S.; Fu, H.; Gotoh, Y.; Greenberg, M.E. Akt phosphorylation of BAD couples survival signals to the cell-intrinsic death machinery. *Cell* **1997**, *91*, 231–241. [CrossRef]
99. Michell, B.J.; Griffiths, J.E.; Mitchelhill, K.I.; Rodriguez-Crespo, I.; Tiganis, T.; Bozinovski, S.; de Montellano, P.R.; Kemp, B.E.; Pearson, R.B. The Akt kinase signals directly to endothelial nitric oxide synthase. *Curr. Biol.* **1999**, *9*, 845–848. [CrossRef]
100. Ho, F.M.; Lin, W.W.; Chen, B.C.; Chao, C.M.; Yang, C.R.; Lin, L.Y.; Lai, C.C.; Liu, S.H.; Lian, C.S. High glucose-induced apoptosis in human vascular endothelial cells is mediated through NF-κB and c-Jun NH2-terminal kinase pathway and prevented by PI3K/Akt/eNOS pathway. *Cell Signal.* **2006**, *18*, 391–399. [CrossRef]
101. Gao, F.; Gao, E.; Yue, T.L.; Ohlstein, E.H.; Lopez, B.L.; Christopher, T.A.; Ma, X.L. Nitric oxide mediates the antiapoptotic effect of insulin in myocardial ischemia-reperfusion: The roles of PI3-kinase, Akt, and endothelial nitric oxide synthase phosphorylation. *Circulation* **2002**, *105*, 1497–1502. [CrossRef]
102. Lanahan, A.A.; Lech, D.; Dubrac, A.; Zhang, J.; Zhuang, Z.W.; Eichmann, A.; Simons, M. Ptp1b is a physiologic regulator of vascular endothelial growth factor signaling in endothelial cells. *Circulation* **2014**, *130*, 902–909. [CrossRef]
103. Pipp, F.; Heil, M.; Issbrucker, K.; Ziegelhoe_er, T.; Martin, S.; Van Den Heuvel, J.; Weich, H.; Fernandez, B.; Golomb, G.; Carmeliet, P.; et al. Vegfr-1-selective vegf homologue plgf is arteriogenic: Evidence for a monocyte-mediated mechanism. *Circ. Res.* **2003**, *92*, 378–385. [CrossRef]
104. Heil, M.; Ziegelhoe_er, T.; Pipp, F.; Kostin, S.; Martin, S.; Clauss, M.; Schaper, W. Blood monocyte concentration is critical for enhancement of collateral artery growth. *Am. J. Physiol. Heart Circ. Physiol.* **2002**, *283*, H2411–H2419. [CrossRef]
105. Ziegelhoeffer, T.; Fernandez, B.; Kostin, S.; Heil, M.; Voswinckel, R.; Helisch, A.; Schaper, W. Bone marrow-derived cells do not incorporate into the adult growing vasculature. *Circ. Res.* **2004**, *94*, 230–238. [CrossRef]

106. Ricard, N.; Zhang, J.; Zhuang, W.; Simon, M. Isoform-Specific Roles of ERK1 and ERK2 in Arteriogenesis. *Cells* **2019**, *9*, 38. [CrossRef]
107. Voyvodic, P.L.; Min, D.; Liu, R.; Williams, E.; Chitalia, V.; Dunn, A.K.; Baker, A.B. Loss of syndecan-1 induces a pro-inflammatory phenotype in endothelial cells with a dysregulated response to atheroprotective flow. *J. Biol. Chem.* **2014**, *289*, 9547–9559. [CrossRef]
108. Siebel, C.; Lendahl, U. Notch signaling in development, tissue homeostasis, and disease. *Physiol. Rev.* **2017**, *97*, 1235–1294. [CrossRef]
109. Krishnasamy, K.; Limbourg, A.; Kapanadze, T. Blood vessel control of macrophage maturation promotes arteriogenesis in ischemia. *Nat. Commun.* **2017**, *8*, 1. [CrossRef]
110. Yang, C.; Guo, Y.; Jadlowiec, C.C.; Li, X.; Lv, W.; Model, L. Vascular endothelial growth factor-A inhibits EphB4 and stimulates delta-like ligand 4 expression in adult endothelial cells. *J. Surg. Res.* **2013**, *183*, 478–486. [CrossRef]
111. Kerr, B.A.; West, X.Z.; Kim, Y.W. Stability and function of adult vasculature is sustained by Akt/Jagged1 signalling axis in endothelium. *Nat. Commun.* **2016**, *7*, 10960. [CrossRef]
112. Kang, J.; Yoo, J.; Lee, S.; Tang, W.; Aguilar, B.; Ramu, S. An exquisite cross-control mechanism among endothelial cell fate regulators directs the plasticity and heterogeneity of lymphatic endothelial cells. *Blood* **2010**, *116*, 140–150. [CrossRef]
113. Morrow, D.; Cullen, J.P.; Liu, W. Sonic hedgehog induces notch target gene expression in vascular smooth muscle cells via VEGF-A. *Arterioscler. Thromb. Vasc. Biol.* **2009**, *29*, 1112–1118. [CrossRef]
114. Tian, D.Y.; Jin, X.R.; Zeng, X.; Wang, Y. Notch signaling in endothelial cells: Is it the therapeutic target for vascular neointimal hyperplasia? *Int. J. Mol. Sci.* **2017**, *18*, 1615. [CrossRef]
115. Balligand, J.L.; Feron, O.; Dessy, C. eNOS activation by physical forces: From short-term regulation of contraction to chronic remodeling of cardiovascular tissues. *Physiol. Rev.* **2009**, *89*, 481–534. [CrossRef]
116. Bennett, B.D.; Zeigler, F.C.; Gu, Q.; Fendly, B.; Goddard, A.D.; Gillet, N. Molecular cloning of a ligand for the EPH related receptor protein-tyrosine kinase Htk. *Proc. Natl. Acad. Sci. USA* **1995**, *92*, 1866–1870. [CrossRef]
117. Bae, J.H.; Schlessinger, J. Asymmetric tyrosine kinase arrangements in activation or autophosphorylation of receptor tyrosine kinases. *Mol. Cells* **2010**, *29*, 443–448. [CrossRef]
118. Pitulescu, M.E.; Adams, R.H. Regulation of signaling interactions and receptor endocytosis in growing blood vessels. *Cell Adhes. Migr.* **2014**, *8*, 366–377. [CrossRef]
119. Nakayama, A.; Nakayama, M.; Turner, C.J.; Höing, S.; Lepore, J.J.; Adams, R.H. Ephrin-B2 controls PDGFRb internalization and signaling. *Genes Dev.* **2013**, *27*, 2576–2589. [CrossRef]
120. Himanen, J.P. Ectodomain structures of Eph receptors. *Semin. Cell Dev. Biol.* **2012**, *23*, 35–42. [CrossRef]
121. Lisabeth, E.M.; Falivelli, G.; Pasquale, E.B. Eph receptor signaling and ephrins. *Cold Spring Harb. Perspect. Biol.* **2013**, *5*, a009159. [CrossRef]
122. Deindl, E.; Buschmann, I.; Hoefer, I.E.; Podzuweit, T.; Boengler, K.; Vogel, S.; van Royen, N.; Fernandez, B.; Schaper, W. Role of ischemia and of hypoxia-inducible genes in arteriogenesis after femoral artery occlusion in the rabbit. *Circ. Res.* **2001**, *89*, 779–786. [CrossRef]
123. Horbelt, D.; Denkis, A.; Knaus, P. A portrait of Transforming Growth Factor β superfamily signalling: Background matters. *Int. J. Biochem. Cell. Biol.* **2012**, *44*, 469–474. [CrossRef]
124. Evans, R.a.; Tian, Y.C.; Steadman, R.; Phillips, A.O. TGF-β1-mediated fibroblast–myofibroblast terminal differentiation—the role of smad proteins. *Exp. Cell. Res.* **2003**, *282*, 90–100. [CrossRef]
125. Kadomatsu, K.; Tomomura, M.; Muramatsu, T. cDNA cloning and sequencing of a new gene intensely expressed in early differentiation stages of embryonal carcinoma cells and in mid-gestation period of mouse embryogenesis. *Biochem. Biophys. Res. Commun.* **1988**, *151*, 1312–1318. [CrossRef]
126. Weckbach, L.T.; Groesser, L.; Borgolte, J.; Pagel, J.I.; Pogoda, F.; Schymeinsky, J.; Muller-Hocker, J.; Shakibaei, M.; Muramatsu, T.; Deindl, E. Midkine acts as proangiogenic cytokine in hypoxia-induced angiogenesis. *Am. J. Physiol. Heart Circ. Physiol.* **2012**, *303*, 429–438. [CrossRef]
127. Weckbach, L.T.; Preissner, K.T.; Deindl, E. The Role of Midkine in Arteriogenesis, Involving Mechanosensing, Endothelial Cell Proliferation, and Vasodilation. *Int. J. Mol. Sci.* **2018**, *19*, 2559. [CrossRef]
128. Novotny, W.F.; Maffi, T.; Mehta, R.L.; Milner, P.G. Identification of novel heparin-releasable proteins, as well as the cytokines midkine and pleiotrophin, in human postheparin plasma. *Arter. Thromb.* **1993**, *13*, 1798–1805. [CrossRef]

129. Weckbach, L.T.; Muramatsu, T.; Walzog, B. Midkine in inflammation. *Sci. World J.* **2011**, *11*, 2491–2505. [CrossRef]
130. Gungor, C.; Zander, H.; Effenberger, K.E.; Vashist, Y.K.; Kalinina, T.; Izbicki, J.R.; Yekebas, E.; Bockhorn, M. Notch signaling activated by replication stress-induced expression of midkine drives epithelial-mesenchymal transition and chemoresistance in pancreatic cancer. *Cancer Res.* **2011**, *71*, 5009–5019. [CrossRef]
131. Huang, Y.; Hoque, M.O.; Wu, F.; Trink, B.; Sidransky, D.; Ratovitski, E.A. Midkine induces epithelial-mesenchymal transition through Notch2/Jak2-Stat3 signaling in human keratinocytes. *Cell Cycle* **2008**, *7*, 1613–1622. [CrossRef]
132. Orr, A.W.; Sanders, J.M.; Bevard, M.; Coleman, E.; Sarembock, I.J.; Schwartz, M.A. The subendothelial extracellular matrix modulates NF-kappaB activation by flow: A potential role in atherosclerosis. *J. Cell Biol.* **2005**, *169*, 191–202. [CrossRef]
133. Horiba, M.; Kadomatsu, K.; Nakamura, E.; Muramatsu, H.; Ikematsu, S.; Sakuma, S.; Hayashi, K.; Yuzawa, Y.; Matsuo, S.; Kuzuya, M. Neointima formation in a restenosis model is suppressed in midkine-deficient mice. *J. Clin. Investig.* **2000**, *105*, 489–495. [CrossRef]

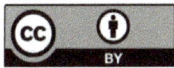

© 2020 by the authors. Licensee MDPI, Basel, Switzerland. This article is an open access article distributed under the terms and conditions of the Creative Commons Attribution (CC BY) license (http://creativecommons.org/licenses/by/4.0/).

MDPI
St. Alban-Anlage 66
4052 Basel
Switzerland
Tel. +41 61 683 77 34
Fax +41 61 302 89 18
www.mdpi.com

Cells Editorial Office
E-mail: cells@mdpi.com
www.mdpi.com/journal/cells

www.ingramcontent.com/pod-product-compliance
Lightning Source LLC
LaVergne TN
LVHW070401100526
838202LV00014B/1367